PRACTICAL IMMUNOLOGY

Practical Immunology

LESLIE HUDSON
PhD BSc ARCS

Department of Immunology
St. George's Hospital Medical School
London, England

FRANK C. HAY
PhD BTech

Department of Immunology
Middlesex Hospital Medical School
London, England

SECOND EDITION

BLACKWELL SCIENTIFIC PUBLICATIONS

OXFORD LONDON EDINBURGH BOSTON MELBOURNE

© 1976, 1980 by
Blackwell Scientific Publications
Editorial offices:
Osney Mead, Oxford OX2 0EL
8 John Street, London WC1N 2ES
9 Forrest Road, Edinburgh EH1 2QH
52 Beacon Street, Boston,
    Massachusetts 02108, USA
214 Berkeley Street, Carlton
    Victoria 3053, Australia

First published 1976
Second edition 1980

Typeset by
Santype International Ltd.,
Salisbury, Wiltshire
Printed and bound in Great Britain
by Morrison & Gibb Ltd., Edinburgh

DISTRIBUTORS

USA
    Blackwell Mosby Book Distributors
    11830 Westline Industrial Drive
    St Louis, Missouri 63141

Canada
    Blackwell Mosby Book Distributors
    120 Melford Drive, Scarborough,
    Ontario M1B 2X4

Australia
    Blackwell Scientific Book
    Distributors
    214 Berkeley Street, Carlton
    Victoria 3053

British Library
Cataloguing in Publication Data

Hudson, Leslie
    Practical immunology. – 2nd ed.
    1. Immunology
    I. Title   II. Hay, Frank Charles
    574.2′9   QR181

    ISBN 0-632-00353-7

Contents

2   The lymphocyte: its rôle and function   24

3   Lymphocytes and effector cells   52

vii

8   Affinity chromatography 203

9   Immunochemical methods 226

11 Hybridoma cells and monoclonal antibody 303

Appendixes

Index 350

Foreword to First Edition

Immunology might well claim to be the most popular and the most glamorous of the biological sciences today. I suspect that there has been a sharper increase in the number of research workers in immunology over the last two decades than in any other scientific discipline.

Applied immunology, plus the intangibles we lump together as the rising standard of living, has virtually rid the world of smallpox, yellow fever, diphtheria and poliomyelitis and helped in many other fields. Its prestige lingers on as the major tool of preventive medicine but, as one whose first immunological paper was published more than fifty years ago, I have seen a complete switch in the contemporary importance of immunology—but not a diminution.

Immunology today is a science in its own right. The enthusiasm of younger workers like the authors of this book, is primarily directed toward understanding; medical applications of the new knowledge will be wholeheartedly welcomed but they are not central. For me, and to some extent all of us in immunology, the excitement is in the lead that our subject is giving toward a real understanding of the form and strategy of living process. Thanks to the *recognizability* of the significant molecules, antibody, antigen and the like, we have been able to apply the new techniques of molecular biology to the elucidation of one of the essential bodily functions. We are leading the field, for nowhere else have genetics, biochemistry and every other basic science that can help, been so effectively applied to living function. It is the first step toward a sophisticated understanding of what we are and how we became so.

This book is basically an introduction to the techniques and ideas on which immunology is based to one who grew up with the older, predominantly medical approach, the new version can be sensed everywhere in the authors' approach.

I wish them every success.

F.M. Burnet

Basel, Switzerland

Acknowledgements to Second Edition

Our original notion in the compilation of this book was based on the lazy hope that such a small collection of 'core' techniques would change little, and so would entail little future revision. How wrong we were! In addition to a general revision, we have had to rewrite many of the sections dealing with the isolation of immunoglobulins, affinity chromatography, ELISA, and of course, add a complete new chapter on hybridomas and monoclonal antibodies.

We are extremely grateful to our many friends and colleagues who have suggested or discussed our revisions. In particular, we wish to thank Roger Budd, Hansha Bhayani, Janette Flint, Jens Jensenius, Alan Johnstone, Meinir Jones, David Male, Alison Mawle, Lynn Nineham, Graham Rook, Colin Shapland, Yasmin Thanavala, and John Whateley.

Our special thanks are due to Margaret Williams and Queenie Jaywardena for their excellent secretarial assistance.

Acknowledgements to First Edition

This book was started while we were carrying out research for our doctorates in the department of Professor Ivan M. Roitt. He both encouraged and, indeed, stimulated us to become interested in the teaching of immunology. Our grateful thanks are also due to Dr Giorgio Torrigiani for initiating us into the world of immunochemistry.

We wish to thank our colleagues Siraik Zakarian, Harald von Boehmer, Andrew Kelus, Hansruedi Kiefer, Clive Loveday, Jan Obel, Marcus Nabholz, Richard Pink and Jonathan Sprent both for their helpful discussions and in many cases for allowing us to use their unpublished material. We are particularly grateful to Sir Macfarlane Burnet for writing the foreword to this book.

Without the valuable assistance of Lynn Nineham and Anthony Finch it would have been impossible for us to gather all the information and data required for this book. In addition, we wish to acknowledge the tenacity with which Penny Hamilton-Jones converted our pages of hieroglyphs into typewritten sheets.

We have written this book for the use of those individuals, from the undergraduate to post-doctoral level, with a sound theoretical knowledge of immunology, who wish to extend their knowledge by experimentation.

We have been made painfully aware of the interdependence of the branches of immunology in writing this book. It proved extremely difficult to find a point at which to begin. The approach finally adopted was one from the view of cellular biology rather than the classical immunological approach which starts with antibody, a mediator produced half-way through the immune response, and leads to the logical gymnastics of proceeding backwards, to the cellular basis of this response, and forwards, to the secondary mechanisms initiated by antibody–antigen interaction. We believe that the development of the book from the basic 'lymphocyte unit' to the complete immune system avoids the fast approaching dichotomy between cellular immunology and immunochemistry.

Introduction and Additional Reading

Reading to accompany this book

ROITT I.M. (1980) *Essential Immunology.* 4e. Blackwell Scientific Publications, Oxford.

STEWARD M.W. (1976) *Immunochemistry.* 2e. Chapman & Hall, London.

PLAYFAIR J.H.L. (1979) *Immunology at a Glance.* Blackwell Scientific Publications, Oxford.

For the advanced student

BELLANTI J.A. (1978) *Immunology II.* 2e. W.B. Saunders, Philadelphia.

BENACERRAF B. & UNANUE E.R. (1979) *Textbook of Immunology.* Williams & Wilkins, Baltimore.

BRYANT N.J. (1978) *Laboratory Immunology and Serology.* W.B. Saunders, Philadelphia.

GLYNN L.E. & STEWARD M.W. (eds.) (1977) *Immunochemistry: An Advanced Textbook.* John Wiley, Chichester.

HOLBOROW E.J. & REEVES W.G. (eds.) (1977) *Immunology in Medicine.* Academic Press, London.

KABAT E.A. (1976) *Structural Concepts in Immunology and Immunochemistry.* 2e. Holt, Rinehart & Winston, New York.

MISHELL B.B. & SHIIGI S.M. (1980) *Selected Methods in Cellular Immunology.* Freeman, San Francisco.

NISONOFF *et al.* (1975) *The Antibody Molecule.* Academic Press, London.

THALER M.S., KLAUSNER R.D. & COHEN H.J. (1977) *Medical Immunology.* Lippincott, Philadelphia.

WEIR D.M. (ed.) (1978) *Handbook of Experimental Immunology.* 3e. Blackwell Scientific Publications, Oxford.

Many of the techniques described in this book involve radioactive isotopes; it is therefore essential that individuals be familiar with some manual dealing with the 'Code of Practice against Radiation Hazards'.

Recurrent publications, for the advanced student and specialist

Advances in Immunology. Academic Press, London and New York

Contemporary Topics in Immunobiology. Plenum Press, New York

Contemporary Topics in Molecular Immunology. Plenum Press, New York

Perspectives in Immunology. Academic Press, London and New York

Immunological Reviews. Munksgaard, Copenhagen

Major Journals for Immunologists

Cellular Immunology
Clinical and Experimental Immunology
European Journal of Immunology
Human Immunology
Immunochemistry
Immunological Communications
Immunology
Immunology Letters
Infection and Immunity
International Archives of Allergy and Applied Immunology
Journal of Experimental Medicine
Journal of Immunogenetics
Journal of Immunology
Journal of Immunological Methods
Journal of Reproductive Immunology
Lancet
Nature
Parasite Immunology
Proceedings of the National Academy of Science
Scandinavian Journal of Immunology
Science
Thymus
Transplantation

The growth of knowledge within the field of immunology has been so immense within the last five years that we would recommend that those individuals who wish to keep up to date with the current literature should consult either:

Current Titles in Immunology, Transplantation and Allergy. MSK Books Ltd, London; or

Current Contents (Life Sciences). Institute for Scientific Information, Philadelphia, USA.

1   Initial preparations

1.1 **INTRODUCTION TO PRACTICAL IMMUNOLOGY**

It would be very expensive to purchase immunological reagents in the quantities required for some of the procedures described in the book. With time, patience and experience it is possible to prepare all the reagents you will require. We have designed the book such that reagents used at later stages will already have been prepared in the earlier chapters. Accordingly this introductory section is not included in the logical sequence of the book. A full explanation of all the techniques and their applications is given in later chapters.

1.2 **ANTIGENS**

Many are not expensive and so may be purchased commercially.

1.2.1 **ERYTHROCYTES**

Sheep erythrocytes (SRBC) are used widely in immunology both as antigens and indicator cells. They should be purchased in Alsever's solution (See Appendix II), and have a shelf life of 3–4 weeks at 4°.

Horse RBC are sold commercially as oxalated whole blood (See Appendix II). Their shelf life at 4° is only 2 weeks.

1.2.2 **SOLUBLE ANTIGENS** (ammonium sulphate precipitation)

Fowl gamma globulin ($F\gamma G$). This is a very powerful antigen, (a strong immunogen) especially in mice, and is usually prepared as an ammonium sulphate precipitate of whole chicken serum. It is not strictly γ globulin but is serum depleted mainly of albumin.

1.2.2a **Preparation of $F\gamma G$**

Materials and equipment

Ammonium sulphate
Dilute ammonia solution
Chicken (adult, preferably cockerel)
UV spectrophotometer

1

Method

1 Dissolve 1000 g ammonium sulphate in 1000 ml distilled water at 50°, allow to stand overnight at room temperature and adjust the pH to 7·2 with dilute ammonia solution or sulphuric acid.

2 Bleed chicken by cardiac puncture (Section 2.5.1) and separate the serum from the clotted whole blood.

3 Dilute serum 1 : 2 with saline and add saturated ammonium sulphate solution (prepared in 1) to a final concentration of 45% (v/v.).

4 Stir at room temperature for 30 min.

5 Spin off precipitate (1000 g for 15 min at 4°).

6 Wash precipitate with 45% saturated ammonium sulphate and re-centrifuge.

7 Redissolve the precipitate in the same volume of PBS as the original serum.

8 Centrifuge to remove any insoluble material.

9 Re-precipitate the γ-globulin using a final concentration of 40% saturated ammonium sulphate.

10 Spin off the precipitate and wash with 40% saturated ammonium sulphate.

11 After centrifuging the washed precipitate, re-dissolve in a minimum volume of PBS.

12 Dialyse the FγG against 5 changes of PBS at 4°. Centrifuge off any precipitate.

13 Prepare a 1 : 20 dilution of the FγG and determine the absorbance at 280 nm using a UV spectrophotometer.

Calculation of protein content. At 280 nm, an OD of 1·0 (1 cm cuvette) is equivalent to an FγG concentration of 0·74 mg ml^{-1}.

Example: if OD at 1 : 20 = 0·95,
$$F\gamma G \text{ concentration} = 0.95 \times 0.74 \times 20$$
$$= 14.1 \text{ mg ml}^{-1}.$$

Technical notes

1 Calculation of volume of saturated solution required to achieve a required concentration of ammonium sulphate:

volume saturated solution (ml) to be added per 100 ml volume,

$$= \frac{100(S_f - S_i)}{1 - S_f},$$

where S_f = final saturation (fraction, not per cent),
S_i = initial saturation (fraction, not per cent).

2 To minimize excessive volumes of solution when working in bulk, add solid ammonium sulphate according to the nomogram on the front inside cover.

3 18% sodium sulphate may be used to precipitate a crude γ-globulin fraction of serum. Unlike ammonium sulphate however, its

degree of saturation changes markedly with temperature (cf. Section 7.1). All centrifugation must be at room temperature.

1.2.2b   **Keyhole limpet haemocyanin (KLH)**

This is the respiratory pigment of the keyhole limpet and is prepared as an ammonium sulphate precipitate. We suggest you obtain it commercially (Appendix II). It is a very strong immunogen in mice. Because this antigen tends to self associate to form large complexes it is difficult to assign an accurate molecular weight.

1.2.2c   **Mouse γ globulin**

Materials and equipment

20 mice—any strain, or outbred (Section 1.8.2 and Appendix II)
Ether
Saturated ammonium sulphate solution, pH 7·2
UV spectrophotometer

Method

1   Anaesthetize the mice with ether and exsanguinate by severing the axillary vessels under the arm with a pair of scissors (Fig. 2.1.).
2   Collect the blood into glass tubes and allow it to clot.
3   Free the clot from the walls of the tube to aid retraction.
4   Collect the exuded serum and remove any contaminating cells by centrifuging at 150 g for 15 min and then at 350 g for 15 min.
5   Precipitate the gamma globulin with ammonium sulphate as described in section 1.2.2a.

After dialysis determine the protein content of the solution using the following conversion factor: at 280 nm, OD 1·0 (in a 1 cm cuvette) $= 0·69$ mg ml^{-1} gamma globulin.

1.2.2d   **Rabbit γ globulin (RγG) and human serum albumin**

Both should be bought commercially (see Appendix II).

1.2.3   RAPID 'DIALYSIS' OF PROTEINS (desalting)

Dialysis is used either to remove small molecular contaminants or to change the buffering conditions of the solution. The same effect can be achieved rapidly by the use of a Sephadex G-25 column. Small molecules, such as free dinitrophenol, as well as the ions of the original buffer are retarded by the Sephadex while the protein molecules are excluded and can be collected in the effluent, already, equilibrated in the column buffer. Rapid 'dialysis' is often important

3

when the protein is under harsh conditions, where conventional dialysis would be too slow and allow irreversible denaturation.

Materials and equipment

Sephadex G-25, fine (swollen in water containing sodium azide, Appendix II)
Chromatography column (Appendix II)
Blue dextran, $1\% w/v$ in water (see Appendix II)
Peristaltic pump for column

Determination of column void volume

1   Pour the Sephadex into a chromatography column and pack under pressure.
2   Ensure that the surface of the gel is level and pump the water into gel. Close the column.
3   Add 1 ml of blue dextran solution to the surface of the gel. Allow this to enter the gel completely while collecting the effluent into a graduated cylinder. Close the column.
4   Add water to the surface of the gel and continue collecting the effluent until the blue dye just appears. The liquid collected represents the VOID VOLUME of the column.

Repeat the void volume determination for different heights of the gel. Plot a graph of void volume against column height. If you use the same diameter column each time then the void volume may be read off from the graph using the column height.

Molecules in the excluded fraction of Sephadex G-25, e.g. proteins, leave the gel just after the void volume, and their volume is expanded to approximately 1·5 times the original sample volume.

Use of column for protein 'dialysis':

Materials and equipment

Sephadex G-25 column (Section 1.2.3)
1% Blue dextran solution (Appendix II)
Peristaltic pump
Protein solution to be dialysed

Method

1   Determine void volume of the column.
2   Equilibrate the gel with 3 times the void volume of buffer.
3   Apply the sample in a volume not greater than half the void volume.
4   Allow the void volume of buffer to leave the column and collect 1·5 times the original sample volume.

4

If you are using small sample volumes, for example, during radio-iodination of proteins, it is advisable to determine the final sample volume more precisely by using a test volume of blue dextran equal to the original sample volume. This avoids unnecessary dilution.

After one run, the column may be re-equilibrated with 3 times the void volume of buffer, provided the retained material has not ir-reversibly bound to the column, e.g. as with fluorescein isothiocyanate, or altered the gel chemically.

1.3   HAPTEN-CARRIER CONJUGATES

1.3.1   DINITROPHENYL-F$_\gamma$G OR KLH

A hapten is a small molecule which will bind to B cells or pre-formed antibody, but the hapten alone will not stimulate B-cell differentiation to plasma cells and antibody production. The B-cell response to antigen, in the majority of cases, requires cooperation by T cells. As the hapten is small it cannot stimulate two cells simultaneously. Accordingly, if the hapten is conjugated to an im-munogenic protein, then T cells will recognize this protein, or car-rier molecule, and so cooperate with B cells to produce anti-hapten antibody. (Anti-carrier antibody is also produced.) These defined antigens are powerful tools for investigating cell interactions in the immune response.

Probably the most commonly used hapten is dinitrophenyl (DNP) which is conjugated to protein via one of its two reactive forms:

| 2,4-Dinitro-1-fluorobenzene | 2,4-Dinitrobenzenesulphonate.Na |
| (DNFB) | (DNBS) |

Dinitrofluorobenzene is highly reactive with the amino groups of proteins under alkaline conditions where the peptide bond is quite stable. It is used when high substitution ratios are required.

Dinitrophenylation of carrier molecules

a. HIGH SUBSTITUTION RATIOS

Materials and equipment

Keyhole limpet haemocyanin (KLH) (Appendix II)
1M sodium bicarbonate

2,4-Dinitrofluorobenzene (Appendix II)
Sephadex G-25 column (Section 1.2.3)
UV spectrophotometer

Method

1   Dissolve 100 mg KLH in 1 M NaHCO$_3$ (minimum initial concentration 10–20 mg ml^{-1}).
2   Add 0·05 ml DNFB (*Use a pipette bulb and take care as DNFB is an extremely potent skin sensitizing agent*).
3   Mix vigorously for 45 min at 37°.
4   Separate the DNP–KLH conjugate from the free DNFB on a Sephadex G-25 column (Section 1.2.3).
5   Determine the number of DNP groups per KLH molecule using the conversion:
DNP: at 360 nm, OD of 1·0 (1 cm cuvette) is equivalent to 0·067 mmol DNP.
KLH: at 278 nm, OD of 1·0 (1 cm cuvette) is equivalent to 0·00018 mmol KLH. (*Note*. The presence of dinitrophenyl groups on the protein accounts for approximately 40% of the absorbance at 278 nm. This is allowed for in the conversion.)

b. LOW SUBSTITUTION RATIOS

Materials and equipment

Fowl γ globulin (FγG) (Section 1.2.a)
0·15 M potassium carbonate
Dinitrobenzene sulphonate, Na salt recryst (DNBS, Appendix II)
Sephadex G-25 column
UV spectrophotometer

Method

1   Dissolve 100 mg FγG in 5 ml. 0·15 M potassium carbonate.
2   Add 20 mg Na dinitrobenzene sulphonate and mix overnight at 4°.
3   Prepare a column of Sephadex G-25 and equilibrate against PBS (Section 1.2.3).
4   Add the FγG/DNP mixture to the column and pump through, adding more PBS when required.
5   Collect the first visible band to elute from the column. This is the DNP–FγG conjugate. The free DNP is retained at the top of the column.
6   Collect 1·5 times the original sample volume.
7   Dilute two aliquots of DNP–FγG 1 : 20 with PBS.
8   Read one aliquot at 280 nm in the spectrophotometer, and the second at 360 nm.

Calculation of DNP–FγG ratio

DNP: At 360 nm, OD of 1·0 (1 cm cuvette) is equivalent to 0·067 mmol DNP.

FγG: At 280 nm, OD of 1·0 (1 cm cuvette) is equivalent to 0·0029 mmol FγG.

Note. The DNP interferes with the protein OD at 280 nm. This is allowed for in the conversion factors.

The chemical and antigenic properties of carrier proteins are altered after hapten substitutions. FγG, for example, is irreversibly denatured and becomes insoluble at ratios greater than DNP_{40} FγG. With the method described for dinitrophenylation of FγG you should obtain $DNP_{3\ 4}$ FγG. There is good hapten and carrier priming when mice are immunized with this conjugate. With $DNP_{15\ 20}$ FγG, carrier priming is greatly reduced, whereas with $DNP_{30\ 35}$ FγG direct (IgM) plaques alone are detected, there is no switching to indirect (IgG) plaque formation in the antibody response to the hapten (cf. section 3.1.2).

The KLH molecule can accept up to 100 hapten groups before carrier priming is affected.

1.3.2   PARA-AMINOBENZYL HSA

Materials and equipment

p-aminobenzoic acid (PABA) (Appendix II)
1 M hydrochloric acid
1 M sodium hydroxide
0·2 M sodium nitrite
Starch, 10 g l^{-1}
0·5 M potassium iodide
White tile
Human serum albumin and fowl γ globulin (Appendix II and Section 1.2.2a)
Dialysis tubing (Appendix II)
Buffer (0·13 M NaCl; 0·16 M boric acid, adjust to pH 9·0 with 1 M NaOH).

Method

1   Diazotize 50 mg of p-aminobenzoic acid (PABA) in 2 ml 1 M HCl by adding cold 0·2 M sodium nitride dropwise. (Test for end point of reaction, i.e. immediate blue colour—using a mixture of 10 g l^{-1} starch + 0.05 M potassium iodide—on a white tile.)
2   Dissolve 1 g of carrier protein (HSA or FγG) in 20 ml of buffer on ice.
3   Add diazotized PABA slowly to the dissolved protein and maintain the pH at 9·0 by the dropwise addition of 1 M NaOH. Stir for 1·5 hours in the cold.

4   Dialyse against 5 l of PBS for 1–2 days, with 2–3 changes of PBS, to remove the free hapten.

5   Store at $-20°$ at a protein concentration of 10–20 mg ml^{-1}.

1.4   ANTISERA

Antigens are more immunogenic when presented in an insoluble form or with an adjuvant. The most commonly used adjuvant is Freund's complete adjuvant into which soluble antigen is combined as a stable water-in-oil emulsion. The mode of adjuvant action is unclear but it is probable that the slow release of the antigen from the emulsion 'depot' acts as a prolonged series of small injections. In addition, a proportion of the subsequent antibody production occurs within the granuloma induced by the *Mycobacterium tuberculosis* in the adjuvant.

1.4.1   FREUND'S ADJUVANT

Freund's complete adjuvant is a mixture of oil (Bayol F) and detergent (mannide mono-oleate) containing *Mycobacterium tuberculosis*. The incomplete adjuvant is a mixture of oil and detergent alone. The complete and incomplete adjuvant may be purchased commercially (Appendix II).

For obvious reasons, this adjuvant is not clinically acceptable for human use and indeed great care should be exercised to avoid personal contamination during its experimental use. Although Freund's adjuvant was first described almost 40 years ago, it is still the most effective non-specific immunopotentiator known. The relative abilities of some common adjuvants to stimulate humoral or cell-mediated immunity have been extensively investigated by Bomford (see references at end of chapter).

Every laboratory has its own method of raising antisera. Those we describe below work, and are rapid.

1.4.2   RABBIT ANTI-MOUSE γ GLOBULIN

Materials and equipment

Mouse γ globulin (Section 1.2.2c or Appendix II)
Freund's complete adjuvant (Appendix II)
Glass syringe with Luer lock
Large rabbits

Method

1   Dissolve 500 μg of mouse γ globulin (Section 1.2.2c) in 1 ml saline.

2 Add protein dropwise to 1 ml of Freund's complete adjuvant. Homogenize with a syringe and needle to a white cream after adding each drop.

3 Continue homogenizing until a stable water-in-oil emulsion is obtained. Check this by gently placing one drop from the syringe onto saline. *If the emulsion is stable the first or second drop will not disperse.*

4 Inject approximately 1 ml of the emulsion intramuscularly into each hindquarter of the rabbit. (*Many investigators favour a foot pad injection regime. Theoretically this is advantageous as there is good lymphatic drainage to the local nodes, in practice, however, it is not advisable especially if the rabbits are housed over wire grilles.*)

5 Two weeks later repeat the injections. (*If the granuloma ulcerates after the second injection of antigen in Freund's complete adjuvant, we suggest you omit the* M. tuberculosis *from this second injection in your general immunization schedule.*)

6 After two further weeks take a 5 ml sample bleed from the central ear artery.

7 Transfer the blood to a glass tube and allow it to clot at 37° for 1 h. Loosen the clot from the tube to aid retraction.

8 After incubation, store at 4° until serum is expressed.

9 Test the antiserum in an interfacial ring test.

1.4.3 INTERFACIAL RING TEST

Materials and equipment

Test serum (e.g. from previous section)
Durham tubes (Appendix II)
Mouse γ globulin (10–20 mg ml^{-1}) (Section 1.2.2c or Appendix II)

Method

1 Place 0·1 ml of serum in a small rimless (Durham) test tube.

2 Carefully layer over 0·1 ml of the original mouse gamma globulin sample in PBS (10–20 mg ml^{-1}).

If a visible precipitate is not formed within 1–2 min you must continue boosting the animal with alum-precipitated antigen.

1.4.4 ALUM PRECIPITATION OF ANTIGENS

Materials and equipment

Protein antigen
1 M sodium bicarbonate
0·2 M aluminium potassium sulphate
Phosphate buffered saline, PBS (Appendix I).

9

Method

1 For each 10 ml of protein solution add 4·5 ml of 1 M sodium bicarbonate.

2 Add 10 ml of 0·2 M aluminium potassium sulphate while stirring. Add slowly to minimize frothing.

3 Leave for 15 min.

4 Spin off precipitate (300 g for 15 min) and wash three times with PBS by centrifugation.

5 Re-suspend the insoluble protein to the required concentration (3 mg ml^{-1} for rabbits; 4 mg ml^{-1} for mice).

Boost the rabbit with 300 μg alum precipitated protein given subcutaneously, until a good precipitating serum is obtained. Exsanguinate the rabbit by cardiac puncture and separate the serum. Heat inactivate the serum at 56° for 45 min and store at $-20°$.

Strictly one should obtain a pre-immunization serum sample to use as a control for this antiserum. However, as antisera are often pooled it is convenient to use a large pool of normal rabbit serum (NRS) instead (Appendix II).

1.4.5 RABBIT ANTI-FOWL γ GLOBULIN (FγG)

Prepare as described in Section 1.4.2 with antigen prepared in Section 1.2.2a.

1.4.6 RABBIT ANTI-HUMAN WHOLE SERUM AND SERUM ALBUMIN (HSA)

Prepare antisera as described in Section 1.4.2.

1.4.7 GOAT OR SHEEP ANTI-RABBIT γ GLOBULIN

It is rarely convenient to raise such antisera under normal laboratory conditions. This may, however, be done commercially as a customer request (see Appendix II). Usually 1–1·5 litres of sterile, heat inactivated antiserum, and a sample pre-immunization serum is supplied per animal. Use the immunization schedule as given for rabbits (Section 1.4.2).

1.5 HAPTEN-CARRIER PRIMED MICE

Hapten-carrier primed mice should be used 2–3 months after the original priming if memory B lymphocytes are required.

Materials

Saturated ammonium sulphate, pH 7·2
Carrier protein or hapten-carrier conjugate (Section 1.3)
Bordetella pertussis (Appendix II)

Method

1   Alum precipitate each carrier or hapten-carrier conjugate as described in Section 1.4.4, and adjust the final protein concentration to 4 mg ml^{-1} in PBS.
2   Mix 0·1 ml of alum precipitated antigen with 4×10^9 *B. pertussis* organisms (0·1 ml of standard 'Whooping Cough' vaccine).
3   Inject mouse intraperitoneally.

1.6   **PREPARATION OF FLUOROCHROME CONJUGATED ANTISERA**

Again it is advisable to prepare and standardize these labelled proteins before actually starting the experiments in the book.

1.6.1   CONJUGATION TECHNIQUE

Materials and equipment

Antiserum
Saturated ammonium sulphate pH 7·2
0·25 M, pH 9·0 carbonate/bicarbonate buffer (Appendix I)
Sephadex G-25 column
UV spectrophotometer
Fluorescein isothiocyanate

Method

1   Precipitate the antiserum with 40% saturated ammonium sulphate as described in Section 1.2.2a.
2   Dialyse the γ-globulin fraction of the antiserum against 0·25 M, pH 9·0 carbonate–bicarbonate buffer using a Sephadex G-25 column (see Section 1.2.3).
3   Determine the protein concentration of the solution (see Section 1.2.2c) and adjust to 20 mg ml^{-1}.
4   Add 0·05 mg fluorescein isothiocyanate per mg of total protein.
5   Mix overnight at 4°.

11

6 Separate the conjugated protein from the free fluorochrome by passing the mixture down a G-25 Sephadex column equilibrated with PBS.

Conjugation with tetramethylrhodamine isothiocyanate (Appendix II) is done under the same conditions but it is necessary to separate rhodamine-conjugated antisera from free rhodamine on ion-exchange columns (Section 7.3).

1.6.2 CALCULATION OF FLUOROCHROME: PROTEIN RATIO

This should be done routinely every time a new conjugate is made. The presence of the fluorochrome interferes with the OD of the protein at 280 nm; this is allowed for in the formula:

$$\text{fluorescein: protein ratio} = \frac{2\cdot87 \times \text{OD 495 nm}}{\text{OD}_{280\,\text{nm}} - 0\cdot35 \times \text{OD}_{495\,\text{nm}}}.$$

Unless you use crystalline rhodamine for conjugation, which we do not recommend, it is not possible to make the same correction when calculating the rhodamine and protein ratio:

$$\text{rhodamine: protein ratio} = \frac{\text{OD}_{515\,\text{nm}}}{\text{OD}_{280\,\text{nm}}}.$$

If you intend to use the conjugate to stain fixed material the fluorochrome to protein ratio should be low (1·5 : 1), however, antisera used to stain viable cells, where the specific and non-specific fluorescence is much weaker, should have a higher conjugation ratio (2–4 : 1).

1.6.3 FRACTIONATION OF FLUOROCHROME CONJUGATED ANTISERA

The fluorochrome to protein ratio calculated above is only an average determination, some protein molecules will have more fluorochrome and others less. As each fluorochrome molecule is added to the protein molecule there is a net decrease in charge. Accordingly, conjugated antisera may be fractionated by ion exchange chromatography using an elution gradient of increasing ionic strength. See Section 7.3.3 and Fig. 1.1 for method, results and theoretical considerations.

12

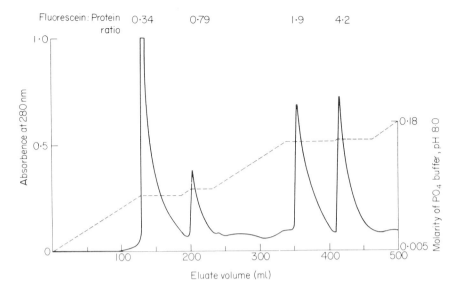

Fig. 1.1. Elution of homogeneously conjugated fluorescein–anti-rabbit IgG from DEAE-cellulose

Fluorescein-conjugated IgG goat anti-rabbit IgG was applied to an ion-exchange column of DEAE-cellulose equilibrated with 0·005 M, pH 8·0 phosphate buffer and eluted with a stepwise gradient of increasing buffer molarity (----). Limit buffer 0·18 M, pH 8·0 phosphate. Antibody activity against rabbit IgG was detected in each peak by Ouchterlony immunodiffusion (Section 5.3.3b).

The stepwise gradient was established using an Ultrograd gradient device and level sensor (Appendix II). The molarity of the eluting buffer is increased by the Ultrograd until eluted protein is detected by the level sensor. At this point, the molarity of the buffer is maintained automatically until elution is complete when the molarity is once more increased to obtain the second and subsequent peaks.

1.6.4   INDIRECT v. DIRECT IMMUNOFLUORESCENCE

Indirect immunofluorescence using an unlabelled antiserum detected by a second, fluorochrome conjugated antiserum is much more sensitive than direct immunofluorescence where one antiserum alone is used. Accordingly, if you have only a transmitted light UV microscope, we suggest that you use only the former technique. However, the direct technique is more rapid and gives excellent results with an incident light UV microscope (Appendix II).

The techniques of fluorochrome conjugation can be used with human, goat, sheep and rabbit antisera. They are, however, unsatisfactory for the conjugation of mouse alloantisera because of denaturation of the antibody molecules. In addition, mouse alloantisera can only be used as direct conjugates when staining mouse lymphocytes. This problem has recently been circumvented using a

13

dinitrophenylated alloantiserum (Section 10.8.5) which was detected by a fluorescein-conjugated goat anti-DNP–ovalbumin serum (see Section 10.8.7).

1.6.5   STANDARDIZATION OF FLUOROCHROME CONJUGATED ANTISERA

This must be done before attempting the experiments described later in the book. You must determine the titration range over which the antiserum gives a plateau of staining values and then work on this plateau.

Protocol for rabbit anti-mouse Ig indirect immunofluorescent staining

The details of the staining technique are given in Section 2.5.1. Use the same protocol for standardization of rabbit anti-chicken Ig sera (Section 1.4.5).
1   Incubate mouse thymocytes and lymph node cells with a series of dilutions of the unconjugated antiserum starting at 1 : 5 (see Fig. 1.2).
2   Detect the antibody with fluorescein-labelled goat or sheep anti-rabbit gamma globulin (1 mg ml^{-1}).

Remember to include a NRS control.

Evaluation of results: Plot a graph of percentage staining for each antiserum dilution as shown in Fig. 1.2. As can be seen from Fig. 1.2 at low dilutions there is an elevated percentage staining, or prozone, before the plateau. This is probably caused by non-specific sticking of serum proteins at high concentrations (cf. staining with NRS). Obviously the best dilution at which to use this antiserum would be between 1 : 10 to 1 : 15. One can be sure of being on the plateau but still economize in the use of antiserum (see also Section 2.5.1 for details of immunofluorescent staining).

1.6.6   SPECIFICITY OF IMMUNOFLUORESCENT STAINING

Antisera are biological materials and not chemical reagents. Accordingly, many antisera or control sera do not behave as expected. You should be aware of the limitations on the use of antisera, especially in a sensitive system such as immunofluorescence. We have listed some of the pitfalls of this technique and their correction. You must, of course, ensure that the microscope is working properly.

14

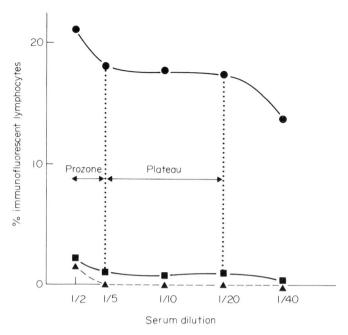

Fig. 1.2. Indirect immunofluorescent staining of mouse thymus and lymph node lymphocytes

● ——● Lymph node cells with rabbit anti-mouse Ig.
■ ——■ Thymus cells with rabbit anti-mouse Ig.
▲ - - - ▲ Thymus cells with normal rabbit serum.

Lymph node cells showed no prozone with normal rabbit serum. The binding of the rabbit antiserum was detected by a fluorescein-conjugated goat anti-rabbit IgG serum.

1 Everything staining everywhere

It is probable that one of the antisera is recognizing species or cell-surface determinants other than immunoglobulin. If both control and anti-Ig slides show total staining then the lack of specificity is probably due to the conjugate. If only one of the slides shows high staining it is probably one of the unconjugated sera. We suggest that you absorb the offending serum with liver membranes as follows:

a Force chopped mouse liver through a tea-strainer or a 63 μm steel sampling sieve into tissue culture medium on ice.
b Wash the membrane suspension 10–15 times by centrifugation (500 g for 20 min at 4°) until the optical density of the supernatant is below 0·1 ($E_{280\ nm}^{1·0\ cm}$).
c Mix a volume of the packed-cell membranes with an equal volume of the serum to be absorbed.
d Leave the suspension to mix at 4° overnight on a rotator.
e Spin off the cell membranes (500 g for 20 min at 4°) and re-test the antiserum.

15

2 No staining anywhere

Almost certainly you have forgotten to add the conjugate. If you are sure you added the conjugate then you have forgotten the positive unconjugated antibody or it does not bind in any case. It is rare for conjugates to become completely inactive during storage.

This may also be due to the UV microscope, a transmitted-light microscope is good for stained sections but epi-illumination is required for cell-surface immunofluorescence. Finally, ensure that the eye-pieces are of the correct magnification for the lens system— the intensity loss with $\times$ 12·5 compared with $\times$ 6·3 eye-pieces often makes the difference between nothing and superb fluorescence.

3 Everything staining with bright stars

Your conjugated antiserum is either contaminated with bacteria or has been frozen or thawed too many times thus producing immune complexes. Ultracentrifuge the conjugate to remove the contamination.

Whenever possible, store antisera at 4° with a preservative (either sodium azide or merthiolate), if it is not possible to use a preservative, store at $-20°$ in small aliquots.

4 Negative control serum giving positive staining

Strictly, the negative control serum must be taken from the animal before immunization. Staining either indicates non-specific binding (perhaps due to a high protein concentration) or the presence of antibodies not elicited by immunization. It is not valid to attempt to absorb out this reactivity, you must immunize another animal.

5 Uptake of exogenous proteins onto cell surfaces

In later sections, cells will be cultured in medium containing a serum supplement. Rat serum, for example, gives good *in vitro* maintenance of mouse cells but cross-reacts with anti-mouse sera. (Even FBS can be a problem in this way.) If required, we suggest that you ensure that your antisera stain specifically by absorbing them in the following manner:

Method for absorbing antisera with insolubilized antigens

Materials

Saturated ammonium sulphate, pH 7·2
Fetal bovine serum or rat serum (whichever serum supplement is giving cross-reactivity)
Saline (Appendix I)
2·5% v/v glutaraldehyde in aqueous solution

Method

1 Precipitate the γ-globulin fraction of the serum (Section 1.2.2a) and re-dissolve the precipitate in a minimum volume of PBS.

2 Dialyse the re-dissolved precipitate against PBS either overnight in dialysis tubing or by passing it through a Sephadex G-25 column equilibrated with PBS (see Section 1.2.3).

3 Measure the protein concentration of the sample and adjust to 20 mg ml^{-1}.

4 Add glutaraldehyde dropwise to the protein solution while stirring (use 0·5 ml of a 2·5% aqueous solution of glutaraldehyde for each 100 mg of protein to be insolubilized). A gel should form almost immediately.

5 Allow the gel to stand for 3 hours at room temperature and then disperse in PBS using a Potter homogenizer.

6 Wash the gel with PBS by centrifugation (500 g for 20 min) until protein cannot be detected in the undiluted supernatant by UV spectroscopy (O.D. less than 0·01; $E_{280\,nm}^{1\cdot0\,cm}$).

7 Mix an equal volume of the immunoadsorbent gel with the anti-Ig sera. Mix at 4° overnight.

8 Spin off the immunoadsorbent (500 g × 20 min) and store the antiserum at −20° until used.

It is obviously important to ensure specificity of the antisera under these conditions as one may simply be examining the uptake of proteins from the serum supplement of the tissue culture medium. It is important to use an insoluble immunoadsorbent to avoid the formation of soluble complexes in the absorbed antiserum.

1.7 **BASIC CELL TECHNIQUES**

1.7.1 PREPARATION OF LYMPHOCYTES FROM BLOOD

Many different methods have been described for separating white cells from erythrocytes. Differential centrifugation on a density gradient gives high purity lymphocyte preparations and is rapid.

Mouse and human lymphocytes

DIFFERENTIAL CENTRIFUGATION

Blood is layered onto a density gradient formulated such that only the red cells form a pellet.

Materials required

Triosil 75 (available commercially, and is sterile) (Appendix II)
Ficoll (Appendix II)

17

Method

1   Prepare a 9·2% Ficoll solution in distilled water and autoclave.
2   Mix 43·4 ml of Ficoll solution and 6·6 ml of Triosil 75.
3   Use 5 ml of blood with 2 ml of the gradient mixture and centrifuge at 300 g for 15 min at 4°. *The white cells should not enter the gradient, but remain at the plasma/density gradient interface as a white band.*
4   Remove the medium above the gradient and wash the lymphocytes three times by centrifugation (150 g for 10 min at 4°).

This technique will work with heparinized blood.

Commercial preparations of the density gradient are prepared gravimetrically and give more reproducible results. There are many suppliers, for example, Lymphoprep (Appendix II).

1.7.2   DEFIBRINATION OF BLOOD

Materials required

100 ml bottles
Glass balls (Appendix II)
Blood without anticoagulant
1 M hydrochloric acid

Preparation in advance

1   Wash the glass balls overnight in 1 M HCl and then wash three times with a detergent.
2   Wash the balls thoroughly with distilled water and dry them in an oven.
3   Add 3 g of the glass balls to each 100 ml bottle and autoclave at 138 kPa (20 p.s.i.) for 20 min.

A 100 ml bottle can be used to defibrinate 50 ml of blood.

Method

1   Add blood to bottles and mix by inverting until the clot has completely formed (10–20 min). Do not allow the blood to clot without mixing.
2   Allow the clotted blood to stand for 30 min and remove the serum which will contain free cells.

CHICKEN LYMPHOCYTES

Although dextran sedimentation techniques are available to prepare chicken leucocytes, they give very poor cell yields. Fortunately chicken erythrocytes are much larger than the white cells and so separation by differential centrifugation is possible without a density gradient. In addition, chicken polymorphonuclear cells tend to clump readily under normal conditions and so these are also removed from the plasma.

Materials

Chicken blood containing heparin

Method

1   Cool the blood to 4°.
2   Centrifuge at 150 g for 3 min at 4°.
3   Reduce the centrifugal force to 35 g, and continue spinning for a further 10 min at 4°.

The supernatant plasma will contain lymphocytes virtually free of all other cells. It is essential to use blood containing heparin, as citrated saline reduces the viscosity of the plasma and reduces cell yield and purity. Because cockerel blood has a lower viscosity than hen blood due to its lower lipid content, a loose buffy coat often forms during centrifugation, this should be re-suspended by gentle stirring.

1.7.3   PREPARATION OF LYMPHOCYTES FROM SOLID LYMPHOID ORGANS

Lymphocyte suspensions may be prepared from the spleen, lymph nodes, bursa or thymus by teasing the organs apart with forceps. Either squeeze the organ with broad forceps so that cells are forced into tissue culture medium, or tease the organ with fine forceps over a fine wire mesh or tea strainer.

Cell suspensions prepared in this way vary in their viability: thymus usually 95%, spleen 80–90% and lymph node 70–80%. It is therefore necessary to remove the dead cells using the technique described in Section 10.9.1, Technical note.

1.7.4   REMOVAL OF PHAGOCYTIC CELLS

Macrophages can be removed from a cell suspension using either their adherence or phagocytic properties.

a. ADHERENCE TO SEPHADEX

Materials and equipment

Cells for depletion.
Sephadex, G10 (Appendix II)

Tissue culture medium (Appendix I) containing 10% fetal bovine serum (FBS)
Syringe barrel, 20 ml

Method

1   Hydrate the Sephadex in PBS and settle for 10 min to remove 'fines'.
2   Autoclave in glass bottles at 138 kPa (20 p.s.i.) for 15 min.
3   Pack 10 ml of sterile Sephadex into a 20 ml syringe barrel fitted with a sintered plastic disc, and wash with 10 ml of warm tissue culture medium.
4   Add a maximum of 2×10^8 cells in 1 ml and allow them to become included into the column bed.
5   Wash out the non-adherent cells with 20 ml of warm tissue culture medium, collect the effluent and concentrate the cells by centrifugation (150 g for 10 min at 4°).

Although adherent cells are also removed by filtration through glass beads or fibres, the resulting cell suspensions show a greater depletion of B lymphocytes compared to the technique described above.

b. PHAGOCYTOSIS OF IRON POWDER (for removal of actively phagocytic cells)

Materials and equipment

Iron powder (Appendix II). Wash in ethanol and water. If the cells are sterile autoclave as above.
Eclipse magnet (or one equally powerful) (Appendix II)
Cell suspension in medium containing 5% fetal bovine serum (FBS)
10 ml conical plastic tubes

Method

1   Adjust the cell suspension to $2–3 \times 10^7$ lymphocytes ml^{-1}.
2   Add 4 mg of iron powder and mix thoroughly.
3   Incubate at 37° for 30 min, mixing occasionally.
4   Stand the plastic tube on one of the poles of the magnet and leave at 4° for 10 min.
5   Remove the cells in suspension (with the tube still standing on the magnet) and transfer to a second plastic tube.
6   Re-settle the cells on the magnet for a further 10 min at 4°.

These are not preparative techniques. Macrophages containing, or coated with, iron powder are not functional.

PERITONEAL EXUDATE CELLS

Macrophages containing up to 50% lymphocytes may be prepared by washing the peritoneal cavity of mice or guinea-pigs. For many purposes it is possible to elicit larger numbers of macrophages by producing a local inflammatory response, for example, with starch, sodium trioleat, or paraffin oil, etc. You must remember, however, that macrophages elicited with starch, etc., will have engulfed particles and so not be completely 'normal'.

Materials

Mice or guinea-pigs
1% starch in saline
Tissue culture medium (Appendix I)
Repelcote (for siliconized glassware—Appendix II)
1% neutral red in saline.

Method

1   Inject 2 ml of starch solution into the peritoneal cavity of the mouse (25 ml with guinea-pigs).
2   Kill the animal after 3 days.
3   Inject 2–5 ml of tissue culture medium into the peritoneal cavity and gently press the abdomen to bring the cells into suspension (100 ml for guinea-pigs).
4   Open the abdominal skin of the mouse and hold up the centre of the peritoneum with forceps.
5   Make a small hole in the peritoneum and remove the medium with a pipette.
6   Finally open the mouse fully and suck out all the medium. *To handle these peritoneal exudate cells you must either use siliconized glassware or plastic.*
7   Estimate the number of phagocytes by the uptake of a 1% neutral red solution (haemocytometer count).
Note. A normal mouse will yield 5×10^6 peritoneal exudate cells, up to 50% of which will be lymphocytes.

ALTERNATIVE METHOD (especially for macrophage migration inhibition test, Section 10.12.1)

Materials

Guinea-pigs
Bayol F (Appendix II)
Tissue culture medium with 10% FBS (Appendix I)
1% neutral red in saline

Method

1 Inject 30 ml of mineral oil (Bayol F) into the abdominal cavity of the guinea-pig.

2 Kill with chloroform 3–6 days later and inject 100–150 ml tissue culture medium into the abdominal cavity.

3 Knead the animal's abdomen and remove the fluid with a 50 ml syringe.

4 Separate the oil from the tissue culture medium in a separating funnel or measuring cylinder.

5 Wash cells three times by centrifugation and estimate the number of phagocytes by neutral red uptake.

The exudate should contain approximately 75% phagocytes and 25% leucocytes.

1.8   ANIMALS

You will use mainly rabbits and mice throughout this book; the former to raise antisera, and the latter as experimental animals.

1.8.1   RABBITS

These do not need to be inbred, but should be as large as possible to give the maximum yield of blood and serum (you should get 100–120 ml blood, 60–75 ml serum per rabbit at exsanguination).

1.8.2   MICE

Many of the experiments described later can be performed with outbred mice. However, with cell transfer experiments inbred mice are essential.

The common strains of inbred mice are widely available from commercial dealers (Appendix II). As individuals within each strain have a much more restricted gene pool it is best to use them for investigational use whenever possible.

COMMON INBRED STRAINS

C3H }
CBA } These mice may be used for all the experiments described.
C57Bl }

BALB/c Although widely used for other purposes, it is best to avoid these mice for cell transfer experiments as their lethal X-ray dose is below that required for good immunosuppression.

DBA/2 } These strains are used for certain experiments described.
AKR   } However, they are uncommon and expensive.

22

NZB   Immunologically this is a very interesting mouse strain as it is subject to spontaneous immunopathological disorders (Section 4.4).

Nu/Nu   This strain is congenitally athymic (or nearly so!) and has largely replaced the 'B' mouse (Section 10.6). As you may expect, they are difficult to keep and are expensive. Nude strains are now available that are congenic with BALB/c and C57Bl.

1.8.3   X-IRRADIATION OF MICE

Mice are routinely immunosuppressed by 800–850 R total body irradiation. Under these conditions you should have only the occasional death by 7 days' post-irradiation without bone marrow therapy. Early X-ray death is usually due to gut damage, accordingly X-ray resistance may be increased by starving the mice 24 hours before irradiation.

For conventional animal rooms it is recommended that irradiated mice, whether given bone marrow therapy or not, should be maintained on antibiotics for the first few weeks post-irradiation.

Antibiotic regime: in drinking water, *ad libitum*: 1 g Neomycin; 100 mg polymixin to 10 l distilled water.

Dose response curve of X-ray induced immunosuppression is determined in Section 10.4.1.

FURTHER READING

BOMFORD R. (1980) The comparative selectivity of adjuvants for humoral and cell mediated immunity. *Clin. Exp. Immunol.* **39**, 426, 435.

GREEN C.J. (1979) *Animal Anaesthesia.* Laboratory Animals Ltd, London.

HERBERT W.J. (1978) Laboratory animal techniques for immunology. In *Handbook of Experimental Immunology* 3e, ed. D.M. Weir. Blackwell Scientific Publications, Oxford.

MARRETTA J. & CASEY F.B. (1979) Dependence of guinea pig IgE and IgG, immune responses on the inclusion of potassium in the preparation of alum adjuvant. *J. Immunol. Methods* **31**, 188.

NAIRN R.C. (1976) In *Fluorescent Protein Tracing* 4e. Churchill Livingstone, Edinburgh.

ROSE N.R. & FRIEDMAN H. (1976) *Manual of Clinical Immunology.* American Society for Microbiology.

SELA M. (ed.) (1973 *et seq.*) *The Antigens*, vols. 1–5. Academic Press, London.

THOMPSON R.A. (ed.) (1977) *Techniques in Clinical Immunology.* Blackwell Scientific Publications, Oxford.

WILLIAMS C.A. & CHASE M.W. (1967 *et seq.*) *Methods in Immunology and Immunochemistry.* Academic Press, London.

——— (1972) *The UFAW Handbook on the Care and Management of Laboratory Animals* 4e. Churchill Livingstone, Edinburgh.

2　The lymphocyte: its rôle and function

2.1　WHAT IS A LYMPHOCYTE?

Having caught measles as a child you became sick. As you obviously survived you are no longer afraid of catching measles, although you may catch chickenpox. The protection afforded by the immune system is specific to those dangerous antigens you have previously experienced and survived! The basic unit of this SPECIFIC IMMUNE RESPONSE is the LYMPHOCYTE. Throughout the book you will encounter the lymphocyte and its precursors being acted upon and reacting to, not dangerous antigens such as viruses or bacteria, but to artificial antigens of a much more defined and informative nature. Fortunately lymphocytes react as readily to 'artificial' antigens as 'natural' ones.

Lymphocytes differentiate from precursor cells (derived from the yolk sac, bone marrow and fetal liver) which migrate to the so-called CENTRAL LYMPHOID ORGANS, i.e. the thymus and the bursa (or its equivalent in mammals). When their differentiation is complete lymphocytes migrate to and populate the peripheral lymphoid organs, i.e. blood, spleen, lymph nodes, Peyer's patches, lymphoid appendix, etc. At this stage the animal is usually immunologically mature and able to respond to antigenic challenge.

The mouse has been invaluable in immunological research as an animal model for the clinically important 'human situation'. Its convenience as a research tool is obvious, and consequently its immune system is probably the best known in the Animal Kingdom. The anatomical and morphological aspects of Chapter 2 should not be by-passed as a thorough knowledge is essential, both to obtain material for further study, and to understand the cell traffic through the lymphoid compartments in any immune response.

2.2　LYMPHOID ORGANS OF THE MOUSE

Fig. 2.1 shows the major lymphoid organs of the mouse and their cellular composition. There is a continuous traffic of recirculating

Fig. 2.1 (facing page) **The major lymphoid organs of the mouse**
One of the major lymphoid organs not obvious in the drawing is the blood. It contains $5-11 \times 10^6$ lymphocytes ml^{-1}.

The data given in the figure for the lymphocyte content of the various organs were derived from BALB/c and CBA mice of about 4–8 weeks' old. The cell content is known to vary with age (especially the thymus), strain, sex, health and immune status of the individual.

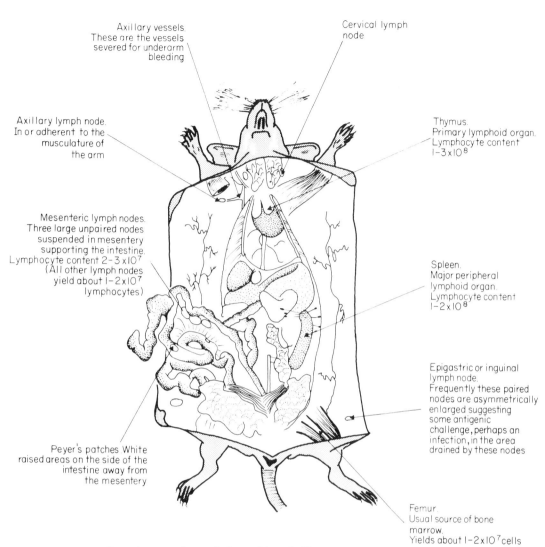

Axillary vessels.
These are the vessels
severed for underarm
bleeding

Cervical lymph
node

Axillary lymph node.
In or adherent to the
musculature of
the arm

Thymus.
Primary lymphoid organ.
Lymphocyte content
$1-3 \times 10^8$

Mesenteric lymph nodes.
Three large unpaired nodes
suspended in mesentery
supporting the intestine.
Lymphocyte content $2-3 \times 10^7$
(All other lymph nodes
yield about $1-2 \times 10^7$
lymphocytes)

Spleen.
Major peripheral
lymphoid organ.
Lymphocyte content
$1-2 \times 10^8$

Epigastric or inguinal
lymph node.
Frequently these paired
nodes are asymmetrically
enlarged suggesting
some antigenic
challenge, perhaps an
infection, in the area
drained by these nodes

Peyer's patches White
raised areas on the side of the
intestine away from
the mesentery

Femur.
Usual source of bone
marrow.
Yields about $1-2 \times 10^7$ cells

Lymphocyte sub-populations of lymphoid organs

Organ	% T lymphocytes	% B lymphocytes	% 'Null' cells
Thymus	97	1	2
Lymph node	77	18	5
Spleen	35	38	27
Blood	70	24	6
Thoracic duct lymph	80	19	1

Definition of cells in figure

T lymphocyte. Thymus-derived small lymphocyte, detected by presence of
Thy.1 antigen and absence of Ig on surface membrane.

B lymphocyte. Bursa-equivalent-derived small lymphocyte, detected by
presence of Ig and absence of Thy.1 antigen on surface membrane.

'Null' cell. Small mononuclear cell, no Thy.1 or Ig on surface membrane
may or may not be a cell of the lymphoid series, and probably of more
than one cell lineage.

small lymphocytes from the blood into the other peripheral lymphoid organs such as the spleen, lymph nodes, etc. From here the cells enter the other tissues and finally return to the blood via the lymphatic vessels, e.g. thoracic duct. You should remember that the intact immune response involves great changes in the 'trafficking' pattern of antigen reactive lymphocytes. When specific small lymphocytes are confronted with antigen they will leave this recirculating pool, and congregate at the site of the greatest antigen concentration.

2.3 THE SMALL LYMPHOCYTE

Cells will be stained for morphological examination from mouse thymus (a central lymphoid organ) and blood (a very important peripheral lymphoid organ).

2.3.1 MORPHOLOGY OF THYMUS AND BLOOD LEUCOCYTES

2.3.1a **Blood film**

Materials and equipment

Mouse
Microscope slides (cleaned overnight in acetone : ethanol 50 : 50 v/v)
95% methanol in water

Method

1   Warm the mouse, either under a lamp or by immersing its tail in hand hot water.
2   Grasp the mouse firmly by the nape of the neck and cut 1 cm from the end of its tail.
3   Squeeze one drop of blood from the tail and place at one end of a clean slide.
4   Use a second, 'spreader' slide and touch the extreme edge of the drop of blood. Hold this slide at about 45°.

26

5 Allow the blood to flow along the edge of the spreader slide and then push it away from the drop to obtain a film of cells (ideally in the shape of a bunsen flame).

6 Wave the slide in the air to dry it rapidly.

7 Fix in 95% methanol for 2 min.

With practice a serviceable, if not perfect, blood film can be produced. It is necessary to vary the size of the drop of blood and the amount taken up on the spreader slide to obtain an optimal distribution of cells.

2.3.1b **Smears of cell suspensions**

The blood plasma is viscous and so protects the cells from damage as they are smeared. Smears are more difficult to obtain from single-cell suspensions taken from organs. Although a cytocentrifuge provides an easy answer (Section 3.1.1b), it is possible to obtain excellent preparations by simply suspending the cells in neat serum and smearing them as in the previous section.

Materials and equipment

Organs from mouse in previous section
Phosphate buffered saline (PBS) (Appendix I)
Fetal bovine serum (FBS)
Clean microscope slides as previous section
95% methanol in water

Method

1 Kill the mouse by cervical dislocation and remove the spleen, mesenteric lymph nodes and thymus into Petri dishes containing PBS or tissue culture medium.

2 Cut up the organs with scissors and store pieces on ice for later use (Section 2.4).

3 Tease one lobe of the thymus apart with forceps into 1 ml of fetal bovine serum (FBS), squeezing gently until cells leave the thymus.

4 Place one drop of the cell suspension on a clean slide and smear with a second slide as before (Section 2.3.1a).

5 Dry the slide in the air and fix in 95% methanol for 2 min.

6 Wash the slide in running tap water for 30 minutes to remove the FBS.

Again, the concentration of the cells in the suspension and the volume used must be varied to obtain a good smear.

To examine the morphological details of the prepared cells, it is necessary to stain them. Pleasing results can be obtained with May–Grünwald/Giemsa staining.

MAY–GRÜNWALD/GIEMSA STAINING

Materials and equipment

Cell smears from previous sections
Giemsa buffer (Appendix I)
May–Grünwald stain (Appendix II)
Giemsa stain (Appendix II)
Staining racks and troughs
Neutral mounting medium (DePeX—Appendix II)
(Note: the stains must be freshly diluted)

Method

1 Immerse the fixed cells in buffer for 5 min.
2 Transfer to May–Grünwald stain (diluted 1 : 2 with buffer) for 5 min.
3 Rinse the slides in buffer and blot dry.
4 Stain in Giemsa solution (diluted 1 : 5 with buffer) for 15 min.
5 Rinse in the buffer.

If the cells are overstained (too blue) allow them to stand in the buffer. Finally dry the slides in air and examine them under the microscope. If permanent preparations are required the cells may be mounted in a neutral mounting medium under a coverslip. (Use DePeX. Canada Balsam, although sold in a neutral form, eventually decolourizes the stained cells.)

Examination of cell smears

During smearing white cells tend to move differentially to the red cells and so you will find them at the edges and extreme end of the film. Fig. 2.2 shows the typical morphology of cells encountered in stained mouse blood. Although you should be familiar with their appearance you will rarely look at stained cells in modern immunology, because small lymphocytes have the disadvantage of all looking alike.

The stained cells from the thymus are much more homogeneous than those of the blood, the majority have the morphological appearance typical of small lymphocytes (Fig. 2.2).

Most of the cellular experiments described in this book use living cells, and so the reader should ensure that he is able to recognize the different white cells under a phase contrast microscope. To this end we suggest that cell counts should be performed on cell suspensions prepared from the second thymus lobe, lymph nodes and spleen of the mouse just killed. The order of examining organs has been so arranged to allow practice in recognizing small lymphocytes in homogeneous suspension before counting the spleen cell suspension, which is much more heterogeneous.

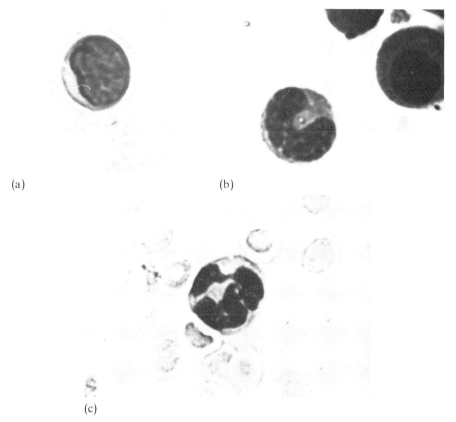

(a)

(b)

(c)

Fig. 2.2. Morphology of blood leucocytes concerned in the immune response
(a) Small lymphocyte. ($\times$ 2500)
(b) Monocyte. ($\times$ 1500)
(c) Polymorphonuclear leucocyte. ($\times$ 1500)

2.4   VIABLE LYMPHOCYTE COUNT

It must be emphasized that at all the following stages in the book, the experimentor will be handling living cells. Maximum *in vitro* viability is usually maintained if the cells are kept at 0°, i.e. in melting ice. Guinea-pig lymphocytes, however, are the exception to this rule; they should not be cooled below room temperature.

Cells that are to be used in an experiment must be removed freshly from the animal, and the experiment completed, or the cells put into culture or transferred *in vivo* as quickly as possible. In general, living cells will not survive overnight in a refrigerator.

The plasma membrane of a viable cell does not permit the entry of non-electrolyte dye substances. This phenomenon is used to distinguish dead from living lymphocytes. Many dyes are suitable for this purpose, for example, trypan blue or eosin in dilute, physiological solution. However, we have found that nigrosin has invariably been the least toxic dye for estimation of cell viability (See Fig. 2.3).

29

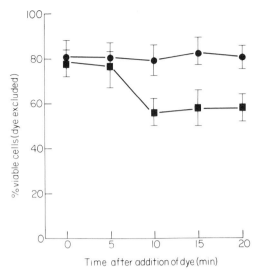

Fig. 2.3. Cell viability in trypan blue and nigrosin dyes
An aliquot of mouse lymph node cells in phosphate buffered saline was
mixed with an equal volume of 0·2% trypan blue (■———■) or nigrosin
dye (●———●) and incubated at 37° for 3 min to facilitate dye uptake into
dead cells. The suspensions were then returned to 0° (time 0) and the
percentage of viable cells determined at the time points shown on the graph.

Although the cell viability decreased rapidly over the first 10 min in
trypan blue, it remained at a plateau value of 60% for the next 60 min (full
data not shown). The material released from the dead cells bound to the
trypan blue and formed a precipitate.

2.4.1   DYE EXCLUSION TEST

Materials and equipment

Organs from mouse in Section 2.3.1b
Phosphate buffered saline (PBS) (Appendix I)
Nigrosin dye (Appendix II)
Nylon wool
2 ml syringe barrels
Centrifuge, refrigerated (Appendix II)
Haemocytometer—improved Neubauer ruling, preferably rhodium
plated

Method

1   Tease the remaining thymus lobe, spleen and lymph nodes into
5 ml aliquots of PBS in a petri dish standing on ice.
2   Loosely pack 1 ml of nylon wool into each of the syringe barrels,
and wash with 5 ml of PBS.
3   Filter each cell suspension through a nylon wool column and
wash out with 2 ml of PBS. *Filtration removes cell aggregates and
gives a single-cell suspension. This step is required for all* in vitro
techniques encountered later.

30

Whenever lymphocytes are used for in vivo *or* in vitro *study they are usually washed by centrifugation to remove any adherent exogenous material. In addition, dead cells are often disrupted during centrifugation and so the percentage cell viability increases during this washing procedure. It is included here merely to concentrate the lymphocytes for further handling.*

4 Centrifuge all lymphocyte suspensions at 150 g for 10 min at 4°.

5 Remove the supernatant using a Pasteur pipette connected to a water vacuum pump. Keep the pipette at the meniscus at all times to avoid turbulence and cell loss.

6 Resuspend the cells in 5 ml of PBS.

7 Mix 0·1 ml of each cell suspension with 0·1 ml of 0·2% nigrosin solution and incubate at room temperature for 5 min.

8 Count the number of viable (unstained) lymphocytes using a haemocytometer and a phase-contrast microscope.

9 Dead cells may be removed as described in Section 10.9.1 technical note 1.

Technical note
Prepare a 2% stock solution of nigrosin and dilute with sterile saline for use.

2.4.2 CELL COUNTS WITH A HAEMOCYTOMETER

When counting lymphocyte suspensions it is most convenient to use a ×40 objective and to count in the central, triple-ruled area of the haemocytometer (this area is used for red-cell counting in haematology). Count the cells in the large triple-ruled squares until a minimum of 100 unstained (viable) lymphocytes have been counted (see Fig. 2.4).

Calculate the number of viable cells as follows:

Number viable lymphocytes $\text{ml}^{-1} =$

$$\frac{\text{Number lymphocytes counted}}{\text{Number triple-ruled squares}} \times 25 \times 10^{4}$$
$$\times \text{ original dilution (if any)}$$

2.5 LYMPHOCYTE SURFACE MEMBRANE

In a normal animal, the majority of the circulating lymphocytes spend their time apparently doing nothing, they are resting or G_0 cells. As will be seen later, these dormant cells are specifically activated after contact with antigen. Antigen contact occurs as a specific surface event at the plasma membrane and generates a signal which causes nuclear de-repression. The cell enters the cell cycle and divides, it can eventually form a clone of effector cells all of the same specificity.

31

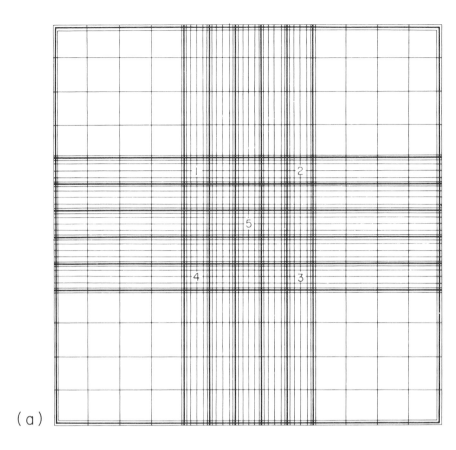

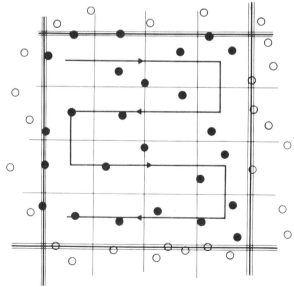

(a)

(b)

The initial observations on the basis of antigen stimulation will be made on avian lymphocytes, birds in general are immunologically convenient animals as you are about to prove. The next two experiments might appear pointless without previous knowledge, however, you will make observations that are basic to cellular immunology.

2.5.1 IMMUNOFLUORESCENT STAINING OF LYMPHOCYTE MEMBRANES

Preparation required: the antisera used in this experiment must be standardized for chicken blood as described for the mouse system in Section 1.6.5.

Materials and equipment

1 cockerel, about 2–4 months old
Heparin (25,000 units ml^{-1})
Tissue culture medium (Appendix I) containing 20 mM sodium azide
Nylon wool
2 ml syringe barrels
Haemocytometer
Rabbit anti-fowl γ-globulin (anti-Ig) (Section 1.4.5)
Fluorescein-conjugated goat or sheep anti-rabbit γ-globulin (anti-Ig) (Sections 1.4.7 and 1.6)
Mounting medium: 70% glycerol, 30% glycine-saline buffer, pH 8·6 (Appendix I)

CELLS

This procedure must be done with the aid of an assistant.

Method

1   Invert the chicken over the edge of the bench with its head facing downwards. Hold legs and wings with one hand and the head with the other.
2   Take 0·1–0·2 ml of heparin into the syringe. *Although a convenient volume, this is a vast excess.*
3   Insert the syringe needle into the chicken at the internal apex of the clavicles ('wish bone') keeping the syringe horizontal. A slight

Fig. 2.4 (opposite page). Improved Neubauer ruling haemocytometer
(a) For high-density lymphocyte populations count in the central, triple-ruled area, in the order shown.
(b) Enlarged view of square 1. Cells falling across the top and left border lines of a square are considered to be in that square, whereas cells on the bottom and right borders are excluded. The diagram shows 25 cells in an area of $\frac{1}{25}$ mm^2, depth of chamber 0·1 mm. Count at least 100 cells per sample.

33

negative pressure should be exerted on the syringe as it enters the bird so that blood will enter rapidly when the heart is pierced.

4   Exsanguinate the chicken. (Ensure that the blood is mixed thoroughly with the heparin in the syringe. Kill chicken by cervical dislocation if required.)

5   Remove the syringe needle and put the blood into tubes on ice.

6   Turn the chicken over and make an incision in the dorsal surface (back) of the neck.

7   Reflect the skin and identify the thymus lobes running beside the carotid artery on either side of the neck.

8   Remove two or three lobes into a Petri dish containing tissue culture medium on ice.

9   At the other end of the chicken, make an incision dorsal to cloaca, between the tail and the vent.

10   Dissect with forceps until a large sac-like organ is seen, this is the bursa. Remove into tissue culture medium.

Lymphocyte suspensions must now be prepared from all these tissues. These cells are living and so it is essential to work on ice or at 4° throughout.

11   Prepare lymphocytes from the blood as described in Section 1.7.1.

12   Cut open the bursa and tease out 4 or 5 of the internal plicae (flaps).

13   Tease out the thymus lobes.

14   Filter the thymus and bursa suspensions through nylon wool to remove aggregates (Section 2.4.1).

15   Wash all cells three times in tissue culture medium by centrifugation (150 g for 10 min at 4°).

16   Resuspend all cells in 10 ml of medium and count the number of viable lymphocytes per ml (Section 2.4).

17   Pipette out two aliquots of approximately 10^7 lymphocytes of each cell suspension and centrifuge to obtain a pellet (150 g for 10 min at 4°).

18   Add 0·1 ml of the required dilution of rabbit anti-chicken Ig or 0·1 ml of the control NRS dilution to one aliquot of each cell type. (Antiserum standardized as in section 1.6.5).

19   Incubate for 30 minutes on ice.

20   Wash twice by centrifugation (150 g for 10 min at 4°) to remove the unbound protein.

21   Add 0·1 ml of the fluorescein-conjugated goat or sheep anti-rabbit Ig (1 mg ml^{-1}) to all cell pellets.

22   Incubate for 30 minutes at 4°.

23   Wash three times by centrifugation to remove the unbound conjugate (150 g × 10 min at 4°).

24   Resuspend, and add 1 drop of glycerol-glycine mounting medium to the dry cell pellet and mix thoroughly.

25   Put one drop of cell suspension on a microscope slide and ring the coverslip with nail varnish.

ASSESSMENT OF POSITIVE CELLS

Examine the mounted cells under an incident light UV microscope. Identify positive (stained) and negative (unstained) lymphocytes under the UV and tungsten light respectively (see Fig. 2.5). Dead cells have a bright homogeneous fluorescence.

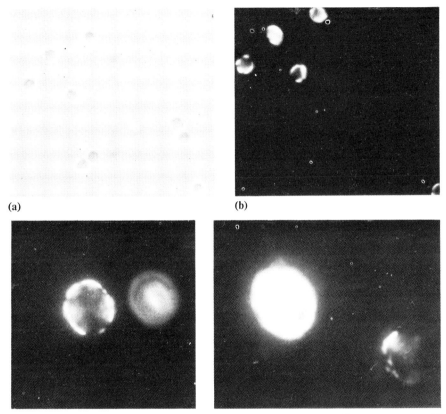

(a)   (b)

(c)   **Fig. 2.5. Lymphocytes showing cell membrane immunofluorescence**   (d)

(a) Mouse lymph node lymphocytes viewed under tungsten light.

(b) Same microscope field under incident UV light. Cells have been stained with a direct conjugate of rhodamine and rabbit anti-mouse light chain. As can be seen, fluorescence is limited to only a proportion of the cells seen in (a).

(c) Lymphocyte stained with rhodamine conjugated anti-light chain and visualized under UV light. The patchy ring staining is typical of viable lymphocytes. The fluorochrome conjugated antiserum is unable to cross the cell membrane and so only reacts with surface determinants, seen here in optical cross-section. The patching is not inhibited at 4° or in the presence of metabolic inhibitors, for example, sodium azide (20 mM final concentration) and is thought to be due to local cross-linking of membrane determinants.

(d) A dead cell showing bright homogeneous intracytoplasmic fluorescence; such cells should be excluded from all counts of stained (positive) cells.

35

For each microscope field: count the number of fluorescing lymphocytes under UV light and then the total number of lymphocytes in the field under tungsten light. Count a total of 200 cells under the tungsten light and calculate the percentage of fluorescing (positive) lymphocytes for each preparation. Record the results as in the example below.

Example of experimental record:

Anti-Ig staining of chicken lymphocytes: thymus, bursa, blood.
Animals: 2-month-old White Leghorn cockerel
Tissues: 50 ml heparinized blood
       3 thymus lobes
       4 bursal plicae

Cell counts:

	No. of lymphocytes ml^{-1}	Total vol.	Vol. per aliquot for staining
thymus	$3\cdot3 \times 10^7$	10 ml	0·3 ml
bursa	$4\cdot5 \times 10^6$	10 ml	2·2 ml
blood	$3\cdot0 \times 10^7$	10 ml	0·4 ml

Antiserum: Rabbit anti-chicken Ig—identification number and dilution. NRS—identification number and dilution.
Results:

	Anti-Ig		NRS	
Cells	*Stained lymphocytes* Total counted	% positive	*Stained lymphocytes* Total counted	% positive
thymus	$\dfrac{13}{210}$	6	$\dfrac{0}{230}$	0
bursa	$\dfrac{201}{240}$	84	$\dfrac{2}{210}$	1
blood	$\dfrac{73}{208}$	35	$\dfrac{0}{210}$	0

Although the thymus and bursa contain immature lymphocytes, a large proportion of the bursa cells (B lymphocytes) already express surface immunoglobulin. The association of anti-immunoglobulin surface immunofluorescence with B, but not T, lymphocytes has been confirmed by repeating the above experiment with mature lymphocytes from the peripheral blood of neonatally thymectomized (B lymphocytes) or bursectomized (T lymphocytes) chickens (Section 10.5). In the former, B lymphocytes (as evidenced by anti-immunoglobulin surface fluorescence) can reach virtually 100%, whereas in the latter immunoglobulin bearing cells are greatly reduced or absent.

From independent experiments, using antisera specific for T and B lymphocyte surface antigens, it has been found that the blood of mature chickens contain 60% T lymphocytes, 35% B lymphocytes and 5% 'null' (carrying neither T or B antigens) cells. The percentage of B lymphocytes defined in this way is usually within a few per cent of the cells carrying surface immunoglobulin.

The immunoglobulin bearing cells in the thymus of the chicken examined above probably represent B lymphocytes 'trafficking' through the blood vessels around the thymus, there is no evidence that the thymus can give rise to cells carrying immunoglobulin constant region determinants.

(The control of conjugate alone can be avoided as explained in the technical notes in section 1.6.6.)

The experiment as described will take a whole day without previous experience. The experiment may be shortened using a directly conjugated anti-chicken immunoglobulin serum, however, under these conditions the fluorescence will only be detected with an incident light UV microscope.

Technical notes

1   When working with low cell numbers it is possible to pellet the stained cells in a Beckman Microfuge tube immediately prior to the addition of the mountant (centrifuge at 150 g for 5 min at 4°).
2   Rhodamine conjugated antisera quench much more slowly than fluorescein conjugated antisera.

2.6   **ANTIGEN-BINDING LYMPHOCYTES**

We are now going to describe a basic technique by which antigen-binding lymphocytes can be visualized. The applicability of this approach is limited principally by the experimental design to ensure that non-specific binding is avoided. It is, however, difficult in this type of experiment to include a good specificity control. The approach adopted here is to show that the number of antigen-binding lymphocytes increases after immunization.

2.6.1   SHEEP RBC ROSETTES

You will perform a rosette inhibition experiment with anti-mouse Ig at the same time as determining the number of antigen-binding lymphocytes.

Preparation required

1   Immunize a mouse 7 days before the experiment with 10^8 sheep erythrocytes (SRBC) given intraperitoneally.

2 The anti-mouse γ-globulin and NRS must be absorbed with mouse liver and RBC, as well as sheep RBCs, to be sure they are free of anti-species activity. (See Section 2.9.1.)

Materials and equipment

Normal and SRBC immunized mice
Sheep erythrocytes (SRBC)
Tissue culture medium (Appendix I)
Rabbit anti-mouse γ-globulin (anti-Ig) (Section 1.4.2)
Normal rabbit serum (NRS) (Appendix II)
Nylon wool
2 ml syringe barrels
2 ml plastic tubes

Method

1 Kill the mice, prepare spleen-cell suspensions by teasing and filter through nylon wool (Section 2.4).
2 Remove phagocytic cells (Section 1.7.4).
3 Wash the cells 3 times by centrifugation (150 g for 10 min at 4°).
4 Count the number of viable lymphocytes ml^{-1} (Section 2.4) and adjust to 3×10^7 ml^{-1}.
5 Label tubes and add 0·1 ml aliquots of the lymphocyte suspensions as shown in the protocol.

Protocol

Tube	Lymphocytes from:	Antiserum incubation before rosetting:
1	immune spleen	none
2	normal spleen	none
3	immune spleen	anti-mouse γ globulin
4	immune spleen	NRS

6 Add 0·1 ml of the appropriate sera to tubes 3 and 4. (Use the optimal dilution for immunofluorescence. Alternatively you may wish to do a full titration curve of rosette inhibition.)
7 Incubate tubes 3 and 4 at 4° for 30 min.
8 Add 0·1 ml SRBC suspension ($2·4 \times 10^8$ SRBC ml^{-1}) to tubes 1 and 2. Mix well.
9 Centrifuge tubes 1 and 2 at 150 g for 10 min at 4°.
10 Add 0·3 ml of the 0·05% acridine orange solution if UV microscope is available (if not use tissue culture medium) to tubes 1 and 2 and resuspend the cells on a vertical rotor turning at 8–10 rev min^{-1} for 5 min. (Alternatively, you may resuspend the cells using a Pasteur pipette. This, however, reduces the number of rosettes.)
11 Repeat the addition of SRBC, centrifugation and resuspension

for the cells pre-treated with antisera (i.e. tubes 3 and 4). This time, however, add only 0·2 ml of acridine orange solution (or tissue culture medium).

12 Count the number of rosettes in each suspension using a haemocytometer and a microscope with transmitted light. Count at least 4 samples per tube.

If you are using a microscope with UV light, live cells may be seen at the centre of the rosette by their green fluorescence (dead cells are deep red). If a UV microscope is not used then 0·1 % toluidine blue may be used to visualize nucleated cells. Do not count rosettes with more than one lymphocyte, or clumped red cells without lymphocytes.

See Fig. 2.6.

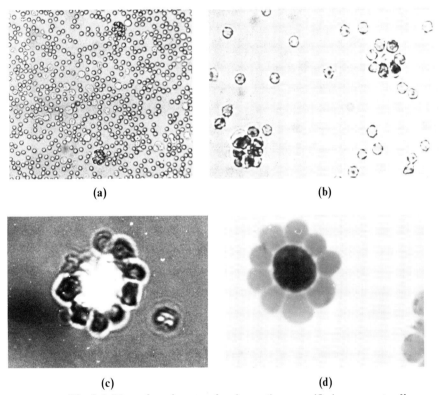

(a) (b)

(c) (d)

Fig. 2.6. Mouse lymphocytes showing antigen-specific immunocytoadherence with sheep erythrocytes

(a) Antigen-specific lymphocytes will bind sheep erythrocytes to their surface to form rosettes, two are shown in this field.
(b) At 4° the erythrocytes bind as a single layer.
(c) The nucleus of the lymphocyte at the centre of this rosette has been stained with acridine orange and is visualized under UV and tungsten light.
(d) The morphology of the rosette-forming cell may be seen after Giemsa staining of a cytocentrifuge preparation.

A rosette may be arbitrarily defined as a single lymphocyte binding 5 or more erythrocytes. If rosettes are incubated at 37°, in the absence of metabolic inhibition, erythrocyte 'caps' will form (cf. Section 2.8.1).

39

Calculation and evaluation of results:

a Calculate the number of rosettes ml^{-1} of suspension and from this the number of rosettes per million (10^{-6}) lymphocytes.

b Compare the number of rosettes per 10^6 lymphocytes from the normal and immune animals (tubes 1 and 2) and calculate the factor of immunization.

c You should find that all of the rosettes are blocked by the anti-immunoglobulin serum. Knowing that the RBC binding is a specific immunological event, you should be able to suggest a role for the immunoglobulin demonstrated in Section 2.5.1 on the surface of some lymphocytes. (Although chicken lymphocytes were stained in Section 2.5.1 the same staining characteristics can be shown for mouse lymphocytes.)

2.7   T AND B LYMPHOCYTE RECEPTORS

In immunology the terms receptor and binding site are often erroneously considered to be interchangeable. Although a receptor is certainly a binding site, the term imparts some biological significance to the binding event in initiating some positive or negative effect. The cell surface antigen and mitogen receptors undoubtedly deserve this status, however, it remains to be shown whether the so-called Fc and complement receptors deserve this distinction.

2.7.1   RANGE OF RECEPTORS

2.7.1a   ANTIGEN RECEPTORS

In sections 2.5.1 and 2.6.1 we made the following observations:

1   A sub-population of lymphocytes carry immunoglobulin molecules at their surface as demonstrated by indirect immunofluorescence.

2   The specific binding of antigen to lymphocytes may be blocked by anti-immunoglobulin antisera.

The evidence available here and from other sources suggests that this sub-population of lymphocytes—in fact B lymphocytes—use these immunoglobulin molecules as receptors for antigen. Combination of antigen with these receptors initiates all the phenomena associated with B effector cells described in later chapters and it is in such a receptor that the whole specificity of the immune response is invested.

Many cells (mast cells, monocytes, polymorphonuclear leucocytes, lymphocytes, etc.) carry receptors for the Fc region (see Fig. 7.19) of immunoglobulin molecules. Although there is a weak, easily reversible binding of native IgG to such cells, the strength of binding is greater with IgG antibody complexed either with antigen (Section 2.7.3) or aggregated by heat.

In a similar manner it is possible to demonstrate a site for the binding of activated C3 (in the form of antigen-antibody-complement complexes) to lymphocytes. The available evidence suggests that C3 binding is independent of Fc binding.

Although the role of Fc and C3 receptors on phagocytic cells (Section 6.5.1) in initiating immune elimination (Section 4.1) is clear the physiological significance of such receptors on T and B lymphocytes remains to be established.

2.7.2   LYMPHOCYTE RECEPTORS FOR ANTIGEN

There is ample immunological and biochemical evidence that B lymphocytes have IgM (monomeric) and IgD molecules integrated into their surface membrane as antigen receptors. Although these molecules have extensive homology with serum immunoglobulin, as shown, for example, by their serological cross-reactivity, the membrane bound molecules have chemically modified Fc regions (for example, membrane bound IgM has an extra peptide of 25 hydrophobic amino acids), to allow them to exist (and function) in the highly hydrophobic environment of the membrane.

The nature of the T lymphocyte receptor is still unclear. Their only uncontroversial attribute is that they apparently share idiotypic determinants (same shape of antigen binding site) with B lymphocyte receptors. The nature of the framework residues carrying the antigen combining site is not known.

Almost an equal number of papers have been published in the past showing that immunoglobulin constant region determinants were present or absent on T-lymphocyte surfaces. Although we are no nearer the true identity of the T lymphocyte receptor, the finding that the T lymphocyte antigen, Thy.1, shares limited sequence homology with one of the immunoglobulin heavy chain domains, may explain these anomalous findings.

2.7.3   DEMONSTRATION OF Fc RECEPTORS ON LYMPHOCYTES

Materials
Mice
Sheep erythrocytes (SRBC) (Appendix II)

Anti-SRBC serum, mouse or rabbit (Section 5.4.1b)
Saline (Appendix I)
Tissue culture medium (Appendix I)
Tris-ammonium chloride (Appendix I)

Method

1 Wash SRBC three times in saline by centrifugation (300 g for 5 min).
2 Resuspend pellet to 2×10^8 cells ml^{-1} (approximately 1% v/v) in tissue culture medium.
3 Incubate aliquots of the erythrocytes with the antiserum dilutions in a total volume of 0·5 ml (shown in the protocol) for 30 min at 37°.

Protocol

		Tube number		
	1	2	3	4
Sheep RBC (2×10^8 ml^{-1})	0·5 ml			$\longrightarrow$
Final antiserum	1 : 5	1 : 10	1 : 20	1 : 40

4 Wash each aliquot of SRBC three times in tissue culture medium by centrifugation and resuspend to 1 ml.
5 Take a sample from each aliquot of SRBC and examine under a microscope. Discard all aliquots showing visible agglutination.
6 Prepare cell suspensions from thymus, lymph nodes and spleen (Section 1.7.3) and wash three times in tissue culture medium by centrifugation (150 g for 10 min at 4°).
7 Count lymphocytes and adjust to 5×10^6 cells ml^{-1} (Section 2.4).
8 Mix 0·1 ml of each lymphocyte suspension with 0·2 ml of sensitized SRBC. *Use SRBC suspension with the lowest antiserum dilution not giving agglutination.*
9 Incubate at room temperature for 60–90 min.
10 Add acridine orange or toluidine blue dye (Section 2.6.1).
11 Determine the number of rosettes ml^{-1} as in Section 2.6.1.
12 Lyse a sample of each mixture with an equal volume of tris-ammonium chloride and count the number of viable lymphocytes ml^{-1} (Section 2.4).
13 Calculate the percentage of lymphocytes forming Fc rosettes (cf. fig. 2.7).

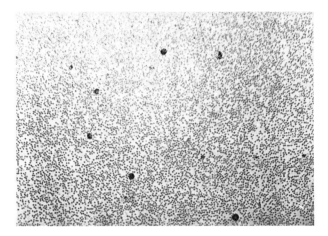

Fig. 2.7. Fc receptors on lymphocytes detected by sheep erythrocyte-antibody complexes.
The Fc of the antibody–erythrocyte complex binds to the Fc binding site on the lymphocyte forming a rosette which can be easily seen, even at low magnification.

The majority of the Fc binding lymphocytes are B cells, although recent evidence indicates that 3% of T small lymphocytes and 40% of antigen-activated T cells have Fc binding sites that can be detected by this technique.

2.8 MOBILITY OF THE LYMPHOCYTE SURFACE MEMBRANE

It should now be clear that the membrane-bound immunoglobulin on lymphocytes (demonstrated in Section 2.5.1) is a specific antigen receptor. It is present in the greatest concentration on the surface of those cells derived from the bursa. (Hence the reason for using chicken, and not the normal mouse model, in Section 2.5.1. Although mammals must possess a functionally equivalent site for B-cell differentiation it has not yet been definitely identified.)

Mouse bone marrow behaves as though it were a source of B cells (Section 4.2) and so, operationally at least, it has some of the attributes of a bursa.

With the techniques so far used you can now make some observations on the characteristics of this receptor molecule, and on the characteristics of nucleated cell membranes in general.

2.8.1 CAPPING OF LYMPHOCYTE RECEPTORS

Materials and equipment

Mouse spleen or lymph node suspension on ice
Tissue culture medium with and without sodium azide, 20 mM
(Appendix I)

43

Rabbit anti-mouse immunoglobulin serum (Section 1.4.2)
Fluorescein conjugated goat or sheep anti-rabbit γ globulin (Sections 1.4.7 and 1.6).

Method

1   Prepare a spleen or lymph node suspension in the usual way (Section 2.4), using tissue culture medium WITHOUT sodium azide.
2   Wash the suspension 3 times by centrifugation (150 g × 10 min at 4°).
3   Count the viable lymphocytes and dispense aliquots of 10^7 cells into each tube shown in the protocol. Centrifuge (150 g × 10 min at 4°) to obtain a cell pellet.

Protocol

| Tube number | Antiserum added | Incubation | | Medium |
		Temperature	Time	
1	anti-mouse Ig	4°	30 min	with azide
2	NRS control	4°	30 min	with azide
3	anti-mouse Ig	37°	5 min	without azide
4	anti-mouse Ig	37°	10 min	without azide
5	anti-mouse Ig	37°	15 min	without azide
6	anti-mouse Ig	37°	20 min	without azide
7	anti-mouse Ig	37°	30 min	without azide
8	anti-mouse Ig	37°	60 min	without azide

4   Add 0·1 ml of anti-mouse Ig or NRS to tubes 1 and 2. (The antiserum must be diluted with medium containing sodium azide, 20 mM final concentration. The sera should have been standardized for immunofluorescent staining, Section 1.6.5.)
5   Incubate tubes 1 and 2 on ice for 30 min.
6   Add the same dilution of anti-mouse Ig to tubes 3–8, however, this time dilute the antiserum with medium WITHOUT sodium azide.
7   Incubate tubes 3–8 in a water bath or incubator at 37°.
8   Remove tube from the 37° incubator at the intervals shown in the protocol and fill them with medium containing sodium azide, 20 mM, and stand on ice.
9   At the end of the incubation period of tubes 1 and 2, fill these with medium containing azide and store on ice.
10   At the end of the total incubation period (60 min), wash all cell suspensions (tubes 1–8) twice by centrifugation (150 g × 10 min at 4°).

44

11   Incubate all cell aliquots with 0·1 ml of goat or sheep anti-rabbit Ig conjugate (1 mg ml^{-1} final dilution) for 30 min at 4°. (Again the diluted conjugate must contain sodium azide.)

12   Wash cells 3 times by centrifugation (150 g × 10 min at 4°).

13   Resuspend the cell pellet in glycerol/glycine-saline mounting medium and observe the fluorescing lymphocytes, preferably with an incident light microscope.

Observations

Tube 1: Here you should see the normal 'broken ring' immunofluorescence already seen for mouse lymphocytes (Fig. 2.5).

Tube 2: This is the control and should be zero. If not proceed as in Section 1.6.6.

Tubes 3–8: You should observe staining as shown in Fig. 2.8 with

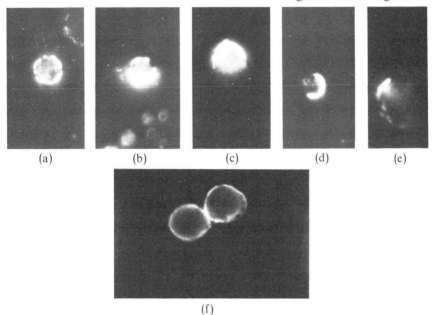

(a)　　　(b)　　　(c)　　　(d)　　　(e)

(f)

Fig. 2.8. Capping of lymphocyte receptors

If lymphocytes are treated with divalent anti-immunoglobulin antibodies the surface immunoglobulin determinants are cross-linked to form aggregates visible as a patchy ring of surface fluorescence (a).

At 37° and in the absence of metabolic inhibitors these patches coalesce (a–d) to form a 'polar cap' (e) which within 30 min is usually pinocytosed or shed into the medium. (Photograph (e) is at twice magnification of the others.)

Monovalent Fab anti-immunoglobulin antibodies are not able to cross-link the determinants and so ring staining is obtained (f), even at 37°. Pinocytosis still occurs on a limited scale even though patch and cap formation is not induced.

Surprisingly, ring staining is obtained when mouse T cells are stained with directly conjugated anti-Thy.1 serum (Section 10.8.5) presumably because of the low density of Thy.1 determinants.

NB. Recent evidence indicates that the blocking of cap formation by sodium azide is reversed by the presence of glucose.

a progressive clustering of the fluorescence to a polar 'cap'. With some anti-Ig sera this cap is then endocytosed and appears as pinpoints of fluorescence within the cell. With other antisera which do not induce endocytosis the stained membrane components are shed into the medium at 37° in the absence of respiratory inhibitors (e.g. sodium azide).

Refer to Fig. 2.8 before counting the stained cells in this experiment.

Data required

Determine the percentage of cells in each suspension showing (a) broken ring and (b) capped staining. If your antiserum induces endocytosis, determine the percentage of cells containing ingested fluorochrome.

Plot a graph against time for each set of data.

2.8.2   EXPERIMENTS WITH 'CAPPED' LYMPHOCYTES

The next experiments outlined are a refinement of the basic principle observed above. We will show: (a) the receptors have indeed been removed from the lymphocyte membrane (and that there has not been, for example, simply a dissociation of the antibody-receptor complex); (b) this capping is induced only by multivalent crosslinking agents; (c) lymphocytes are able to resynthesize their receptors.

a Naked lymphocytes. Attempt to re-stain the denuded lymphocytes with an anti-Ig serum conjugated with another fluorochrome to that used in Section 2.8.1.

b Repeat the 'capping' experiment using the monovalent Fab fragment of rabbit anti-mouse Ig serum. You will prepare this later in the book so the experiment may be conveniently postponed until then (Section 7.7.1).

c Resynthesis studies on lymphocytes *in vitro* are time consuming and require the ability to work under clean, if not sterile, conditions. Such experiments are, however, well worth the effort and we will describe one in detail.

2.8.3   RESYNTHESIS OF SURFACE RECEPTORS

Basically, the cells after being capped, and shown to have lost their surface Ig by shedding or endocytosis, are put into *in vitro* culture and allowed to re-synthesize their receptors. Using endogenous labelling with radioactive amino acids it is possible to show that these newly synthesized receptors are inserted into the membrane *de novo*. Such an experiment is, however, beyond the range of this book

46

because specific precursors are not available and identification of the labelled Ig requires a detailed knowledge of membrane chemistry.

Materials and equipment

Mouse spleen or lymph node suspension
Tissue culture medium with antibiotics (Appendix I)
100 ml flat glass or plastic bottles
Fetal bovine serum
37° incubator for cells
Anti-mouse Ig, directly conjugated with (a) fluorescein or (b) rhodamine
Gas cylinder; 5% CO_2 in air

Method

1 Stain 10^8 lymphocytes as described in Section 2.5.1 using fluorescein-labelled anti-mouse Ig, but use medium without sodium azide.

2 Wash the capped cells and 10^8 normal cells in tissue culture medium containing antibiotics and 5% FBS.

3 Count and adjust the cell suspensions to 10^6 viable lymphocytes ml^{-1}.

4 Put 20 ml aliquots of the cell suspensions into the 100 ml bottles and gas for 60 sec with a mixture of 5% CO_2 in air. Cap bottles tightly.

Remove the cells from culture at the times shown in the protocol given below, and stain the cells with rhodamine conjugated anti-mouse Ig (Section 2.5.1). You must use medium containing 20 mM sodium azide during the staining procedure to stop further capping.

Protocol

Cells in culture		
2×10^7 stained cells culture number	2×10^7 normal cells culture number	Time in culture
1a	1b	0
2a	2b	1 hour
3a	3b	2 hours
4a	4b	4 hours
5a	5b	5 hours
6a	6b	6 hours
7a	7b	7 hours
8a	8b	overnight

5 Stain (rhodamine anti-Ig conjugate) and prepare all the cells for examination under the UV microscope (Section 2.5.1).

47

Technical notes

1   As both rhodamine and fluorescein have been used as tracer molecules it is essential that the UV microscope should be able to excite at each required wavelength.

2   Because of the complexity of the experiment we suggest that you use only direct immunofluorescent staining. A transmitted light UV microscope therefore cannot usually be used.

3   Ensure that your antisera do not cross-react with components of the serum supplement used in the cultures (Section 1.6.6) otherwise you may simply be looking at the rate of uptake of material from the medium.

Data required

1   Determine the percentage of cells showing any surface fluorescence with the fluorescein conjugated antiserum. Plot a graph against time, this represents the rate at which receptors are lost either by endocytosis or shedding.

2   Determine the percentage of cells showing any surface fluorescence with the rhodamine conjugated antiserum. At the very early stages of this experiment you will see cells with double green and red caps—what causes this? Plot a graph against time of the percentage staining, omitting those cells which have double-staining caps. This curve represents the re-appearance of new Ig receptors.

At each stage you should correct for the normal loss of Ig receptors from the surface of B cells cultured *in vitro*; presumably this is due to less than ideal physiological conditions. Accordingly the proportions of cells resynthesizing Ig at each stage of the experiment should be expressed as a percentage of the cells still carrying Ig from the normal, uncapped cultures:

$$\% \text{ resynthesis} = \frac{\% \text{ cells bearing Ig in capped cultures}}{\% \text{ cells bearing Ig in normal cultures}} \times 100.$$

It is rare for the resynthesis of receptors to be so complete that the percentage of Ig-bearing cells returns to the value found for the normal mouse spleen at the beginning of the experiment.

Note

You should not confuse this loss of membrane components by shedding with normal membrane turnover. The former is a greatly accelerated process induced by cross-linking agents and presumably by antigen *in vivo*. It may be envisaged as a process by which the cell 'de-blocks' itself ready for further antigen stimulation after receptor regeneration.

DIFFERENTIAL MOBILITY OF MEMBRANE COMPONENTS

This experiment requires techniques and antisera that will be met with later in the book. It is a refinement of the two previous experiments, we include it simply as it is an extremely useful research tool.

2.9.1 CAPPING OF UNRELATED MEMBRANE COMPONENTS

In Section 2.8 you showed that surface components of the membranes of nucleated cells could be made to change their distribution by the use of bi-functional cross-linking agents; in the experiment described the cross-linking agent was an anti-immunoglobulin molecule. We now wish to show that this redistribution of surface components is specific to the cross-linking agent used. In other words, an anti-Ig antiserum will cause Ig receptors to cap but will leave all other unrelated components undisturbed.

Materials and equipment

Mouse lymph node or spleen lymphocytes
Tissue culture medium with and without sodium azide, 20 mM
Directly conjugated rabbit anti-mouse Ig (fluorescein)
Directly conjugated rabbit anti-mouse lymphocyte serum (rhodamine)
UV microscope—to allow the use of the direct conjugates this should have incident UV illumination
(It is complex and soul-destroying to perform the same experiment by indirect immunofluorescence.)

Initial preparation of antisera

We are going to stain the same cell with both antisera; it is therefore essential to ensure that the antisera do not cross-react.

1 Prepare a suspension of mouse thymus cells in medium.
2 Wash 3 times by centrifugation (150 g × 10 min at 4°).
3 Add an equal volume of rabbit anti-mouse Ig to the dry cell pellet.
4 Mix at 4° overnight, then spin off the cells at 300 g for 20 min at 4° and store the antiserum at $-20°$.
   You should know by now why we are able to use thymus lymphocytes to absorb this antiserum, even though we expect it to stain lymph node or spleen lymphocytes later.
5 Prepare the γ-globulin fraction of mouse serum using 40% saturated ammonium sulphate (Section 1.2.2c) and insolubilize with glutaraldehyde (Section 1.6.6).

49

6   Mix an equal volume of insolubilized mouse γ-globulin with the rabbit anti-mouse lymphocyte serum. Mix overnight at 4° or at 37° for 3 h.

7   Spin off the antiserum (500 g × 20 min at 4°) and store at −20°. *We are using a vast excess of immunoadsorbent to ensure complete adsorption.*

Technique

1   Incubate 10^7 lymphocytes with fluorescein-conjugated anti-mouse Ig serum at a suitable dilution (Section 1.6.5) for 30 min at 37°. The medium must not contain azide.

2   Spin the cells down in medium containing sodium azide final concentration 20 mM (150 g × 10 min at 4°) and incubate with rhodamine conjugated rabbit anti-mouse lymphocyte serum (the antiserum should have been standardized for immunofluorescent staining, Section 1.6.5) for 30 min at 4° in the presence of 20 mM sodium azide.

3   Wash the cells by centrifugation and prepare them for examination under the UV microscope (Section 2.5.1).

Observations

You should see cells with green caps and red bodies, showing that the re-distribution has affected the Ig molecules alone.

Here only one antiserum was used under 'capping' conditions. We suggest you repeat the experiment using the antisera as a mixture under 'capping' conditions and observe the localization of the two caps, one relative to the other.

The basic ability to selectively remove cell surface components as defined by bi- or multivalent cross-linking agents has very wide applicability. One could, for example, investigate whether two cell surface components are distinct by causing one or the other to cap, co-capping would then indicate a close association between the two components. In addition one can overcome the problem of steric hindrance between two surface components by simply capping one away.

2.10   **SUMMARY AND CONCLUSIONS**

The lymphocyte is a cell destined for great things after contact with antigen. Before antigenic stimulation most lymphocytes are dormant. They have, however, an array of surface receptors which in the case of B lymphocytes are immunoglobulin molecules of the same antigenic specificity as the antibody the cell will secrete when it is 'turned on'. T lymphocytes also have receptor molecules but they have yet to be characterized.

50

The immunoglobulin receptor molecules do not have a fixed distribution in the cell membrane but can be drawn together by cross-linking agents, for example anti-Ig. However, such blocked receptors are removed from the cell surface either by endocytosis or shedding. This may be a physiological process, probably occurring after antigenic contact, to allow the cell to resynthesize new receptors.

We have greatly simplified the processes of lymphocyte differentiation and triggering. Both of these areas are only poorly understood at present. In the spleen, for example, representatives of many stages of B lymphocyte differentiation are known to coexist. Upon contact with antigen many virgin cells, with different size and charge characteristics to small lymphocytes, are triggered to differentiate to plasma cells and antibody synthesis.

FURTHER READING

KAPLAN J.G. (1979) *The Molecular Basis of Immune Cell Function.* Elsevier/North Holland, Amsterdam.

LOOR F. & ROELANTS G.E. (eds.) (1977) *B and T lymphocytes in Immune Recognition.* J. Wiley, Chichester.

MARCHALONIS J.J. (ed.) (1975) *The Lymphocyte: Structure and Function.* Marcel Dekker, New York.

3   Lymphocytes and effector cells

You now have a good knowledge of the lymphocyte, its morphology, membrane characteristics and ability to react with antigen via its surface receptor. The lymphocyte is, of course, only the beginning of the whole process. Under the influence of antigen the lymphocyte changes drastically. Concurrent with the easily observable morphological changes, the lymphocyte nucleus becomes derepressed, the cell enters the cell cycle and begins to divide to produce daughter cells all of the same specificity. Each initially stimulated cell can form a CLONE of effector cells all reacting with the same antigen. Eventually as the immune response declines the effector cells are no longer active and are replaced by a clone of small lymphocytes or MEMORY cells. All these cells have the same antigenic specificity as the original lymphocyte and so where previously we had only one cell we now have a whole clone of progeny. This increased number of initiator cells after a primary contact with antigen is sufficient to explain all the characteristics of the secondary or ANAMNESTIC response seen upon a second contact with the same antigen. Accordingly, as discussed in the previous chapter, when one has measles and recovers, there are well-established and enlarged clones of memory cells sufficient to meet any secondary contact with the measles virus. The immunity is specific to the same or closely related antigens, i.e. cross-reacting viruses or antigens. The reader will realize, without requiring to do the experiment, that this is the basis of vaccination. The subject is given a controlled exposure to a killed or avirulent strain of the pathogen to stimulate his immune system and prepare it to confront the virulent pathogen.

Some of the techniques required to measure the effector function of lymphocyte progeny are rather complex and time consuming. They are dealt with in the chapter on Advanced Techniques (Chapter 10).

SPECIFIC EFFECTOR CELLS

There are two major sub-populations of lymphocytes: T and B (see Section 2.7). It is convenient to use this division in examining their effector functions. B cells normally transform to PLASMA CELLS after antigenic stimulation. Plasma cells produce antibody for secretion at the rate of $1-3 \times 10^3$ molecules $\sec^{-1}$. T lymphocytes become BLAST CELLS after antigenic stimulation and do not produce antibody for secretion. The specific effector function of these cells, e.g. the killing of foreign cells, is brought about by direct cell contact. It should be noted that the properties demonstrated for T blasts and effector cells have been shown to have *in vivo* relevance in only a few instances. Accordingly, although the rôle of B cells *in vivo* is well understood, the same is not true for T cells.

The intact immune response is never limited to one cell type. The Mantoux Reaction, for example, although taken as the classical example of T-cell mediated immunity, involves many cell types. The whole area of cell dynamics *in vivo* is still poorly understood and many basic experiments are still required. With the techniques of *in vitro* cell fractionation (Section 8.2) combined with *in vivo* reconstitution (Section 10.6), the reader may wish to attempt many of these experiments himself.

3.1 B-EFFECTOR CELLS

Most of the assays described in this section are carried out on plasma cells *in vitro* or their soluble products, i.e. antibody.

3.1.1 PLASMA CELLS AND ANTIBODY PRODUCTION (Anti-FγG)

Preparation in advance

Prime mice 7–8 days before the experiment with 400 μg of alum precipitated FγG (Sections 1.2.2 and 1.4.4) plus *B. pertussis* (Section 1.5).

Demonstration of plasma cells

This can be done either on spleen sections or with single-cell suspensions smeared on microscope slides.

3.1.1a FROZEN SECTIONS

Materials and equipment

FγG immune mouse
Acetone
Solid carbon dioxide (Dry ice)
Freezing microtome

Method

1   Add small pieces of solid CO_2 to acetone in an insulated metal container until bubbling stops.

53

2 Kill the mouse and chop the spleen transversely into 5 pieces.

3 Drop the spleen fragments into the freezing mixture.

4 Mount one of the fragments on a microtome chuck and cut 5 μm sections. These must be air dried and can then be stored at $-70°$ for up to 3 months.

3.1.1b.   ISOLATED CELLS

Materials and equipment

FγG immunized mouse
Tissue culture medium at 4° (Appendix I)
Fetal bovine serum (FBS) (Appendix II)

Method

1 Kill the mouse, remove the spleen and prepare a cell suspension in tissue culture medium.

2 Allow the aggregates to settle for 10 min at 1 g. *Do not filter the cells through nylon wool because you are going to look at large cells which are easily damaged and trapped in nylon wool.*

3 Wash the cells twice with medium (150 g for 10 min at 4°).

4 Count the cells and adjust to 2×10^7 ml^{-1}.

5 Add an equal volume of fetal bovine serum to the cell suspension.

6 **Prepare cell smears on a Shandon cytocentrifuge. Spin at 400 rpm for 20 min.** It will be necessary to vary the number of drops of cell suspension used to obtain a good smear, however, the total volume of liquid should be maintained at 4 drops per well.

7 Dry the smears thoroughly and fix in 95% methanol (Section 2.3.1b).

It is possible to prepare these smears as described for small lymphocytes in Section 2.3.1b but the plasma cells are large and fragile so you must not use a 'spreader' slide. Simply shake the slide to spread out the drop and air dry before methanol fixation.

3.1.1c   STAINING OF SECTIONS OR CYTOSMEARS FOR
ANTIBODY-PRODUCING CELLS

We will show that there are antibody-producing cells present, and that much of this antibody is specific for the immunizing antigen.

Materials required

Frozen sections or smears from FγG immunized mice
Fluorescein conjugated rabbit anti-mouse Ig (Sections 1.4.2 and 1.6)
Guinea-pig liver powder (Appendix II)
Phosphate buffered saline (PBS) (Appendix I)

54

There is a serious problem of non-specific adsorption of conjugated antisera to fixed material, in contrast to the very low background associated with viable cell immunofluorescence. You should use antisera with a low substitution ratio (Sections 1.6.2 and 1.6.3) and in addition absorb the antiserum with liver powder as follows:

1   Dilute the antiserum 1 : 5 with **PBS** and absorb 1 ml with 100 mg of pig liver powder (use *pro rata*).
2   Mix for 30 min at 4° and spin off the liver powder (500 g × 20 min at 4°).

This absorption must be done at the beginning of each staining session.

Preparation of pig liver powder

Materials and equipment

Pig liver
0·14 M saline
Acetone
Waring blender

Method

1   Remove blood from the isolated liver by an intravenous infusion of saline.
2   Chop liver into pieces and homogenize with 4 volumes of saline using a Waring blender.
3   Concentrate and wash in saline by centrifugation (600 g for 45 min at 4°).
4   Remove large aggregates by filtering through a pad of glass wool or muslin.
5   Centrifuge filter effluent at 600 g for 45 min at 4° and resuspend pellet in acetone.
6   Filter through a Buchner funnel and wash with acetone until the preparation is white on drying.
7   Grind up into a powder and store at 4° under desiccation.

3.1.1d   STAINING TECHNIQUE

1   Dilute two aliquots of the absorbed antiserum to a final dilution of 1 : 10 and 1 : 20 with **PBS**.
2   Apply one drop of each conjugate dilution (1 : 5, 1 : 10 and 1 : 20) to separate spleen sections or cytosmears.
3   Incubate for 20 min at room temperature.
4   Wash off the excess antiserum. This can be done by putting the slides in a tray (face up!) and flooding them with PBS. Washing can be made more effective by placing the tray over a magnetic stirring

platform with the mixing bar at the extreme end of the tray from the slides. Mix slowly for 10 min.

5   Change the PBS and mix for a further 10 min.

6   Add one drop of mounting medium (Section 2.5.1) and add a coverslip. Ring with nail varnish.

7   Examine the slides under a UV microscope (either transmitted or incident light).

We have described a direct immunofluorescence technique; if you use indirect immunofluorescence only the conjugate need be absorbed with liver powder.

Plasma cells should be easily visualized as shown in Fig. 3.1. (You may have problems in staining spleen sections because of secreted antibody which may be trapped. This is not a problem with the cytosmears.)

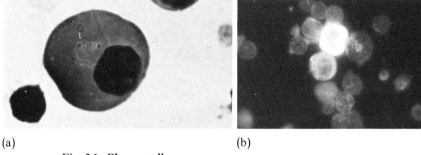

(a)   (b)

Fig. 3.1. Plasma cells
(a) May–Grünwald–Giemsa staining of a cytocentrifuge preparation. (× 984)
(b) Plasma cell stained with fluorescein-conjugated anti-mouse IgG.

3.1.1e   ANTIGEN BINDING

To show that this intracellular antibody is antigen-specific it is necessary to incubate other spleen sections or cell preparations with FγG and then detect the localized antigen with a fluorescein-conjugated rabbit anti-FγG.

Materials required in addition to previous experiment

Fluorescein conjugated anti-FγG (Sections 1.4.5 and 1.6)
Fowl γ globulin (Section 1.2.2a)

Again you should absorb the conjugate with liver powder (Section 3.1.1c) and in addition absorb the FγG as this is also 'sticky'.

1   Dilute absorbed FγG to 1 mg ml^{-1} and put one drop onto each of 3 sections or cytosmears of FγG-immune spleen.

2   Incubate for 20 min at room temperature.

3   Wash away the unbound antigen with PBS (Section 3.1.1d).

4   Add one drop of 1 : 5, 1 : 10, 1 : 20 fluorescein conjugated

anti-FγG to each slide respectively and incubate for 20 min at room temperature.

5   Wash away the excess conjugate, blot dry and mount (Section 3.1.1d).

6   Examine the preparations under a UV microscope.

Technical note

It is important to ensure that the rabbit anti-FγG does not cross-react with mouse immunoglobulin. Refer to Section 1.6.6, note 1, and in addition absorb with glutaraldehyde insolubilized mouse γ-globulin, Section 1.6.6, note 3.

3.1.2   ENUMERATION OF ANTIBODY SECRETING CELLS *IN VITRO*

We have shown in the previous section that plasma cells synthesize intracytoplasmic antibody. Further, it is possible to show that these cells synthesize antibody for secretion and this can be used to quantitate the number of antibody-producing cells in an organ. The basic assay which we will describe was developed by Jerne and Nordin (see refs.) to detect cells producing antibody against erythrocyte antigens. Spleen cells from immune mice are incubated in an agar gel with the immunizing erythrocytes. After the addition of complement the erythrocytes in the locality of the plasma cells are lysed producing holes or plaques in the erythrocyte suspension.

Preparation required

1   Immunize 2 mice with 2×10^8 sheep erythrocytes given intraperitoneally 5 days before the experiment.

2   Agar underlay. Make up 1·4% Difco Bacto Agar in Hank's saline (Appendixes I and II). Heat the agar until it is free from lumps and add enough to a 5 cm plastic Petri dish to just cover the bottom. *An underlay is used to ensure that the base of the assay dish is reasonably flat, so pouring must be done on a levelled surface.*

3   Agar overlay. Prepare 0·7% agar solution in Hank's saline containing 0·5 mg ml^{-1} of DEAE-dextran (final concentration) *DEAE-dextran is used to prevent anti-complementary activity of the agar.* (Appendix II).

Materials required

SRBC immunized mice
2–4-week-old sheep blood in Alsever's solution (Appendix II)
Agar overlay

57

Petri dishes containing agar underlay
Hank's saline (Appendix I)
Water bath, 45°
Guinea-pig serum, complement (Appendix II)

Method

1   Wash sheep erythrocytes in Hank's saline (three times at 300 *g* for 10 min). Adjust to 20% v/v.
2   Remove spleens from mice and tease with forceps on ice.
3   Suck spleen suspensions in and out of a Pasteur pipette to disperse the cells. (Do not filter cells through nylon wool and do not use a syringe and needle for cell dispersion.)
4   Adjust to a total volume of 2·5 ml in Hank's saline.
5   Dilute 1 ml of the spleen cell suspension 1 : 10 and 1 : 100 with Hank's saline.
6   Pipette out 0·8 ml of overlay into small glass test tubes in a 45° water bath. Use a warm pipette.
7   Add 0·25 ml of the original or diluted spleen cell suspensions to each assay dish according to the protocol (below).
8   Place dish on a levelled surface.
9   Add 0·15 ml SRBC suspension to each overlay tube just before use, mix well by flicking the end of the tube.
10   Add overlay to dish and mix thoroughly with the spleen cells.
11   Allow agar to harden and add 1·0 ml of a 1 : 10 dilution of guinea-pig serum as a source of complement.
12   Incubate dishes at 37° for 1–1·5 hours. If the plaques are not clear when the dishes are removed from the incubator, allow them to stand at room temperature for about 30 min before counting. Counting is easier and more accurate if you use a low-power binocular microscope and draw lines on the bottom of the dish.

Only direct plaques (mainly IgM antibody) are detected by the method described above because of the high haemolytic efficiency of this antibody class. To detect IgG plaques it is necessary to increase the number of molecules binding to any one site (1 molecule of IgM can initiate the complement cascade for RBC lysis but 2 adjacent

Protocol

	Dish number		
	1	2	3
Spleen cell suspension	0·25 ml		→
(initial dilution)	(neat)	(1 : 10)	(1 : 100)
Agar overlay |	|0·8 ml		→
SRBC (20%) |	|0·15 ml		→
Fraction of spleen assayed	1/10	1/100	1/1000

molecules of IgG are required), plaques must therefore be developed with an antiserum against mouse Ig. This method of detecting socalled 'indirect' plaques can be used to assay all the mouse IgG subclasses if appropriate antisera are available.

INDIRECT PLAQUES

Materials and equipment

As in the previous experiment, plus rabbit anti-mouse γ-globulin (anti-Ig) (Section 1.4.2).

Method

1 Prepare a plaquing mixture as in the preceding method (steps 1–10) but instead of adding complement, add 1·0 ml of a 1 : 10 dilution of rabbit anti-mouse Ig and incubate at 37° for 45 min.
2 Wash away the developing antiserum by flooding the plate twice with Hank's saline.
3 Add 1 ml of 1 : 10 dilution of guinea-pig serum. Incubate for 45 min at 37°.

Again, the plaques may be clearer if the plates are left at room temperature for 30 min before counting. Under experimental conditions it is necessary to titrate the developing antiserum until the maximum number of plaques are obtained. The direct or 'IgM' plaques are then subtracted from the total to give the number of 'IgG' plaques.

The technique as described can be used to enumerate antibody-producing cells in any species, however, in the case of chicken antibody-producing cells you must use a homologous serum as a source of complement. Chicken antibody does not fix mammalian complement. Alternatively develop both IgM and IgG plaques using rabbit anti-chicken immunoglobulin class specific antisera and guinea-pig complement.

The haemolytic plaque method can be extended using antigen coupled to erythrocyte indicator cells. This, of course, allows more widespread application of the technique, especially in the Cunningham modification, which is described in Section 10.1.

SUGGESTED EXPERIMENTAL DESIGN

(This may be a class experiment, each group being responsible for one point on the dose-response curve.)

Dose range of sheep RBC: 4×10^5, 4×10^6, 4×10^7, 4×10^8, 4×10^9. (SRBC in Alsever's solution are usually sold at approximately 4×10^9 cells ml^{-1}.)

Replicates: 5 mice per group

Assay time: 5 days after priming

Data: **Example of treatment and presentation of plaque data.** Spleens assayed at a final dilution of $1 : 1000$; 0.25 ml of cell suspension per plate.

Calculate the number of plaque-forming cells per spleen for each mouse and then calculate the geometric mean for each group (Section 4.1.2c) as shown in Fig. 3.2.

The geometric, rather than the arithmetic mean is normally used for this type of data as the proliferative response of the cells to the antigen occurs exponentially and so the error of the system will also occur exponentially. Conventionally, the plaque-forming cells (PFC) are assayed as a proportion of the whole spleen as the total PFC do not always correlate with the number of lymphoid cells per spleen.

Plot a graph of the number of plaques per spleen against the antigen dose used, plot both direct and indirect plaques (Fig. 3.3). In Fig. 3.3 the limits of one standard deviation above and below the geometric mean are given, this describes the scatter of the data. (See Section 4.1.2b for discussion of standard deviation.)

Technical notes

1   We have chosen day 5 for the assay as a compromise for this system. At high SRBC doses (10^6–10^9) the peak of the direct PFC response is at 4 days; at lower doses (10^4–10^5) the peak of the response is at day 5. However, the indirect plaques peak at day 5–6.
2   At lower SRBC doses the route of immunization is important. At 10^4 SRBC and below, intravenous injection gives a greater number of PFC than an intraperitoneal injection. However, above 10^5 SRBC both routes of administration give approximately the same number of plaques.
3   In all future experiments use the spleen dilution giving 2–300 plaques per assay plate.

3.1.3   REVERSE PLAQUE ASSAY USING PROTEIN A
COATED SHEEP ERYTHROCYTES

This assay is particularly useful for the enumeration of total immunoglobulin secreting cells. The secreted immunoglobulin is bound by protein A coated onto indicator erythrocytes (see Section 8.5.2 for

	PFC per spleen (1000 × number per plate)		
	Direct plaques (×10^5) (geometric mean and limits of one standard deviation)		Indirect plaques (×10^5) (geometric mean and limits of one standard deviation)
Antigen dose (SRBC)			
4×10^5	1. 2·00		1. 0·460
	2. 1·89	1·91	2. 0·390	0·386
	3. 2·20	2·01	3. 0·290	0·416
	4. 1·61	1·82	4. 0·400	0·357
	5. 1·90		5. 0·410
4×10^6	1. 2·06		1. 1·30
	2. 2·89	2·48	2. 1·29	1·27
	3. 3·02	2·80	3. 1·16	1·31
	4. 3·10	2·19	4. 1·40	1·23
	5. 1·68		5. 1·23
4×10^7	1. 3·06		1. 1·46
	2. 4·10	3·32	2. 1·59	1·54
	3. 3·70	3·55	3. 1·62	1·71
	4. 2·98	3·10	4. 2·10	1·39
	5. 2·90		5. 1·10
4×10^8	1. 3·19		1. 7·30
	2. 4·01	3·36	2. 1·04	2·17
	3. 3·86	3·59	3. 2·87	3·09
	4. 2·84	3·14	4. 1·20	1·53
	5. 3·04		5. 1·85
4×10^9	1. 6·10		1. 2·26
	2. 1·73	2·21	2. 1·96	1·78
	3. 3·30	3·03	3. 1·34	2·10
	4. 1·03	1·61	4. 1·11	1·51
	5. 1·46		5. 2·70

Fig. 3.2. Haemolytic plaque data
The geometric mean and standard deviation of each group was calculated as described in Section 4.1.2c.

species specificity of immunoglobulin adsorption by protein A), which are then lysed by the addition of a developing anti-immunoglobulin serum plus complement.

Preparation in advance

Coating of sheep erythrocytes with protein A

Materials and equipment

Sheep erythrocytes in Alsever's solution (Appendix II)
0·14 M sodium chloride in water (saline)

Protein A (Appendix II) (2 mg ml^{-1}) in saline
Chromic chloride (0·1 mg ml^{-1}) in saline
Phosphate buffered saline, PBS (Appendix I)

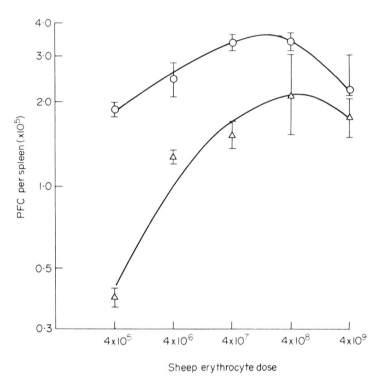

Sheep erythrocyte dose

Fig. 3.3. Dose response curve of direct and indirect plaque-forming cells against sheep erythrocytes
PFC: plaque-forming cells.
RBC: sheep erythrocytes.
○——○ direct plaques.
△——△ indirect plaques.

Method

1　Wash sheep erythrocytes six times by centrifugation (300 **g** for 10 min at room temperature).
2　Add 1 ml of protein A solution (2 mg ml^{-1} initial concentration) to 1 ml of packed erythrocytes.
3　Add 6 ml of chromic chloride solution (0·1 mg ml^{-1}) dropwise. After mixing add 10 ml saline and incubate overnight at 4°.
4　Wash the erythrocytes three times by centrifugation (300 **g** for 10 min at room temperature) and resuspend to 10% v/v in PBS.
　Coated erythrocytes may be used for up to 2 weeks.

Assay

Materials and equipment

Cell suspension for assay
Protein A coated erythrocytes (prepared as above)
Phosphate buffered saline, PBS (Appendix I)
Agarose, 1.8% w/v in distilled water
Tissue culture medium, thrice concentrated (Appendix I)
Bovine serum albumin, BSA, 7% w/v in PBS.
Anti-immunoglobulin, developing serum
Guinea pig serum, as complement source (Appendix II)
Plastic petri dishes, 50 mm

Method

1   Mix 14 ml agarose solution with 5·5 ml of thrice-concentrated tissue culture medium and 1·5 ml of BSA solution.
2   Aliquot 0·7 ml volumes of agarose mixture into glass test tubes in a water bath at 45°.
3   For each assay dish: add 0·2 ml of lymphoid cell suspension, 0·1 ml of anti-immunoglobulin serum and 0·05 ml of protein A coated sheep erythrocytes to a tube containing 0·7 ml agarose mixture. Mix thoroughly and pour into a plastic petri dish. *Swirl the dish to ensure an even covering of agarose-cell suspension.*
4   Incubate for 1–1·5 hours in a humid 37° incubator gassed with 5% CO_2 in air.
5   Add 1 ml of diluted guinea pig serum, as a complement source (at a predetermined dilution) and continue incubation at 37° until haemolytic plaques are visible (within 30–60 min).
6   Count the number of haemolytic plaques and calculate the number of antibody secreting cells in the original suspension.

Technical notes

1   The optimal dilution of anti-immunoglobulin serum and complement source must be determined as in Section 3.1.2.
2   Illuminate the assay dish with light at a low angle of incidence to aid visualization of the plaques. They will appear as uniform dark holes in a light, birefringent layer of erythrocytes.
3   The cell suspension for assay should be used at a concentration sufficient to give not more than 100–200 plaques per assay dish.

3.1.4   EFFECT OF ANTIBODY *IN VIVO*

In the previous section you saw the lytic effect of antibody plus complement on sheep erythrocytes. It is possible to show an identical effect on bacteria or other foreign cells. However, this is not the only action of antibody and complement in *in vivo* protection. The combination of antibody with foreign material facilitates contact with phagocytic cells, either by binding to the Fc receptor site on macrophages (opsonic adherence), or by the C3 in the antibody/antigen complex binding to the complement receptor on phagocytic cells (immune adherence).

The immune adherence and opsonization effect of antibody *in vivo* will be demonstrated in Section 10.8.3.

3.2   **T EFFECTOR CELLS**

The effector functions of T lymphocytes have been determined almost entirely from *in vitro* studies. It has been possible to dissect out lymphocyte populations and determine the role of each T-lymphocyte subset using antisera against cell surface antigens (undoubtedly the number of subsets and their functional attributes have not yet been exhausted). Briefly, there are at least four functional subsets, and although their function might change with time, at any one instant the cells are apparently monofunctional:

1   T cooperator lymphocytes—provide antigen-specific 'help' for the activation of B lymphocytes (Section 4.2).
2   T cytotoxic lymphocytes—are responsible for direct (cell-mediated) killing of foreign target cells (Section 10.11.6).
3   T lymphokine-secreting lymphocytes—after antigen stimulation, these cells secrete non-antibody factors (see Section 10.12) which affect the function of different cell types, for example, they can induce a mitogenic response in lymphocytes, inhibit the migration of macrophages (Section 10.12.1), cause an increase in vascular permeability, induce a local inflammatory response due to their chemotactic effect (Section 3.2.1) etc. Lymphokines may be produced by more than one subset.
4   T suppressor lymphocytes—can suppress an immune response, either with or without regard to antigen specificity. They are probably negative regulators of immune reactivity (cf. 'helper' T lymphocytes) and are intimately associated with the induction and maintenance of tolerance (Section 4.3).

An antigen-induced T lymphocyte response *in vivo* undoubtedly involves several or all of these subsets acting alone or in concert. The soluble mediators thus produced affect other lymphoid or non-lymphoid cells not involved in the primary antigenic stimulation. The result is a complex series of cell and humoral changes at the site of antigen stimulation.

The best known example of cell-mediated immunity is the Mantoux Reaction obtained by the injection of tuberculin into the skin of an individual previously exposed to the tubercle bacillus either by infection or vaccination. The reaction is characterized by a reddening of the skin and a localized injurious reaction which reaches its height at 24–48 hours, hence the name of delayed-type hypersensitivity.

3.2.1   *IN VIVO* ASSAYS OF DELAYED HYPERSENSITIVITY

The magnitude of a localized delayed hypersensitivity reaction *in vivo* may be assayed by measuring one of the secondary consequences of lymphocyte activation, for example, leakage of intravascular [125]I—albumin into the tissues, increase in foot volume or ear thickness (in mice) or the enlargement of the wattle in male chickens. Unfortunately, many of these assays have poor reproducibility or may be initiated by mechanisms that are not entirely mediated by T lymphocytes.

An extremely elegant assay has recently been described that relies on the localization of isotopically labelled cells at the site of antigen administration. Although the magnitude of the response is low (as with the other assays listed above) the reproducibility is impressive.

Localization of isotopically labelled cells

Initial preparations

Sensitize mice with antigen using a regime known to stimulate good delayed hypersensitivity. For example, paint the skin of shaved mice at three sites using 50 μl dinitrofluorobenzene (10 mg ml^{-1} in a 1 : 1 mixture of acetone: olive oil).

Materials and equipment

Mice, sensitized as above
2.4.   Dinitro-1-fluorobenzene (10 mg ml^{-1}) in acetone-olive oil (1 : 1)
5-Iodo-2'deoxyuridine-[125]I (^{125}I-UdR) (Appendix II)
0·14 M Saline
Gamma counter

1   Paint the left pinna (*outer flap of the ear*) of the DNFB sensitized and normal control mice with 5 μl DNFB in acetone and olive oil (as above).
2   Paint the right ear of all mice with 5 μl acetone and olive oil alone.
3   After 10 hours inject 0·1 μl of saline containing 2 μCi ^{125}I-UdR into the tail vein of each mouse. (*Warm the mouse under a heat lamp for 10 min before injection.*) Before removing the needle, inject a small volume of saline intradermally at the injection site. (*This will collapse the vein and prevent leakage from the punctured vessel.*)

65

4   After 16 hours, kill the mice by cervical dislocation and cut off the left (antigen treated) and right (control) pinnae at the hair line.
5   Count the radioactivity in each pinna using a gamma counter. Calculate the response as follows:

$$\text{Index of response} = \frac{\text{cpm left ear}}{\text{cpm right ear}}$$

Technical note

If the mice have been primed with cellular or soluble antigens, elicit the secondary response with a 10 μl intradermal injection into the pinna.

3.2.2   GRAFT REJECTION

The cell-mediated immune response is very important in the apparently high artificial system of transplant rejection. Although the mechanisms of rejection of whole organ grafts are many and varied, cell-mediated immunity is known to be instrumental in the rejection of foreign skin grafts. This is the easiest system in which to demonstrate the basic principles of cell-mediated immunity. Much of the research work, and many of the experiments described in this book, rely on the use of inbred strains of mice; however, the basic phenomenon of skin graft rejection can be shown between outbred mice of contrasting skin colour. (Inbred mice have been brother–sister mated so that, like human monozygotic twins, individuals are genetically identical. Accordingly, grafts made within a strain or between identical twins,ins are not rejected other than for technical reasons.)

3.2.3a   SKIN GRAFT REJECTION

In the experiment described below tail-skin grafts will be transferred.

Materials and equipment

Mice of contrasting colours
Safety razor blades
4–5 cm glass tubes, internal diameter slightly larger than the mouse's tail
Michel clips

It is necessary to prepare a 'bed' for a skin graft before transplantation. In the technique described below with paired mice, the removal of the donor tail-skin graft automatically prepares the 'bed' for the recipient graft.

66

1 Anaesthetize one of the pair of mice with ether.

2 Hold the mouse's tail over your forefinger with the mouse pointing away from you. Hold the razor blade horizontally on the tail, about 2 cm from the base of the tail, and press slightly to indent the skin. Draw the blade towards you with a slicing action. Do not cut too deeply or the tail will bleed; this will not make a good 'bed' for a recipient graft. Cut off a piece of skin about 0·5 cm long, and leave the skin graft on the blade.

3 Move about 1 cm down the tail and cut a second graft.

4 Replace one of the grafts (autograft) but turn it through 180° so that the hairs are facing the wrong way.

5 Use a gauze swab to press the graft firmly in place to exclude all the air. If there is bleeding around the graft, pressure must be applied until haemostasis is achieved.

6 Anaesthetize the second mouse and prepare two pieces of tail skin for grafting as above.

7 Again return one of the pieces of skin to the donor as an autograft. The skin graft of the first mouse (allograft) can now be placed on the second 'bed', again turning it so that the hairs face the wrong direction. Press the graft firmly in place.

8 The first mouse, which will need to be re-anaesthetized, can now receive the allograft.

9 The grafts are protected with glass tail tubes. These should be about 4–5 cm long and wide enough to slide easily over the mouse's tail. (*The cut edges of the glass must be flame polished to avoid injury to the mouse.*)

10 The tail tube is held in place by a Michel clip placed through the tail bones. (*The tube must not be attached too near the base of the tail or it will become fouled with faeces and urine.*)

11 Remove the tail tubes 24–36 h after grafting.

The grafts should be observed during the following two weeks and the time taken for necrosis and sloughing of the allograft recorded. This should occur within 11–14 days of grafting, although with some strain combinations this can be as soon as day 8. Other than for technical reasons, the autograft should become established, and continue to grow.

3.2.2b IMMUNOLOGICAL NATURE

The immunological nature of graft rejection may be established by observing rejection times in immunized and normal mice. This experiment involves the use of 3 inbred mouse strains and cannot conveniently be performed with outbred mice.

Previous preparation

Recipient mice become immune when they have rejected a primary or first-set skin graft. This immunization by a previous skin graft can be established more conveniently by transferring an allogeneic spleen cell suspension between the two strains to be tested as follows:

1 Prepare a spleen-cell suspension of CBA cells in tissue-culture medium. Wash, and count the cells (Section 2.4).
2 Inject 10^7 CBA spleen cells intraperitoneally into adult BALB/c mice.
3 These BALB/c mice will be immune to CBA cells two weeks after injection.

Materials

Recipient BALB/c mice, normal and previously injected with CBA cells
CBA- and C57BL-strain donor mice.

Method

1 Kill the CBA and C57BL donor mice and remove 2 skin grafts from each strain as previously described (Section 3.2.2a, steps 1–3).
2 Anaesthetize the normal BALB/c recipient mouse and remove 3 sections of tail skin.
3 Return one piece of skin as an autograft, and transplant the CBA and C57BL grafts to the other two 'beds'.
4 Protect the grafted areas by a tail tube held in place by a clip.
5 Repeat the grafting procedure for the immune BALB/c mouse, again protecting the grafted areas with a tail tube.
6 Remove all tail tubes 24–36 h after grafting.

The rejection time for the grafts must now be observed. The normal BALB/c should reject the two allogeneic grafts within 11–14 days. The allografts on the immune BALB/c mouse should show differential survival times. The rejection of the CBA graft should be accelerated, about 7 days, whereas the C57BL graft should stay on for the full 11–14 days.

This experiment again demonstrates that the memory or anamnestic response is specific; both for B cells, as seen previously, and for T cells, as seen here.

This experiment may be varied by using mice in which the immune response has been generally suppressed using anti-lymphocyte serum (Section 10.8.1), or in T-cell deficient mice (either nu/nu or 'B' mice Sections 1.8.2 or 10.6).

3.2.3   HOST REJECTION (graft versus host reaction)

In the previous experiments we saw that an immunologically mature animal was able to reject a foreign skin graft. There are, however, situations in which the graft, rather than the host, is im-

68

munologically competent and so the host is rejected by the graft. Clinically, such reactions have arisen during attempts to reconstitute immunodeficient children, for example, those with severe combined immunodeficiency, by bone-marrow therapy. Human bone marrow, unlike that of the mouse, contains many immunologically competent cells which produce a florid graft versus host (g.v.h.) reaction characterized by fever, rash, diarrhoea, splenomegaly, pancytopenia and death.

The degree of splenomegaly can be used experimentally in neonatal mice or chickens *in ovo* to quantitate the g.v.h. reaction following an injection of adult allogeneic lymphocytes.

Rats used: 4 DA donors.
    21 (DA × Lewis)F_1 hybrids. Donors and recipients.
Recipients given lymphocytes in 0·1 ml into footpad according to table below:
    Right footpad—DA cells (g.v.h. node).
    Left footpad —F_1 cells (control node).
    Lymph nodes assayed at 7th day post-injection.

Number of lymphocytes transferred		Weight of g.v.h. node	Weight of contralateral (control) node	Index of enlargement	Geometric mean
$5·0 \times 10^6$	1	49·43	4·80	10·3	
	2	63·20	5·12	12·3	11·6
	3	59·60	5·80	10·3	
	4	68·35	4·91	14·1	
$2·5 \times 10^7$	1	110·10	7·93	13·9	
	2	98·92	7·19	13·8	15·6
	3	99·54	5·23	19·0	
	4	120·61	7·44	16·2	
$5·0 \times 10^7$	1	89·96	5·83	14·4	
	2	90·25	7·81	11·6	13·0
	3	67·34	7·22	9·3	
	4	75·43	4·10	18·4	
$1·0 \times 10^8$	1	80·31	5·00	16·0	
	2	65·62	8·31	7·9	11·0
	3	81·40	7·20	11·3	
	4	73·60	7·21	10·2	

Fig. 3.4. Graft versus host reaction dose response curve (Data by courtesy of S. Zakarian.)

The g.v.h. reaction can also be induced in adult animals, in the absence of immunosuppression, by injecting parental cells into an F_1 hybrid. Because the histocompatibility antigens are co-dominant the F_1 hybrid will express both parental antigens, and be tolerant to both. Accordingly, parental cells will not be recognized as foreign by the F_1 cells, but the parental cells will recognize and react to the other parental component on the F_1 cells. The g.v.h. reaction can be assayed in rats using lymph node enlargement. Here the g.v.h. reaction is limited to the popliteal lymph node by injecting parental cells into the footpad of an F_1 hybrid (the popliteal node receives the lymph drainage from the footpad area). The lymph node enlargement assay in rats has several advantages over the splenomegaly assay in mice, for example:

1   The index of lymph node enlargement (10–15 times) is much greater than that of splenic enlargement (2–3 times).
2   The contra-lateral node, receiving the same number of SYN-GENEIC cells, provides an excellent internal control for non-specific enlargement.

Materials

Individuals of an inbred strain of rats and F_1 hybrids, e.g. DA, or Lewis and (DA × Lewis)F_1 (Appendix II).

1   Remove the spleens from the parental and F_1 hybrid donors.
2   Tease out, wash and filter the cells (Section 2.4).
3   Count the cells and adjust to the required concentration (see protocol in suggested experimental design Fig. 3.4).
4   Inject 0·1 ml of the parental and F_1 cells into the right and left footpad respectively.
5   After 7 days kill all the recipients and remove the right and left popliteal nodes (the nodes are in the muscle just behind the knee joint—remove the g.v.h. node first as this is the easiest to find cf. Fig. 3.5.)
6   Weigh each pair of nodes and calculate the index of enlargement as follows:

Index of enlargement (I.E.)
$$= \frac{\text{Weight of node receiving parental cells}}{\text{Weight of node receiving } F_1 \text{ cells.}}.$$

An I.E. up to two may be expected from the injection of syngeneic cells alone. The normal range for a g.v.h. situation is 10–15.
7   Calculate the geometrical mean for each group (Section 4.1.2c).
8   Determine the optimum number of parental cells, i.e. the number giving maximum I.E.

The observed increase in lymph node weight during the local g.v.h. reaction is due to an increased number of host, not donor, cells. Presumably, this host response is caused by mitogenic and chemotatic factors, released by the activated donor cells, which induce non-specific inflow and division of host cells (Section 3.2.1).

70

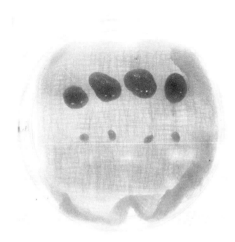

Fig. 3.5. Lymph node enlargement induced during a g.v.h. reaction
Popliteal lymph nodes taken from (DA × Lewis)F$_1$ rats receiving DA cells into the right foot pad (above) and an equal number of F$_1$ cells into the left foot pad (below).

It is possible to assay a host versus graft reaction in this system by transferring F$_1$ cells into parental recipients.

GRAFT VERSUS HOST REACTION IN OTHER ANIMALS

In mice, the degree of lymph node enlargement produced by a local g.v.h. reaction is much less dramatic and reliable. The index of enlargement is in the range of 1·5–3·0. The reasons for this difference between the rat and mouse system are not known.

A g.v.h. reaction may be reliably quantitated in mice and chickens by measuring the degree of splenic enlargement induced by an intravenous injection of allogeneic cells into an immunologically incompetent host. Again, this incompetent situation is achieved by: (a) injecting adult lymphocytes into heavily irradiated adult recipients, (b) by injecting parental cells into a F$_1$ hybrid, or (c) injecting adult cells into a newborn or embryonic recipient. In (c), it is necessary to use a group of age-matched, litter-mate mice as controls, and to inject them with an equal number of adult syngeneic cells. In both experimental and control groups, the g.v.h. spleen weight is expressed as a fraction of the total body weight.

It is also possible to enumerate g.v.h. effector cells in chicken lymphocyte populations by their ability to induce g.v.h. 'pocks' on the chorioallantoic membrane of allogeneic embryos. Each of the assays mentioned above have been extensively reviewed by Simonsen 1962 (see Further Reading at end of chapter).

As will be seen in Chapter 10, the g.v.h. and mixed lymphocyte reactions (Section 10.11.4) have several properties in common, it is not possible, for example, to demonstrate an effect of presensitization on the magnitude of the response to major histocompatibility differences, and in both reactions, specific T-effector cells are generated which are able to lyse appropriate target cells (Section 10.11.6).

3.3   SUMMARY AND CONCLUSIONS

We have described experiments in this chapter showing the B- and T-cell systems responding independently; in the intact immune response this seldom, if ever, happens. In the next chapter we will examine the cellular dynamics involved in the humoral response to antigen, and show that the T-cell system has no little role to play.

FURTHER READING

CALNE R. (ed.) (1973) *Immunological Aspects of Transplantation Surgery.* MTP Press, Lancaster.

JERNE N.K., NORDIN A.A. & HENRY C. (1963) The agar plaque technique for recognising antibody producing cells. In Amos & Koprowski (eds.) *Cell-bound Antibody.* Wistar Institute Press, Philadelphia.

LUCAS D.O. (ed.) (1977) *Regulatory Mechanisms in Lymphocyte Activation.* Academic Press, New York.

SIMONSEN M. (1962) Graft versus Host Reactions. Their natural history and applicability as tools of research. *Prog. Allerg.* **6**, 349.

4   Cellular dynamics *in vivo*

We are now at the stage where we can start to reconstruct the immune system of our animal model and try to gain some understanding of the complex interactions that actually occur in a 'real' immune response. Again, for ease of experimental manipulation, the animal will be responding to highly artificial antigens.

While being intrigued by the wonderful specificity and adaptation of lymphocytes (and their progeny and soluble mediators) we must also consider an area of immunity that shows only 'crude' specificity and virtually no adaptivity. This is innate, non-specific or natural immunity.

4.1   INNATE IMMUNITY

The body has many mechanisms of defence against micro-organisms that are of prime importance but do not concern lymphocytes at all. Indeed many potential pathogens are resisted and destroyed without the lymphoid system becoming aware of their existence.

At the body surface, for example, lactic acid in sweat and the fatty acids in sebaceous secretions, are very potent anti-bacterial agents. In the tissues there are anti-bacterial enzymes, for example, lysozyme—which splits the linkages between N-acetyl glucosamine and N-acetyl muramic acid in the bacterial cell wall. This enzyme is known to facilitate the disruption of bacteria after an antibody and complement-mediated lesion has been formed. Again we see that although the body has many potentially independent mechanisms of defence, they usually act in concert.

4.1.1   PARTICLE CLEARANCE BY THE RETICULO-ENDOTHELIAL SYSTEM

Micro-organisms, or their experimental equivalent of carbon particles, are readily engulfed by circulating and tissue-fixed phagocytes.

Polymorphonuclear leucocytes and monocytes (Section 2.3.1) together with histiocytes or tissue macrophages constitute the RE-TICULOENDOTHELIAL (RE) SYSTEM. The cells of the RE system are all capable of ingesting foreign material and degrading it by means of intracellular enzymes in phagolysosomes.

73

Albino mice
Colloidal carbon (Appendix II)
Acetic acid (1 % v/v glacial acetic acid in water)
Spectrophotometer or colorimeter

1   Warm the mouse at 37° for 15–20 min.
2   Snip the end from the tail and collect one drop of blood onto a microscope slide. Lyse a 20 µl sample in 4·0 ml of acetic acid.
3   Inject 0·1 ml of colloidal carbon into the tail vein. (Inject near to base of tail.)
4   When the mouse's eyes have turned black (within 30 sec) collect one drop of blood and lyse a 10 µl sample in 2 ml of acetic acid.
5   Collect one drop of blood at the following times post-innoculation: 2, 5, 10, 15, 20, 30, 45, 60, 90 min, and lyse a 10 µl sample, before it clots, in 2 ml of acetic acid solution.
6   Observe the colour change of the mouse's eyes. Kill the mouse and examine the lungs, liver and spleen. (If necessary kill and examine a control mouse, not injected with carbon.)
7   Using the original, pre-injection blood sample as a standard, read the density of all the lysed samples.

4.1.2   DATA PRESENTATION

We have decided to use the data from this experiment, in which the underlying biological principles are relatively simple, to illustrate some of the methods of data presentation. However, the comments and methods of presentation are generally applicable.

By inspection of the data in Fig. 4.1, it can be seen that each mouse has a slightly different rate of clearance of carbon particles

Time (min)	0	2	5	10	15	20	30	45	60	90
Mouse	% Transmittance of lysed sample									
1	44	26	29	47	51	89	78	92	100	100
2	0	6	12	19	31	27	42	80	76	100
3	9	21	30	41	49	52	68	89	95	100
4	15	22	28	59	58	74	87	92	100	100
5	0	9	12	33	16	20	31	26	—	—
6	9	18	28	—	44	48	74	86	89	100
Arithmetic mean ($\bar{X}$)	13	17	23	40	42	52	63	78	92	100
Standard deviation (s.d.)	16	8	9	15	15	27	22	26	10	0

Fig. 4.1. Clearance of blood-borne colloidal carbon by the reticuloendothelial system

from the blood. This is due to many biological variables, both un-controlled and uncontrollable, such as age, blood volume, number and activity of phagocytic cells, etc., and also the technical error of the sampling method. We wish to present the data in a way that it can be:

(a) appreciated, to discern any central tendency of the dependent variable (amount of carbon in the blood) relative to the independent variable (time);

(b) analysed, we may ultimately wish to know whether mice treated in different ways vary significantly in their clearance times (see Section 4.1.4).

4.1.2a ARITHMETIC MEAN

This is the simplest description of the data, in that we are all used to using this value. The sample arithmetic mean, $\bar{x}$, may be calculated as follows:

Sample mean $\bar{x} = \dfrac{\sum x}{n}$

where: $\sum x$ = sum of all values of x
n = number of observations.

1 Tabulate your data and calculate the mean transmittance value for each time point as in Fig. 4.1.

2 Plot a graph of (100—mean transmittance value), i.e. the relative amount of carbon remaining in the blood, against time as in Fig. 4.2. (It is conventional to plot the independent variable on the x or horizontal axis and the dependent variable on the y or vertical axis.)

If the sample mean alone is recorded we are losing valuable information describing the distribution of the data around the mean. The simplest description of the spread of the data is the RANGE. However, this depends only on the extreme values of the dependent variable. In most cases the extreme values occur least frequently and so will be the least typical members of the distribution. One therefore defines the STANDARD DEVIATION.

4.1.2b STANDARD DEVIATION

This value gives an estimate of the dispersion of the data which takes into account the frequency with which each value occurs and its distance from the mean.

Standard deviation, s.d. $= \sqrt{\dfrac{\sum (x - \bar{x})^2}{n - 1}}$

where: x = value of each observation
$\bar{x}$ = sample mean
n = number of observations.

75

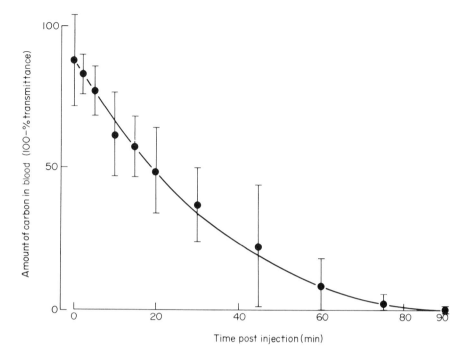

Fig. 4.2. Exponential clearance curve of colloidal carbon
The rate of carbon clearance is proportional to the excess of the residual
blood concentration over a certain threshold value. Although the individual time-points conform reasonably to the curve fitted by eye it is more
accurate to fit a straight line curve to the log transformed data.

The standard deviation of each group of observations is shown as bar
lines above and below the arithmetric mean.

For ease of calculation, this equation may be rewritten:

$$s.d. = \sqrt{\left[\sum x^2 - \frac{(\sum x)^2}{n}\right]\frac{1}{n-1}}$$

This has been calculated for each time point in Fig. 4.1. The sample
mean ± standard deviation uniquely defines each set of data. The
standard deviation (above and below the mean) is shown on the
graph (Fig. 4.2) as horizontal bar lines. It can be shown that 68% of
the data lie within the limits of one standard deviation above and
below the sample mean.

The data in this experiment do not lie in a straight line but
instead form a smooth curve. This is known as an EXPONENTIAL
CLEARANCE CURVE where the rate of carbon clearance is proportional to the excess of the concentration over a certain threshold
value. Fitting such a curve mathematically, especially when the
measurements contain random variation can be a very elaborate
statistical exercise. In addition, we wish to determine the slope of
the curve as this will give us the rate of carbon clearance. It is,

76

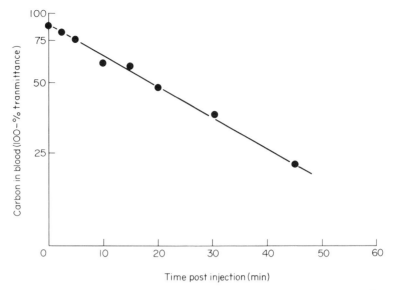

Fig. 4.3. Clearance of colloidal carbon from blood (log transformed data)
After logarithmic transformation the data should conform to a straight line.
At sample times later than 50 min there is a bend in the straight line
showing that other variables are exerting an effect on the rate of clearance.
The slope of the line, i.e. the rate of carbon clearance, is determined only for
those observations before the point of inflection.

therefore, necessary to transform the data logarithmically by plot-
ting it on semi-log graph paper as shown in Fig. 4.3. The points now
approximate to a straight line which can be fitted more accurately
than the exponential curve. Calculate the slope of the line to determine the rate of carbon clearance.

4.1.2c ADDITIONAL NOTES

Geometric mean

In the above data there was less than one log variation at any one
time point. With haemolytic plaque data (Sections 3.1.2 and 4.2),
there is usually much greater variation. Under these conditions an
arithmetic mean is biased towards the extreme values and so a
GEOMETRIC MEAN is used. It is calculated as follows:

Geometric mean, $g = \sqrt[n]{x_1, x_2, \ldots, x_n}$

For ease of calculation this may be re-written as:

$$\log g = \frac{\sum\limits_{i=1}^{n} \log x_i}{n}$$

where: x_i = values of x
n = numbers of observations.

77

Standard error

Many workers represent their data by a mean value $\pm$ the STAN-
DARD ERROR OF THE MEAN. This is a description of the oscilla-
tion of the sample mean around the TRUE or POPULATION MEAN
and is calculated as follows:

Standard error, s.e. $= \dfrac{s.d.}{\sqrt{n}}$

where: s.d. = standard deviation
         n = number of observations.

The standard error is, of course, smaller than the standard deviation and reduces as the size of the sample is increased. It does not,
however, describe the distribution of the data around the sample
mean.

4.1.3   NEUTROPHIL FUNCTION TESTS

In vitro assays are available for only a proportion of the neutrophil
activities shown in Fig. 4.4, for example, chemotaxis, phagocytosis
and microbicidal activity. However, even where tests are available,
the precise parameter being measured, and its *in vitro* relevance, is
not always clear.

The nitroblue tetrazolium reduction assay described below can
be used to measure both phagocytosis (this is the only way in which
the dye enters the cell) and one of the metabolic pathways responsible for microbial killing (hexose monophosphate shunt
activation).

NITROBLUE TETRAZOLIUM (NBT) TEST

The addition of the yellow NBT dye to plasma results in the formation of a NBT-heparin or NBT-fibrinogen complex, which may be
phagocytosed by neutrophils. Normal neutrophils show little incorporation of the complex unless they are 'stimulated' to phagocytic
activity, for example, by the addition of endotoxin. This assay may
be used, therefore, to measure the degree of 'stimulation' of untreated cells or their capacity for phagocytosis after stimulation.

Stimulated neutrophils incorporate the dye complex into phago-
somes and, after lysosomal fusion, intra cellular reduction results in
the formation of blue insoluble crystals of formazan. The percentage
of phagocytic cells may be determined using a light microscope or,
as described below, the total dye reduction may be quantitated
spectrophotometrically after dioxan extraction.

Materials and equipment

Sample of venous blood in heparin (20 iu . ml^{-1})
Distilled water
Phosphate buffered saline (PBS) (Appendix I)

78

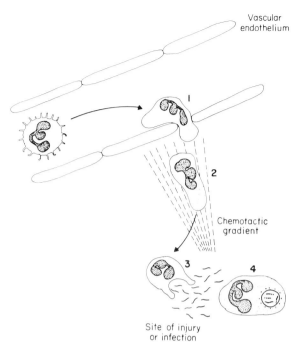

Fig. 4.4. Action of neutrophils

Neutrophils leave the blood and congregate at the site of tissue injury (for example, Section 4.5.3) or infection. Dysfunction in any of the stages shown would adversely affect the ability of neutrophils to perform their rôle as front line defenders against microbial infection. The important stages in the development of an inflammatory response are (1) attachment to, and migration through, the vascular endothelium, (2) locomotion, which may be chemotactic, (3) phagocytosis and (4) digestion of microbes.

E. coli endotoxin (Appendix II) 1 mg ml^{-1} in PBS
4 mM Nitroblue tetrazolium dye (Appendix II) in PBS containing 340 mM sucrose
Dioxan
0·1 M hydrochloric acid
Nylon wool (Appendix II), 100 mg in siliconized pasteur pipette
Water bath, at 70°
Spectrophotometer

Method

1   Obtain blood sample in heparin (20 iu . ml^{-1}) by venepuncture. Use a sample for total and differential leucocyte counts (Section 2.3.1). *The NBT reduction activity of the sample must be determined within 60 min of venesection.*

2   Add 15 μl of endotoxin solution (1 mg . ml^{-1} in PBS, initial concentration) to 1·5 ml of blood and incubate at 37° for 10 min.

3   Add 0·3 ml of freshly prepared NBT dye solution and mix gently.

4 Add blood dropwise to a nylon wool column.

5 Once the sample has entered the column wash twice with 2 ml of PBS and then 2 ml of distilled water. *The distilled water will lyse any residual erythrocytes.*

6 Add two drops of hydrochloric acid to the column, to stop further reduction of the intracellular dye, and wash with 2 ml of distilled water.

7 Remove the nylon wool with forceps and place in 5 ml dioxan (in a *glass* container).

8 Incubate at 70° with occasional vigorous shaking until the nylon wool returns to its original white colour (about 20 min).

9 Centrifuge the dioxan extract to remove any precipitate or nylon fibres (1000 g for 10 min at room temperature).

10 Measure the extinction at 520 nm using a spectrophotometer (use a dioxan standard).

The unstimulated control value is obtained by a parallel incubation of untreated blood, i.e. add 15 μl PBS alone at step 2, then assay as 3–10.

Technical notes

1 All glassware must be siliconized to prevent adherence of phagocytes.

2 Both neutrophils and monocytes ingest NBT by phagocytosis.

3 The conversion factor for the calculation of moles of formazan from extinction coefficient must be calculated for a sample of each batch of dye, after chemical reduction, as below.

DETERMINATION OF CONVERSION FACTOR

Materials and equipment

Ascorbic acid
4 mM Nitroblue tetrazolium in distilled water containing 340 mM sucrose
0·1 M Sodium hydroxide containing 24 mM sodium bicarbonate
Distilled water
Dioxan
Waterbath at 70°
Spectrophotometer

Method

1 Add 150 μmol ascorbic acid to 0·2 ml of NBT solution and mix.

2 Add 2 ml of 0·1 M sodium hydroxide containing 24 mM sodium bicarbonate.

3 Incubate for 10 min at room temperature and add 5 ml distilled water.

4 Centrifuge at 1000 g for 15 min at room temperature.

5 Wash once in water by centrifugation (1000 g for 15 min at room temperature). Remove the supernatant and resuspend the blue insoluble formazan precipitate in 10 ml dioxan.

6 Dilute 1 ml of the suspension with 9 ml dioxan and incubate at 70° for 20 min.

7 Cool to room temperature, and measure the extinction at 520 nm using a spectrophotometer (use a dioxan blank).

8 Calculate the conversion factor from the extinction value.

As a rough guide, the conversion factor should be approximately:

1 extinction unit $\equiv$ 40 n mol of formazan.

CALCULATION OF NBT UPTAKE BY PHAGOCYTES

1 Using the conversion factor determined above, determine the number of moles of formazan extracted from the untreated and endotoxin stimulated blood.

2 Calculate the number of potential phagocytes used per assay (the percentage of the absolute count due to neutrophils and monocytes).

3 Express results as moles of formazan per phagocyte.

Normal range: untreated blood, 0·92–3·62 f mol per phagocyte.
Normal range: endotoxin stimulated blood, 2·52–4·90 f mol per phagocyte.

4.1.4 RETICULOENDOTHELIAL BLOCKADE

The foreign material taken into phagocytic cells is not invariably degraded and lost. It is known that the antibody response to many antigens is macrophage dependent. This may involve some form of 'antigen presentation' to the B cells via the macrophages. This will be discussed in more detail in Section 4.6.

The rate of uptake of foreign material into phagocytes varies under different conditions. It has been shown that an acute malarial infection will cause an RE blockade, presumably because of release and subsequent phagocytosis of malarial organisms, toxins and red cell fragments. This blockade may be mimicked by loading up the R.E. system with colloidal carbon and then observing the clearance of a second material, for example, heat aggregated protein.

Materials and equipment (see also Section 5.2.2a for iodination technique)

Albino mice
Bovine serum albumin
Colloidal carbon (Appendix II)
Gamma counter

1   Heat the BSA solution at 60° for 40 min to form soluble complexes. Centrifuge off any precipitate. Iodinate the soluble aggregated protein as in Section 5.2.2a.
2   Inject groups of 4 mice with 0·1, 0·2 and 0·5 ml of colloidal carbon respectively. (See protocol below.)
3   3 h later inject 5 mg of heat aggregated ^{125}I-BSA intravenously.
4   Collect 20 μl blood samples (Section 4.1.1) at the times shown in the protocol. (Do not lyse the sample.)
5   Determine the radioactivity in each sample by gamma-counting.
6   Calculate the percentage of radioactivity remaining in the blood for each time point and plot a graph of the data as for section 4.1.1.

Protocol

Mouse number:	1	2	3	4	5	6	7	8	9	10	11	12	13	14	15	16
Colloidal carbon, ml.	none ⟶			0·1 ⟶				0·2 ⟶				0·4 ⟶				
^{125}I-BSA	5 mg ⟶															
Sample times (minutes post-BSA injection)	0	20	40	60	0	20	40	60	0	20	40	60	0	20	40	60

Analysis of data

In the above experiment you have compared the activity of phagocytic cells in normal animals with cells in animals undergoing 'RE blockade'. We wish to ask the question: has the blockade been effective, i.e. has the phagocytic ability of the cells been altered after carbon treatment? In this case the answer should be clear by simply inspecting the slopes of the two graph lines. In many experiments, however, the difference between control and experimental animals is not so clear. In such cases it is necessary to use statistical tests to evaluate the significance of the difference between groups.

A full discussion of statistical tests is beyond the range of this book. We suggest you consult the reference (Campbell, 1974) at the end of this chapter and perform a test of significance on the effectiveness of 'RE blockade' on the clearance of aggregated BSA.

In this case, where we are comparing the mean values of two treatments, it is useful to determine the standard error of the mean. As a rule of thumb; if the standard errors of two means do not overlap then the difference between the means is likely to be statistically significant.

Alternative experiments

A. It is relatively simple to demonstrate the ability of the RE system to clear micro-organisms from the blood. For many purposes this may be thought to be a more relevant teaching demonstration.

Materials and equipment

Rabbit
Suspension of *Escherichia coli*
McConkey agar (Appendix II)
Culture broth (Appendix II)

Method

1 Inject the rabbit intravenously with 10^6 *E. coli* organisms.
2 Take 0·5 ml blood samples at the following times post-injection:
0, 5, 10, 20, 30, 60, 90 min.
3 Dilute the blood 1 : 10 and 1 : 100 with broth and plate 1·0 ml
aliquots onto McConkey agar.
4 Sacrifice the rabbit at the end of the experiment and grind up the
lungs, liver and spleen individually in broth. Dilute a sample of each
1 : 1000 and plate 1·0 ml aliquots onto agar as before.
5 Count the number of bacterial colonies (*circular colonies with a
smooth convex surface—red-pink colour on McConkey agar*).
6 Plot a graph of number of colonies against time and calculate
the rate of clearance of micro-organisms from the blood.

B. Determine the clearance rates in normal and immunized animals. This will demonstrate IMMUNE ELIMINATION where the
rate of phagocytosis of bacteria-antibody complexes is accelerated.
An experiment analogous to immune elimination involving hetero-antibody in normal animals is described in Section 10.8.3.

4.2   **T-B COOPERATION**

In the previous sections we have demonstrated the T- and B-cell
systems reacting independently to antigen. However, in the intact
immune response this seldom, if ever, happens. The production of
antibody by B cells depends not only on an interaction with macro-phages (Section 4.6) but also on an interaction with T cells. Accordingly, although T cells never secrete antibody they are essential
for the production of antibody—to many but perhaps not all
antigens—by the process known as COOPERATION.

Cooperation involving T and B cells cannot be demonstrated
using thymus and bursa cells from the chicken. In the mouse the
bursa-equivalent has not been definitely identified but fortunately in
the experiment we will describe the bone marrow behaves as though
it were a source of B cells devoid of T cells, it is therefore operationally equivalent to the avian bursa.

Materials and equipment

6-month-old inbred mice for X-irradiation (Section 1.8)
3–4-week-old inbred mice as thymus and bone marrow donors

Sheep erythrocytes (Appendix II)

X-ray machine or γ-source

Materials for haemolytic plaques (Section 3.1.2)

We will use X-irradiated (immunosuppressed) mice as 'living test tubes' to examine the response of transferred T and B cells, separately and together, to sheep erythrocytes.

Protocol

Group	Number* of mice	Cells for transfer	No. ml i.v.	Sheep cell challenge
A	3	bone marrow	0·1	10^8 i.p.
B	3	thymocytes	0·1	10^8 i.p.
C	3	$\begin{cases} \text{bone marrow} + \\ \text{thymocytes} \end{cases}$	0·1 + 0·1	10^8 i.p.

* For experimental purposes it is necessary to use 4 or more mice per group.

1   Give 9 mice 800 R of irradiation (see notes in Section 1.8.3).

2   Remove the femurs from 6 untreated donor mice.

3   Cut each end off the bones and 'blow out' the marrow with tissue culture medium using a hypodermic syringe with an 18 g needle.

4   Disperse the cells with a Pasteur pipette.

5   Count the cells and adjust to 2×10^8 ml^{-1}.

6   Remove the thymus from each of 4 donors and tease the cells into medium.

7   Wash the cells twice by centrifugation (150 g for 10 min at 4°) count and adjust the cells to 10^9 ml^{-1}.

Reconstitute and challenge the X-irradiated recipient mice as shown in the protocol.

8   After 8 days assay the recipient spleens for direct haemolytic plaques as described in Section 3.1.2.

9   Calculate and tabulate the number of plaque-forming cells per spleen for each group of mice.

Technical notes

1   No control group is included to show that the X-irradiation was successful in suppressing the immune response of the recipient mice.

2   Bone marrow is a relatively poor source of B cells. In the regime described you will obtain a maximum of $4·0$–$6·0 \times 10^3$ plaques spleen^{-1}. More satisfactory results may be obtained using 'B' spleen, prepared either by reconstitution of X-irradiated, thymectomized recipients (Section 10.6) or, more conveniently, by anti-Thy.1 treatment of normal spleen (Sections 10.8.5 and 10.9). Using

2×10^7 'B' spleen cells $+ 10^8$ thymus cells you can expect at least $3 \cdot 0 \times 10^4$ plaques spleen^{-1}.

In this experiment we have demonstrated the basic requirement for T cells in antibody production. The mechanism and specificity of this requirement is shown in later experiments (Section 10.2).

4.3   **TOLERANCE**

In chemical terms all antigens are equal; in immunological terms some are more equal than others. As we do not now question that an animal will react to foreign antigens we must therefore ask why does it not react to itself? Burnet suggested that lymphocytes must go through a 'learning phase' in ontogeny when they learn to distinguish between 'self' and 'non-self'. He postulated that potential antigens present during this 'learning phase' in some way suppress the development of specific antigen reactive clones. Thus the animal will be rendered tolerant to any antigen, 'self' or otherwise, present during the perinatal period. Tolerance is known to exist in both T and B lymphocyte populations but may be demonstrated more simply in assays involving the latter.

Materials and equipment

Neonatal mice
Bovine serum albumin (BSA) (Appendix II)
Freund's complete adjuvant (Appendix II)
Sheep erythrocytes (Appendix II)
Material for Farr assay (Section 5.2.1)
Materials for haemagglutination (Section 5.4.1)

Method

1   Prepare a 10 mg ml^{-1} solution of BSA and centrifuge at 100,000 g for three hours. *Antigens are more immunogenic if they are insolubilized (Section 1.4), conversely they are more tolerogenic if used in a soluble form completely free of aggregates.*
2   Inject 10 1–2-day-old mice with 1 mg of ultracentrifuged BSA intraperitoneally. Keep an equal number of littermates as controls.
3   Inject the mice with the same antigen dose each week for a total of 6 weeks.
4   On the 8th week, inject all mice intraperitoneally with 1 mg of BSA in Freund's complete adjuvant and 10^8 sheep erythrocytes.
5   Bleed all the mice on week 9, separate and store the sera at $-20°$ for testing.

Tests on sera

1   Perform a Farr assay for antigen-binding capacity to BSA as in Section 5.2.2.

2   Perform an haemagglutination test for anti-sheep erythrocyte antibodies (Section 5.4.1).

Data and observations

Calculate and compare the average antigen binding capacity of the sera from tolerized and normal mice. Record and compare end point haemagglutinin titre for each group.

4.3.1   TOLERANCE V. SELECTIVE UNRESPONSIVENESS

It is essential to establish a clear difference between tolerance and selective unresponsiveness. It is useful to reserve the term tolerance for the complete mechanism by which self-unresponsiveness is established and maintained. All experimental attempts to reproduce this mechanism have merely concerned a selective unresponsiveness.

Two mechanisms have been proposed to explain the experimental finding:

1   *Immunoparalysis.* This may be envisaged as a deletion or switching-off of selected T and B, antigen-reactive clones. This mechanism would be passive or recessive and could be over-ridden by the addition of normal antigen-reactive cells. (See also Section 4.6.)

2   *Positive suppression.* In this case the unresponsiveness would be dominant and could suppress the response of normal antigen-reactive lymphocytes. Evidence indicates that suppression may be mediated via a sub-population of T cells. (See references at end of chapter.)

Mitchison has shown that selective unresponsiveness may exist at two levels dependent on the dose of antigen used to induce the unresponsiveness. He termed these two states low- and high-zone *tolerance* (our italics). Low-zone *tolerance* is induced by antigens that fail to immunize with an injection of 1 μg (weak immunogens). High-zone *tolerance* may be established and maintained with repeated injections of antigens in excess of 1 mg. Weigle *et al.* have shown that at low antigen doses T cells alone are rendered unresponsive, whereas both T and B cells are rendered unresponsive at high antigen levels. It has been argued that the depressed antibody response to an immunogenic challenge seen after an injection of a non-immunogenic concentration of the same antigen (low-zone *tolerance*) may in fact be due to a switch away from humoral to cell-mediated immunity. If this were the case, then the initial chal-

86

lenge would have generated 'T-killer' rather than 'T-cooperator' cells. In other words, in this experimental situation, unresponsiveness may simply reflect a change in the immune response away from the parameter being measured.

The two mechanisms for the induction of experimental unresponsiveness mentioned above may or may not operate together, however, it is apparent that whatever mechanism(s) operates to establish and maintain self-tolerance, it must act on all the sectors of the immune response.

4.4   AUTOIMMUNITY

When the normal 'self' tolerance situation is either not established or breaks down, autoantibodies are produced. It is, however, often difficult to establish a causal rôle for autoantibodies in the so-called autoimmune diseases. Indeed, many investigators have suggested that autoantibodies may be 'normal', aiding the disposal of altered self components.

Several clinical situations in which autoantibodies may be detected are described in Sections 5.4.3, 6.3.2b and 6.4. Experimentally, the New Zealand Black (NZB) mouse presents an excellent model for autoimmune disorders. Among several other autoantibodies (e.g. Section 6.4) this strain produces anti-erythrocyte antibodies; these may be detected by a haemagglutination assay.

Materials and equipment

NZB mice (Appendix II)
Rabbit anti-mouse immunoglobulin serum (Section 1.4.2)
Microtitre trays and equipment for haemagglutination (Section 5.4.1)

Method

1   Bleed the mice by severing the axillary vessels (see Fig. 2.1). Collect the blood in heparin.
2   Wash the blood cells three times with PBS by centrifugation (300 g for 10 min) and prepare a 2% suspension.
3   Determine the highest dilution of antiserum giving complete haemagglutination with erythrocytes of individuals of different ages (see Section 5.4.1).

Technical notes

1   The sensitivity of the haemagglutination technique as described can be increased: set the test up as above and after 1 hour incubation at room temperature, centrifuge the plates at 150 g for 1

minute. Then stand the trays at an angle of 45° for 20 minutes, the unagglutinated cells will roll away from the apex of the V. This modification is said to increase the sensitivity by 2 or more dilutions.

2   Specificity controls as in Section 5.4.1.

4.5   HYPERSENSITIVITY STATES

After primary contact with antigen an individual is immunized or primed, and exists in a state of so-called HYPERSENSITIVITY. The types of hypersensitivity states recognized by Coombs and Gell may be listed as follows:

Type 1—Anaphylactic hypersensitivity
Type 2—Cytotoxic hypersensitivity
Type 3—Immune complex-mediated hypersensitivity
Type 4—Delayed (cell-mediated) hypersensitivity

Types 1–3 initially involve the interaction of antibody with antigen. Type 4 is purely cell mediated and involves the reactions of the T-cell system seen throughout the book, it will therefore be excluded from further discussion in this section.

4.5.1   ANAPHYLACTIC HYPERSENSITIVITY

Animals given repeated intravenous injections of soluble antigen become immune but they also tend to die due to a reaction known as ACUTE ANAPHYLAXIS.

4.5.1a   ANAPHYLAXIS in vivo

Guinea-pigs are exquisitely sensitive to anaphylaxis. If primed by an intravenous injection of 1 mg of ovalbumin they will die due to anaphylactic shock upon a second injection 2–3 weeks later. At post-mortem examination the animal will characteristically show intense constriction of the bronchi, thus accounting for death by asphyxia.

4.5.1b   ANAPHYLAXIS in vitro

The sensitivity of guinea-pigs to anaphylaxis may be demonstrated less dramatically but more humanely in vitro.

Materials and equipment

Guinea-pigs
Ovalbumin (Appendix II)
Freund's complete adjuvant (Appendix II)
Hank's saline (Appendix I)
Apparatus as in Fig. 4.5.

88

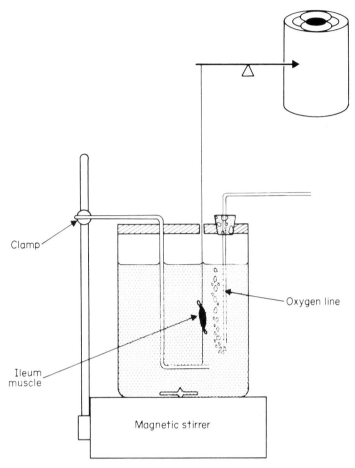

Kymograph or stress transducer

Clamp

Oxygen line

Ileum muscle

Magnetic stirrer

Fig. 4.5. Organ bath and recording apparatus for the demonstration of immediate hypersensitivity *in vitro*
Classically uterine muscle was used for this assay but it has now been replaced by ileum muscle which has a shorter contraction and relaxation time.

Previous preparation

Sensitize the guinea-pigs by an intramuscular injection of 500 μg of ovalbumin in Freund's complete adjuvant 3–4 weeks before the experiment.

Method

1   Kill the guinea-pig and remove the ileum into Hank's saline at 37°.
2   Remove a strip of muscle and mount it in the organ bath at 37° (Fig. 4.5).

3 Allow the muscle to relax for 20–30 min.
4 Add the antigen in solution and observe the contraction of the muscle.

Suggested experiments (use fresh muscle preparation for each experiment):

1 Add increasing concentrations of antigen to the bath starting at 1 μg ml^{-1} (final concentration) in steps of 5 μg. Determine the minimum concentration required to elicit contraction. After contraction, add further antigen in the mg range to stimulate a second contraction. Observe the magnitude of the first and second contractions in relation to the concentration of antigen added.
2 Use bovine serum albumin to test the specificity of the response.
3 Soak muscle from normal animals in sensitized guinea-pig serum for varying times at 37°. Test for passive sensitization.

In man anaphylaxis is known to be mediated by cell-bound IgE antibodies. Unlike membrane bound immunoglobulin receptor molecules (Section 2.7) which are inserted into the membrane after endogenous synthesis, this antibody is attached via its Fc portion to the Fc binding site on the plasma membrane of mast cells. When antigen combines with the IgE antibody the mast cell is caused to degranulate releasing the pharmacological mediators of anaphylaxis, the best known of which is histamine.

4.5.2 CYTOTOXIC HYPERSENSITIVITY

Antibodies to cell-surface components may bring about cell death by promoting phagocytosis via opsonic or immune adherence (Sections 6.5 and 10.8.2) or by the activation of the complement system for direct cell lysis (Section 10.9). The result of cytotoxic hypersensitivity is seen in transfusion reactions or in haemolytic disease of the newborn due to rhesus incompatibility (Section 5.4.6).

4.5.3 IMMUNE COMPLEX-MEDIATED HYPERSENSITIVITY

Circulating immune complexes have been detected in a wide variety of clinical conditions, from chronic parasitic infections, for example malaria, to 'autoimmune' diseases, for example, systemic lupus erythematosus and rheumatoid arthritis. (In rheumatoid arthritis, recent experimental evidence suggests that the immune complexes found in synovial fluid are formed by the reaction of antiglobulin antibodies with self immunoglobulin molecules.)

The formation and deposition of immune complexes usually initiates complement fixation with the consequent release of anaphylatoxins and chemotactic factors (Section 6.6). Anaphylatoxins mediate histamine release and consequently induce increased vascular permeability and oedema. Chemotactic factors attract neutrophils, which release their proteolytic enzymes and cause local tissue destruction at the sites of immune complex deposition in the skin, vascular endothelium, joints and kidney glomeruli.

Immune complex mediated tissue damage is usually a self limiting condition which resolves once the source of antigen for complex formation has been removed.

See Section 9.1 for assay of immune complexes.

Experimentally this condition is characterized by oedema and necrosis at the site of antigen injection in a hyperimmune animal.

4.6   **SUMMARY AND CONCLUSIONS**

Although the innate or non-specific immune system is generally thought to be non-adaptive, recent evidence has shown that macrophages from a hyperimmune animal have an increased rate of phagocytosis *in vitro*. It is therefore possible that a primitive capacity for adaptation may exist at this level, although it is difficult to exclude some long-term effect of soluble mediators derived from the lymphoid system (Section 10.12).

Macrophages are known to be required during antigen stimulation of T and B lymphocytes. For example, the removal of glass-adherent cells from lymphocyte populations reduces the *in vitro* immune response to soluble antigens or allogeneic cells. It is important to note, however, that although the majority of glass-adherent cells are macrophages, this population certainly contains other cells, for example, B lymphocytes.

Most soluble antigens are rapidly degraded after phagocytosis, but not, for example, pneumococcal polysaccharide or D amino acids. Approximately $1-3\%$ of the ingested material is said to remain undegraded and eventually appears on the surface of the macrophage where it may have enhanced immunogenicity.

Feldman and his colleagues have proposed a mechanism to explain the observed correlation between thymus- and macrophage-dependence of antigens. They suggested, with good evidence, that an antigen may become associated with antibody-like molecules on the surface of T cells and, after shedding, the complex may bind to macrophage surfaces. The only major point of controversy within this model is whether the antibody on the T cell is endogenously synthesized or derived from B cells.

From this proposed model it can be seen that a phenomenon analogous to 'RE blockade' (Section 4.1.4) may be the basis of antigenic competition. In this latter situation, antigen presentation to B cells via a common macrophage pathway may form a bottleneck before the two competing antigens can diverge along their specific lymphocyte pathways.

91

It has also been suggested that macrophages may have a role to play in at least one form of tolerance induction. As demonstrated earlier (Section 4.3), soluble, de-aggregated antigens tend to be tolerogenic, but are immunogenic if aggregated, rendered insoluble or given in combination with Freund's complete adjuvant (FCA). Soluble antigens are not readily phagocytosed and so may confront the B cells directly to induce tolerance (this is especially true of T-dependent antigens). Insoluble antigens in FCA are rapidly phagocytosed and so only a relatively small amount eventually reaches the B cell, via the macrophage surface.

The role proposed for macrophages in antigen presentation to B cells is essentially non-specific; in contrast, the role played by T cells is highly specific as will be seen in Chapter 10.

FURTHER READING

ALLEN J.C. (1976) *Infection and the Compromised Host.* Williams & Wilkins, Baltimore.

AMOS *et al* (1979) *Immune Mechanisms and Disease.* Academic Press, London.

BURNET M. (1972) *Auto-immunity and Auto-immune Disease.* MTP, Lancaster, England.

CAMPBELL R.C. (1974) *Statistics for Biologists*, 2nd ed. Cambridge University Press.

NOSSAL G.J.V. (1973) The Cellular and Molecular Basis of Immunological Tolerance. *Essays in Fundamental Biology* Roitt (editor). Blackwell Scientific Publications, Oxford.

PLAYFAIR J.H.L. (1971) Cell Co-operation in the Immune Response. *Clin. exp. Immunol.* **8,** 839.

SIGEL M.M. & GOOD R.A. (1972) *Tolerance, Autoimmunity and Ageing.* C.C. Thomas, Springfield, Illinois.

TURK J.L. (1973) *Immunology in Clinical Medicine.* Heineman, London.

WEIGLE W.O. (1973) *Immunological Unresponsiveness. Adv. Immunol.* **16,** 61.

5 Antibody interaction with antigen

Plasma cells produce antibody—this antibody reacts specifically with antigen and activates secondary mechanisms such as the complement system. In this and in the following chapter we are going to study some of the different ways in which this interaction can be demonstrated.

The combination of antigen with antibody to form a complex is a dynamic equilibrium as the bonds formed in complex formation are non-covalent and reversible. The proportions of each reactant in a complex may also vary as antibodies are at least divalent, and antigens multivalent (i.e. they have many antigenic determinants per molecule). Therefore, the amount of reaction observed depends on the proportions of reactants used.

There are usually two stages in most antigen–antibody reactions. The PRIMARY INTERACTION is the specific recognition and combination of an antigenic determinant with the binding site of its corresponding antibody. There then follows a SECONDARY INTERACTION which activates some effector function. This can be, for example, complement fixation, macrophage binding or simply agglutination and precipitation. It is this secondary manifestation which is usually observed in the laboratory. It must be remembered, however, that this secondary effect is only a reflection of the primary antigen–antibody interaction and does not directly correspond to it, especially with antigens having few antigenic determinants. With monovalent haptens, for example, although the primary interaction occurs there is no precipitation or complement fixation.

5.1 ANTIBODY SPECIFICITY

The specificity of the immune response is manifested at many levels, for example, in combating a virus infection the immune system is able to distinguish one virus from another (Section 1.1). The cellular basis of this specificity is invested in those lymphocyte clones selected and expanded after interaction with the virus antigens. At the molecular level, these lymphocytes are specific by virtue of their surface receptors which, in the case of B cells, are immunoglobulin molecules.

Immunoglobulin molecules react with their specific antigens via precisely the same short-range forces governing any protein–protein interaction (Section 8.1). However, the specific antigen–antibody interaction is quantitatively greater because of the complementary

93

3-dimensional shapes of the antibody combining site and its antigenic determinant. Thus the molecules are able to come closer and react over a greater area.

As the configuration of the antigenic determinant changes the degree of cross-reaction with the original antibody falls rapidly. This is shown experimentally in Section 5.3.2.

5.2   **PRIMARY BINDING REACTIONS**

As we discussed earlier, tests based on secondary mechanisms, such as precipitation (Section 5.3.1), do not necessarily measure the degree of primary binding of antigen to antibody. Fig. 5.1 shows a precipitin curve obtained with horse antiserum. In the region of antibody excess there is very little precipitate; the complexes form but remain soluble. In such cases we need other techniques to measure primary binding such as that outlined below.

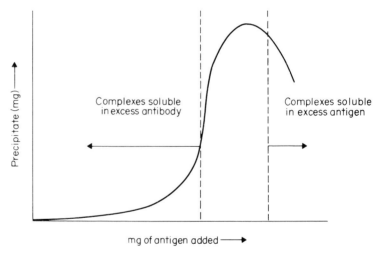

Fig. 5.1. Quantitative precipitin curve of horse antibody with antigen
The point of maximum precipitation is sharply defined because of the solubility of horse antibody–antigen complexes in both antibody and antigen excess. Accordingly the curve has quite a different profile to that found with rabbit antibodies (Fig. 5.6) where the complexes are soluble in antigen excess alone.

5.2.1   AMMONIUM SULPHATE PRECIPITATION (Farr assay)

In Chapter 1 immunoglobulins were prepared from whole serum by precipitation with ammonium sulphate solution. If ammonium sulphate is added to diluted serum to 50% saturation, most of the immunoglobulin is precipitated, while other serum proteins such as albumin, remain in solution. This is the basis of the Farr assay. This test, in its original form, is only suitable for antigens which are soluble in 50% saturated ammonium sulphate solution.

Antigen, often albumin, is radiolabelled and allowed to react with antibody, generally in antigen excess, so that soluble complexes are formed. An equal volume of saturated ammonium sulphate is added and all the immunoglobulin is precipitated. Only that antigen complexed with antibody is precipitated under these conditions. The precipitates are washed with 50% saturated ammonium sulphate solution to remove any free antigen, and then counted for radioactivity. The amount of radioactivity in the precipitate is proportional to the amount of antigen bound by the antibody and so results are expressed in terms of the antigen binding capacity ml^{-1} of serum.

For accurate determinations in research procedures, the results need to be calculated to the same degree of antigen excess for each antiserum. Therefore in the original assay constant amounts of antigen are added to a series of dilutions of serum and the antigen binding capacity determined at each dilution.

Fig. 5.2 shows a typical binding curve. It has become accepted

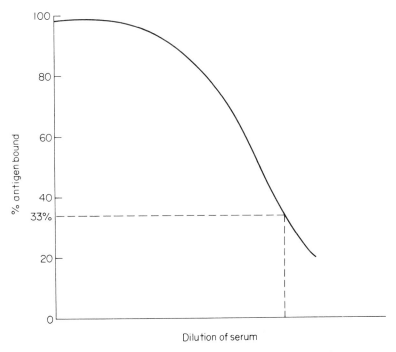

Fig. 5.2. Antigen binding capacity of an antiserum determined by the ammonium sulphate (Farr) assay
In the original Farr assay all results were calculated on the 33% end point and so a full binding curve was required for each serum assayed. In the modified assay a large excess of antigen is used with a single antiserum dilution, thus approaching the total binding capacity of the sample.

that all the results are calculated on the 33% end point, i.e. the dilution of serum which binds 33% of the added antigen. For many purposes a simpler assay can be used in which a large excess of antigen is used at a single antiserum dilution. This modified assay has been used as a research technique in many laboratories and is known to yield reliable results.

5.2.2 MODIFIED AMMONIUM SULPHATE PRECIPITATION ASSAY

Preparation required:

5.2.2a RADIOLABELLING OF ANTIGEN

Radiolabelled antigen can be bought commercially but if required the following iodination procedure is recommended.

NOTE

All the usual precautions for working with radioisotopes should be taken. The iodination procedure must be carried out in a fume cupboard as free ^{125}iodine vapour may be released.

Materials and equipment

Sodium ^{125}iodide, carrier free (Appendix II)
Protein antigen, e.g. albumin 2 mg
Chloramine T, 1 mg ml^{-1} in PBS
Sodium metabisulphite 2 mg ml^{-1} in PBS
Phosphate buffered saline (PBS) (Appendix I)
Sephadex G-25 column, disposable (Section 1.2.3)
Dextran blue dye (Appendix II)
Geiger–Müller counter.

Method

1 Pour a G-25 Sephadex column and calibrate as detailed in Chapter 1 for rapid 'dialysis' (Section 1.2.3).
2 Place 2 mg antigen (albumin) in 0·5 ml phosphate buffered saline in a glass test tube. (Glass is necessary as the iodine may bind to a plastic tube.)
3 Add 500 μCi Na ^{125}I.
4 Add 30 μg Chloramine T.
5 Mix and leave for 2 min at room temperature.
6 Add 60 μg sodium metabisulphite.
7 Place the sample on the Sephadex column and collect the radio-labelled protein after the void volume has left the column. (As an

additional check you may monitor the effluent for the first appearance of radioactivity.) Alternatively, the labelled protein solution can be dialysed extensively against PBS to remove free iodine.

8 Measure the optical density of the labelled protein in a UV spectrophotometer and calculate the protein concentration. For human serum albumin: at 279 nm, an OD of 1·0 (1 cm cell) = 1·88 mg ml^{-1}.

5.2.2b   ASSAY

Materials and equipment

Radiolabelled, ^{125}I, HSA, 2 mg ml^{-1} (Specific activity 20–80 μCi. mg^{-1} protein.)
Test antisera diluted 1 : 10 with **PBS**
Control serum diluted 1 : 10, to determine background binding
Saturated ammonium sulphate solution (Section 1.2.2)
Gamma counter

Protocol summary

Test	Tube number (in duplicate) 1	$2 \cdots n.$
Serum diluted 1 : 10 with PBS	—	20 μl ⟶
^{125}I-albumin 2 mg ml^{-1}	0·1 ml	⟶
	= INCUBATE =	
PBS		0·4 ml ⟶
Saturated ammonium sulphate		0·5 ml ⟶

Repeat for each test antiserum and normal rabbit serum control.

Method

1 Add 20 μl of each diluted serum to tubes—preferably in duplicate. (See protocol summary table.)
2 Add 0·1 ml of ^{125}I-albumin to each tube.
3 Add 0·1 ml of ^{125}I-albumin to two other tubes—cap and leave— these are for determining the specific activity of the albumin.
4 Incubate with occasional shaking at 37° for 2 h (for class purposes acceptable results can be obtained with 15 min incubation) then 2 h in the cold (again this can be reduced if necessary).
5 Add 0·4 ml PBS to each test tube.
6 Add an equal volume of saturated ammonium sulphate solution to each tube and mix rapidly. It is important that thorough mixing is obtained. Allow to stand for 15 min.
7 Spin at 3000 g for 10 min.
8 Remove supernatant and discard.

9   Wash precipitate twice with 50% saturated ammonium sulphate solution by centrifugation.

10   After removing final wash supernatant, count the precipitate and the tubes containing the ^{125}I-albumin alone in a gamma counter.

Calculation of results

$$\text{Specific activity of albumin (cpm } \mu g^{-1}) = \frac{\text{no. cpm in } 0\cdot1 \text{ ml} \times 10}{\text{Protein concentration } (\mu g \text{ ml}^{-1})}$$

$$\text{Antigen content of precipitate} = \frac{\text{no. cpm of antiserum precipitate—no. cpm of normal serum precipitate}}{\text{specific activity of the albumin}}$$

Antigen binding capacity per ml of serum = antigen content of precipitate × 50 × original serum dilution. The antigen binding capacity is expressed as μg albumin bound ml^{-1} of original serum.

The technique can be modified to yield qualitative as well as quantitative information. With ammonium sulphate all the immunoglobulins are precipitated, however, it is possible to induce precipitation by adding an excess of anti-class serum, for example, anti-IgG will precipitate all the IgG and give the antigen binding capacity for IgG antibodies. This can be repeated with specific antisera for each class and subclass. The response in the different classes is found to differ markedly with each type of immunization schedule.

5.2.3   DETERMINATION OF ANTIBODY AFFINITY

So far we have considered antibody–antigen interaction in terms of the quantity of antibody produced. For each antigenic determinant a range of different antibodies are formed, some of which fit the antigen better than others. Those with a better fit will bind the antigen more strongly than the poorer fitting molecules. This leads to the concept of ANTIBODY AFFINITY. Affinity is a measure of the strength of antigen–antibody combination. More correctly affinity refers to the interaction between monovalent antigenic determinants, i.e. haptens, and single antibody combining sites. When dealing with multivalent antigens and antibodies the interaction is more complex and the term AVIDITY is usually used.

Affinity determinations by fluorescence quenching or fluorescence polarization are relatively complex and ideally (i.e. so that the equations used are not approximations) require purified, monoclonal antibody. Steward has developed a technique, based on the Farr assay, which is suitable for affinity or avidity determinations of unselected and unpurified antibody.

98

Mathematical basis (after Steward and Petty, 1972)

The combination of antigen and antibody to form a complex is a reversible reaction:

$$Ab + Ag \underset{Kd}{\overset{Ka}{\rightleftharpoons}} Ab \cdot Ag,$$

where Ka and Kd are the association and dissociation constants, respectively.

The law of mass action can be applied to this reaction with the affinity being given by the equilibrium constant K. As mentioned at the beginning of the section, although the law of mass action is used here, strictly it applies only to homogeneous systems. Antibody is, of course, heterogeneous.

$$K = \frac{Ka}{Kd} = \frac{[Ab \cdot Ag]}{[Ag][Ab]}$$

Remember that Ag refers to monovalent antigenic determinants and independent antibody combining sites. As can be seen the amount of complex formed increases with the K value. As each reactant is expressed in moles . litre^{-1} (mol . l.$^{-1}$), the overall units of K are litres . mole^{-1} (l . mol.$^{-1}$).

If K is determined with respect to total antibody binding sites, Ab_t, the following form of the LANGMUIR ADSORPTION ISOTHERM may be derived from the mass action equation:

$$Ab + Ag \rightleftharpoons Ab \cdot Ag$$

By the law of mass action:

$$\frac{[Ab \cdot Ag]}{[Ab][Ag]} = K \text{ (equilibrium constant)}$$

therefore $[Ab \cdot Ag] = K[Ab][Ag]$ \hfill (1)

Make $[Ab_t] = [Ab \cdot Ag] + [Ab]$

therefore $[Ab] = [Ab_t] - [Ab \cdot Ag]$ \hfill (2)

Substituting (2) in (1)

$[Ab \cdot Ag] = K[Ag]([Ab_t] - [Ab \cdot Ag])$
therefore $[Ab \cdot Ag] = K[Ag][Ab_t] - K[Ag][Ab \cdot Ag]$
$[Ab \cdot Ag] + K[Ag][Ab \cdot Ag] = K[Ag][Ab_t]$
$[Ab \cdot Ag](1 + K[Ag]) = K[Ag][Ab_t]$

Therefore $\dfrac{[Ab \cdot Ag]}{[Ab_t]} = \dfrac{K[Ag]}{1 + K[Ag]}$ \hfill (3)

Make $[Ab . Ag] = b$, then (3) may be re-written as

$$\frac{b}{[Ab_t]} = \frac{K[Ag]}{1 + K[Ag]}$$

$$\frac{b(1 + K[Ag])}{[Ab_t]K[Ag]} = 1$$

$$\frac{1}{b} = \frac{1 + K[Ag]}{K[Ab_t][Ag]}$$

$$= \frac{1}{K[Ab_t][Ag]} + \frac{K[Ag]}{K[Ab_t][Ag]}$$

$$\frac{1}{b} = \frac{1}{K} \frac{1}{[Ab_t]} \frac{1}{[Ag]} + \frac{1}{[Ab_t]} \qquad (4)$$

When $\dfrac{1}{[Ag]} = 0$, in (4), $\dfrac{1}{b} = \dfrac{1}{[Ab_t]}$

As $b = [Ab . Ag] =$ bound Ag concentration, and $[Ag] =$ free antigen concentration, then a plot of $1/b$ against $1/[Ag]$ can be extrapolated to obtain $[Ab_t]$. This is the total of antibody combining sites.

Note

The concentrations expressed in the above equations are molar equivalents, hence, for example, when $[Ab . Ag] =$ bound Ag concentration, this is a molar equivalence and not a weight equivalence.

To return to the mass action equation:

$$K = \frac{[Ab . Ag]}{[Ab][Ag]}$$

If increasing amounts of antigen are reacted with a fixed amount of antibody, a point is reached where half the antibody combining sites are occupied by antigen.

At this point $[Ab] = [Ab . Ag]$

therefore in the mass active equation, $K = \dfrac{[Ab . Ag]}{[Ab][Ag]}$

$$K = \frac{1}{[Ag]}$$

In other words, THE AFFINITY EQUALS THE RECIPROCAL OF THE FREE ANTIGEN CONCENTRATION WHEN HALF THE ANTIBODY SITES ARE OCCUPIED BY ANTIGEN.

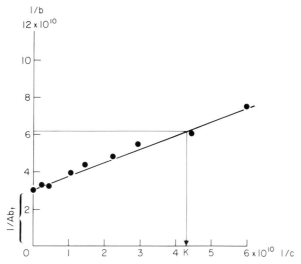

Fig. 5.3. Langmuir plot of reciprocal of bound (1/b) versus reciprocal of free antigen (1/c or 1/Ag) of a serum, from a baboon immunized with human chorionic gonadotrophin.
The regression coefficient, $r = 0.98$. The value for Ab_t obtained by extrapolation to infinite antigen concentration is 3.21×10^{-11} m l^{-1}. Antibody affinity $K = 4.3 \times 10^{10}$ l m^{-1} (Courtesy Dr Y. M. Thanavala).

The value of K can be obtained from the above plot by calculating the value of one half Ab_t and reading off from the graph the value of K (see Fig. 5.3).

In experimental terms this value also can be obtained from a plot of the logarithmic transformations of the Sip's equation as follows:

If $\quad \dfrac{r}{n} = \dfrac{(K[Ag])^a}{1 + (K[Ag])^a}$

where r = moles of antigen bound per mole of antibody
$\qquad n$ = antibody valency
$\qquad a$ = heterogeneity index (see below)

then $\quad \log \dfrac{r}{n - r} = a.\log K + a.\log[Ag]$ $\qquad\qquad$ (5)

For IgG, $n = 2$

therefore moles of antibody $= \dfrac{[Ab_t]}{2}$

and $r = \dfrac{b}{[Ab_t]/2}$ $\qquad$ where $\quad b = [Ab . Ag]$

substituting for n and r in (5),

$\log \dfrac{b}{[Ab_t] - b} = a.\log K + a.\log[Ag]$

101

If $\quad \log \dfrac{b}{[Ab_t] - b}$ is plotted against $\log[Ag]$

when $\quad \log \dfrac{b}{[Ab_t] - b} = 0, \quad K = \underline{\dfrac{1}{[Ag]}}$

The HETEROGENEITY INDEX, a, is a measure of the number of different molecular species of antibody. It can range from a value of 0 to 1. Low values represent a large degree of heterogeneity, whereas monoclonal antibody should theoretically have an index of 1. (See also Pinckard and Weir, reference at end of chapter.)

Outline of experimental technique

A constant amount of antibody is reacted with increasing concentrations of antigen. After equilibration, the concentration of bound antigen is detected in the complex after ammonium sulphate precipitation, and the concentration of free antigen is determined in the supernatant.

If the reciprocal of bound antigen is plotted against the reciprocal of the free antigen concentration and the line extrapolated to $1/[Ag] = 0$, then the reciprocal of the bound antigen will equal the reciprocal of the total antibody combining sites.

Materials and equipment

Radiolabelled, ^{125}I human serum albumin (HSA) (Appendix II) (Section 5.2.2a)
Anti-HSA
Normal rabbit serum, as control
Saturated ammonium sulphate solution
Conical centrifuge tubes, 0·4 ml capacity (Appendix II)
Beckman 152 Microfuge (or equivalent)
Gamma counter

Method

1 Set up 16 tubes as shown in Protocol.

Protocol

Tube number:	1	2	3	4	5	6	7	8
(a) Antiserum or (b) NRS control	50 µl	→						
PBS	50 µl	→						
µg ^{125}I-albumin in 100 µl PBS	2·5	5	10	20	40	80	160	320

2   Mix and incubate for 1 hour at room temperature.
3   Add 0·2 ml saturated ammonium sulphate solution and mix immediately.
4   Incubate for 1 hour at room temperature.
5   Spin the tubes at 10 000 g for 5 min.
6   Remove and keep 0·1 ml of supernatant.
7   Wash precipitate twice with 50% saturated ammonium sulphate.
8   Count the radioactivity in the supernatant samples and precipitates in a gamma counter.

Data required

Free antigen concentration = total radioactivity (cpm) in the supernatant, i.e. radioactivity in sample × 4.

Bound antigen concentration = (cpm antiserum precipitate–cpm control precipitate), for each antigen concentration.

Calculation of results

All the values should be expressed as molar concentrations, 1 pmole of HSA = 0·068 μg.
1   Record and calculate the results as in Fig. 5.4a.
2   Plot $1/b$ (column 9) against $1/[Ag]$ (column 10). Extrapolate the graph line to $1/[Ag] = 0$, i.e. the intercept on the $1/b$ axis, this gives the value of $1/[Ab_t]$.
3   Use the value for $[Ab_t]$ to calculate the values shown in Fig. 5.4b.
4   From Fig. 5.4b, plot

$$\log \frac{b}{[Ab_t] - b} \text{ (column 3) against } \log[Ag] \text{ (column 4)}.$$

The intercept on the $\log[Ag]$ axis, i.e. when

$$\log \frac{b}{[Ab_t] - b} = 0, \quad \text{equals} \quad \frac{1}{K}$$

therefore $K = \dfrac{1}{[Ag]}$

The units of K are litres per mole (1 mol.$^{-1}$).

Low affinity antibodies have K values around 10^4–10^5 1 mol.$^{-1}$, whereas high affinity antibodies often have K values of 10^{12} 1 mol.$^{-1}$.

Tube No.	Column number									
	1	2	3	4	5	6	7	8	9	10
	μg albumin per tube	pmoles of albumin	cpm in supernatant free [Ag]	cpm antiserum precipitate	cpm control precipitate	Bound antigen	Moles of Ag Bound (b)	Moles of free Ag	1/b	1/[Ag]
1	2·5	1 pmole = 0·068 μg				cpm Col. 4 − cpm Col. 5	cpm Col. 6 ÷ specific activity*	cpm Col. 3 ÷ specific activity*	Reciprocal of Col. 7	Reciprocal of Col. 8
2	5									
3	10									
4	20									
5	40									
6	80									
7	160									
8	320									

* Specific activity of antigen = $\dfrac{\text{Counts per min (cpm)}}{\text{Molar concentration of antigen}}$

Fig. 5.4a. Table for calculation of Ab_t

104

Column number: 1	2	3	4
Tube no.	pmoles of antigen	$\dfrac{b}{[Ab_t] - b}$	$\text{Log}\dfrac{b}{[Ab_t] - b}$	Log [Ag]
1			Log_{10} Col. 2	Log_{10} free antigen
2				concentration, i.e.
3				log Col. 8 Fig 5.4a.
4				
5				
6				
7				
8				

Fig. 5.4b. Table for calculation of K

5.2.4   EQUILIBRIUM DIALYSIS

This technique was devised in 1932 as a direct method for studying the primary interactions between antibody and hapten. Unless the valency of the antibody is to be determined, it is possible to work with unpurified antibody, usually as an ammonium sulphate precipitate, as many haptens, but not, for example, oligosaccharides, bind to albumin. The theoretical basis of this method for the determination of K (the average intrinsic association constant between antibody and hapten) is similar to that described in the previous section, however, the manner in which the parameters are determined differ in practice.

Constant amounts of antibody are placed in dialysis sacs or cells and allowed to equilibrate with various concentrations of hapten over a forty-fold range. Free hapten will enter the dialysis sac along its concentration gradient (Fig. 5.5). Some of this hapten will complex with antibody and so will not contribute to the free-hapten concentration. At equilibrium, the free-hapten concentration will be the same on either side of the dialysis membrane, but the total hapten concentration will be relatively greater inside the dialysis sac.

For each experimental point on the binding curve the following samples, each in triplicate, are required:

1   Antibody gamma globulin.
2   Normal gamma globulin, to determine the extent of non-specific binding.
3   Buffer alone, to check that an equilibrium has in fact been established.

Typically each sample of protein or buffer solution (about 0·5 ml) is placed in a small dialysis sac. For each concentration of free

105

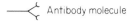 Antibody molecule

O Hapten molecule

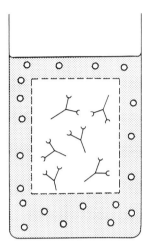 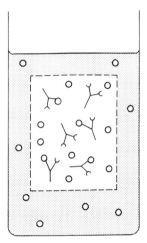

Fig. 5.5. Schematic representation of equilibrium dialysis showing relative distribution of the antibody and hapten molecules at time zero and after the equilibrium is established.
Cell to left shows distribution at the beginning of the experiment, cell to right shows the distribution at equilibrium. There is a greater concentration of hapten molecules in the inner cell of the diagram on the right because of the hapten molecules bound to the antibody.

hapten on the binding curve, the 9 sample sacs can be equilibrated against a single pool of radioactive hapten, usually in a 50 ml bottle. The bottles are left in a water bath with mixing for 24–48 hours and then triplicate volumetric samples are taken from each free hapten solution and each dialysis sac.

The free hapten concentration at equilibrium may be determined directly from the c.p.m. of the samples taken from the bottles. The bound hapten concentration may be calculated as follows:

Antibody-bound hapten, H_b c.p.m. $=$ (HAb c.p.m.)–(H_f c.p.m. + [HN c.p.m. – H_f c.p.m.])
Where:

HAb = cpm of sample from antibody gammaglobulin sac
H_f = cpm of free hapten in bottle.
HN = cpm in sac containing normal gammaglobulin.

The association constant may be calculated with reference to the previous section and Pinckard and Weir (reference at end of chapter).

5.3.1   QUANTITATIVE PRECIPITIN TEST

This test, developed by Heidelberger and Kendall, is the basis of all quantitative studies of antigen–antibody interaction. Increasing amounts of antigen are added to a constant amount of antibody and the weight of precipitate formed in each tube is determined. The procedure outlined below is suitable for most antisera and antigens.

Materials

Antiserum, e.g. anti-human serum albumin (Section 1.4.6)
Human serum albumin (HSA) 1 mg ml^{-1} (Appendix II)
Phosphate buffered saline (PBS) (Appendix I)
0·1 M sodium hydroxide.

Method

1   Add the following μg of antigen to a series of tubes (suitable for centrifugation): 0, 10, 20, 50, 100, 150, 200, 250, 350 and 450. (For antisera with high- or low-antibody content it will be necessary to alter the range of antigen used.)
2   Add PBS to each tube to bring the final volume to 0·45 ml.
3   Add 0·1 ml of antiserum to each tube and mix the reactants.
4   Incubate at 37° for one hour and then at 4° overnight. (Obviously for research purposes these incubations should be extended—up to 10 days at 4°, but for class purposes, with strong antisera, good curves may be obtained with 30 min incubation at 37° and 30 min at 4°.)
5   Spin (3000 g for 5 min) and remove supernatant. An angle-head rotor should be used as the precipitate is formed at the side of the tube. If time is available check each supernatant for free antigen or antibody by a sensitive technique, e.g. single radial immunodiffusion (Section 5.3.3a).
6   Wash the precipitate twice by centrifugation with cold PBS.
7   Redissolve the final precipitate in 0·1 M sodium hydroxide (the volume depends on the cuvettes available).
8   Read the extinction at 280 nm and plot a graph of the optical density of precipitate against the amount of antigen added (see Fig. 5.6).

Calculations

(a) Determine the antibody content per ml of antiserum.
(b) Calculate the number of antigenic determinants on each antigen molecule (i.e. antigenic valency).

107

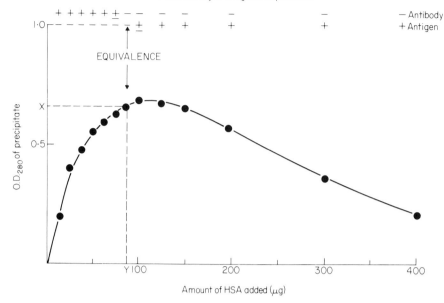

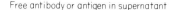

Fig. 5.6. Precipitation curve of human serum albumin (HSA) with anti-HSA
An increasing amount of antigen was added to a fixed concentration of
antiserum and the optical density of the precipitate (in sodium hydroxide)
determined. The supernatant was assayed for the presence of free antibody
or antigen by Ouchterlony single radial immunodiffusion. The equivalence
point (arrowed), when all the antibody and antigen is complexed in the
precipitate, occurs just before the point of maximum precipitation.

To determine the equivalence point exactly, it is frequently necessary to
repeat the assay using closer antigen concentrations around the concentration required to give maximum precipitation.

Theoretical basis of the calculations

Antibody content of the serum

If the supernatant from each tube is examined for the presence of
excess antibody or antigen, there will be one point at which no free
antibody or antigen can be detected. This is the point of EQUI-
VALENCE which occurs just before maximum precipitation (Fig.
5.7). The amount of precipitate increases after the equivalence point
because of continued incorporation of antigen into the complex.
Eventually soluble complexes are formed in antigen excess and the
amount of precipitate decreases. Precipitation is not only dependent
on cross linking, as $F(ab')_2$ fragments precipitate far less readily
with antigen than whole antibody molecules.

In Fig. 5.6, at equivalence, the precipitate contains X μg of total
protein, if this includes Y μg of antigen then there is $(X - Y)$ μg of
antibody. This is the total amount of antibody in the volume of
serum used.

108

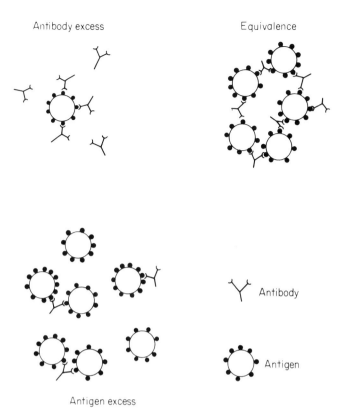

Antibody excess

Equivalence

Antibody

Antigen

Antigen excess

Fig. 5.7. Complexes formed at varying antigen–antibody ratios
Diagrammatic representation of complexes formed between a multivalent antigen and a divalent antibody at:
(a) antibody excess
(b) equivalence
(c) antigen excess.
  In this case maximum precipitation occurs at equivalence when a lattice is formed, producing a complex too large to remain in solution.

Specimen calculation (from Fig. 5.6)

The precipitate was dissolved in 1 ml of 0·1 M sodium hydroxide and optical density measurements were made in 1 cm light path cells.

IgG OD of 1·0 at 280 nm in 1 cm cell = 0·695 mg ml^{-1}
HSA OD of 1·0 at 280 nm in 1 cm cell = 1.886 mg ml^{-1}

  From the graph, at equivalence, OD of precipitate $X = 0.65$. The precipitate contains 87·5 μg HSA, which if dissolved alone in 1·0 ml of sodium hydroxide would give an OD of 0·04. (Calculated from the extinction coefficient.)

Hence, OD of antibody component of the precipitate

= OD precipitate − OD due to HSA
= 0·65 − 0·04
= 0·61.

Hence total antibody content of serum (mg ml^{-1})

$$= \frac{OD \times \text{extinction coefficient}}{\text{sample volume}}$$

$$= \frac{0\cdot61 \times 0\cdot695}{0\cdot1}$$

$$= 4\cdot24 \text{ mg ml}^{-1}.$$

This antiserum has a relatively high antibody content.

Determination of antigenic valency

For this determination some theoretical aspects of the precipitation curve must be considered. When the antigen concentration is low there is a relative antibody excess (see Fig. 5.6). At the other extreme, at high antigen concentrations, there is free antigen and so each combining site of the antibody is occupied. At both these points the complexes are relatively small. At equivalence, however, there is much cross-linking between molecules and large complexes are formed.

Every antigenic determinant is likely to be covered by a separate antibody molecule at extreme antibody excess. If we calculate the amount of antibody in the precipitate at this point, in the same way as above, we can determine the ratio of antibody to antigen and so the relative numbers of molecules of each in the precipitate:

$$\text{i.e.} \quad \frac{\text{Weight of antigen}}{\begin{array}{c}\text{Molecular weight}\\\text{of antigen}\end{array}} : \frac{\text{Weight of antibody}}{\begin{array}{c}\text{Molecular weight}\\\text{of antibody}\end{array}}$$

In a hyperimmune serum the major proportion of antibody will be of the IgG class with a molecular weight of 150,000. The molecular weight of HSA (the antigen in this case) is 68,000.

To obtain the best estimate of antigenic valency the ratio of antibody to antigen in the precipitate should be plotted against the amount of antigen added, as in Fig. 5.8. If the graph line is extended to the antibody : antigen axis the intercept will give the ratio at infinite antibody excess.

Specimen calculation (from Fig. 5.8)

OD of precipitate = 0·15.
OD of HSA (calculated as above) = 0·005 (10 μg).

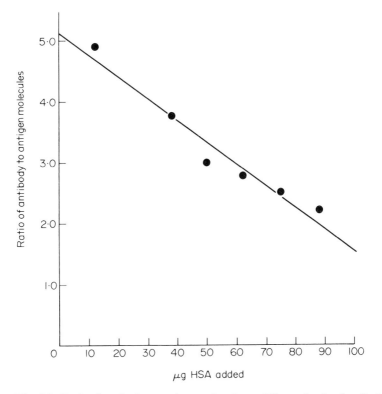

Fig. 5.8. Ratio of antibody to antigen molecules at different levels of antibody excess

The regression line calculated from the antibody to antigen ratios over a range of antigen concentrations, all in antigen excess, gives an intercept of 5·2, indicating that there are five antigenic determinants detected on the HSA molecule by this antiserum. This antiserum differs from that used in Fig. 5.6.

Hence OD of antibody in the precipitate = 0·145 which is equivalent to 101·5 μg ml^{-1} IgG.

Therefore the molar ratios are:

$$\frac{10}{68\ 000} : \frac{101\cdot5}{150\ 000}$$

$$= 0\cdot000147 : 0\cdot000677$$

Therefore the ratio of antibody to antigen molecules = 4·6.

This antiserum recognizes between 4 and 5 determinants on the HSA molecule.

The quantitative precipitin test is particularly useful as it can be carried out without antibody standards; only known concentrations of antigen are required. The shape of the curve varies with different antigens: with protein antigens a sharp peak is usually obtained, but with polysaccharides there is usually a broader peak.

111

In addition different antisera have different properties. Rabbit antisera give the typical curve shown in Fig. 5.6 whereas horse antisera give precipitates which are relatively more soluble in BOTH antigen AND antibody excess (see Fig. 5.1). Both types of precipitin curve may be obtained with human antisera.

5.3.2 DEMONSTRATION OF ANTIBODY SPECIFICITY

The original work of Landsteiner and his colleagues greatly contributed to our understanding of the nature of the interaction between antibody molecules and small chemically defined groupings known as haptens (Section 1.3). In the experiment described below the position of the acidic group on the hapten aminobenzoic acid completely alters the degree of binding of the hapten to the original antibody molecule.

Materials

p. aminobenzoic acid }
m. aminobenzoic acid } Each at 1 mg ml^{-1} in PBS
o. aminobenzoic acid }
p. aminobenzyl-FγG (Section 1.3.2)
anti-p. aminobenzyl-HSA (Section 1.3.2)

Method

1 Determine the equivalence point of the precipitin curve between p. aminobenzyl FγG and anti-p. aminobenzyl HSA (as in Section 5.3.1).
2 Using equivalence conditions, add 0·1 ml (100 μg) of each free hapten to separate tubes to inhibit the reaction.
3 Measure OD of precipitate dissolved in 0·1 M NaOH.
4 Determine the relative effectiveness of each hapten.

Example

Working at equivalence conditions for p. aminobenzyl-FγG with anti-p. aminobenzyl-HSA:

Free hapten	OD of precipitate at 280 nM	Relative binding (to hapten)
none	0·55	—
p. aminobenz.	0·00	100%
m. aminobenz.	0·50	9%
o. aminobenz.	0·60	0%

PRECIPITATION IN GELS

Although the precipitin test gives a great deal of basic information, it is lengthy to perform and requires relatively large quantities of reagents. In addition, it is difficult to compare two antisera or two antigens qualitatively. Many gel precipitation techniques have been developed to overcome these problems.

Previous preparation required

Buffered agar and agar-coated slides may be prepared as described below for use in all the experiments in this section.

BUFFERED AGAR

Materials

Barbitone buffer (Appendix I)
Agar (Appendix II)

1   Mix 2 g of agar with 50 ml of distilled water and dissolve in a boiling water bath. Finally, boil directly over a Bunsen flame to remove all lumps but do not char the agar.
2   Add 50 ml of hot barbitone buffer and mix well. The agar may be stored at 4° for many weeks.

Note

The agar must be bought specifically for electrophoresis; many culture agars are not suitable for this purpose.

AGAR-COATED SLIDES

Materials and equipment:

Glass microscope slides
Agar (Appendix II)

Method

1   Dissolve 0·5 g of agar in 100 ml of distilled water as in the previous section.
2   Pipette the agar solution onto clean, dry slides. Add enough to just cover one surface of the slide.
3   Dry the slides and store at room temperature until required.

Slides are pre-coated with a weak agar solution to hold the final agar gel in place during the washing procedure.

113

Diffusion in gel reactions have been used since 1905 and have been developed into highly sophisticated techniques. Oudin originally used analytical techniques involving the diffusion of antigens into an antibody-containing gel (single diffusion in one direction). Feinberg and later Mancini, Carbonara and Heremans extended this technique by incorporating the antiserum into a thin layer of agar and placing the antigen in wells cut into the agar. As the antigen diffuses radially a ring of precipitation forms around the well and moves outwards, eventually becoming stationary at equivalence. At equivalence, the diameter or area of the ring is related to the antigen concentration in the well. Using standard antigen concentrations a calibration curve may be constructed to determine unknown concentrations of the same antigen.

Materials and equipment

2% agar in barbitone buffer (Section 5.3.3)
Pre-coated slides (Section 5.3.3)
Antiserum, e.g. anti-human IgG
Standard antigen solution, e.g. human IgG (Appendix II)
PBS (Appendix I)
Flat level surface (use a spirit level)
Gel punch (Appendix II)
Humid chamber (plastic box with wet filter paper)

Method

1   Melt the agar in a boiling water bath and transfer to 56°.
2   Dilute the antiserum with PBS. (The optimal dilution will, of course, depend on the strength of the antiserum and antigen as the diameter of the precipitation ring is inversely proportional to the antiserum concentration. In practice, with rabbit antisera to human IgG, we find that a final dilution of approximately 1 : 40 in the agar is suitable for measuring IgG concentrations in the range of 50–200 μg ml^{-1}. However, this should only be used as a guide as a standard curve should be determined for each antiserum.) Typically, add 75 μl of an antiserum to 1·9 ml of PBS and warm to 56°.
3   Add the diluted antiserum to 1 ml of agar at 56° and mix well.
4   Layer the agar onto a precoated slide standing on a levelled surface and allow to set.
5   After the agar has set use a gel punch to cut about 8 wells per slide. The wells should be 2–3 mm in diameter, and must have absolutely vertical sides.
6   Remove the agar plug with a Pasteur pipette attached to a water vacuum pump.

7 Fill each of four wells with standard solutions of 50, 100, 150, and 200 μg ml^{-1} IgG. Use the other wells for the IgG solutions of unknown concentrations. Fill the wells quickly until the meniscus just disappears.

8 Leave the slide in a humid box to equilibrate. (Although a satisfactory standard curve may be obtained by overnight equilibration, the points will better approximate to a straight line if the slide is allowed to equilibrate longer: IgG and IgA 48 h, IgM 72 h. IgG concentrations may also be determined by incubation at 37° for 4 hours.)

Measurement of precipitation rings

The diameter of each ring may be measured either directly using a magnifying glass with a micrometer scale, or, after staining, with a plastic ruler.

Direct measurement

Hold the slide over a black background and illuminate it from the side. Measure the rings from the reverse side through the glass plate, do not rest the magnifying glass on the gel. If the rings are not distinct, soak the slides in 1% tannic acid for 1 min to increase resolution. (This is not a permanent preparation.)

Stained preparations:

1 Wash the slide for 24 h in several changes of PBS to remove free protein from the agar.
2 Cover the slide with good quality filter paper and dry overnight.
3 Remove the filter paper after dampening it slightly.

The slide may then be stained with any protein dye, but we suggest Coomassie blue.

Staining solution

Coomassie brilliant blue 1·25 g (Appendix II)
Glacial acetic acid 50 ml
Distilled water 185 ml

Stain the slide for 5 min and differentiate in the same solution without the dye. *Staining with this dye is completely reversible so do not leave the slide too long in the de-staining solution.*
(The staining solution may be stored for several weeks in a stoppered bottle. The de-staining solution can be regenerated by passing through powdered charcoal.)

Place the dry, stained slides in a photographic enlarger and measure the diameter of the precipitation rings with a ruler. (Strictly, one should estimate the area within the precipitation ring.)

Calculation of results

Fig. 5.9 shows a typical determination. The diameter of the rings was measured and plotted on a linear scale against the log of the antigen concentration. (With a semi-log transformation, the points should approximate to a straight line.)

Although single radial immunodiffusion is now used as a quantitative technique, its first use was to compare the identities of different antigen solutions. If two antigens, placed in neighbouring wells

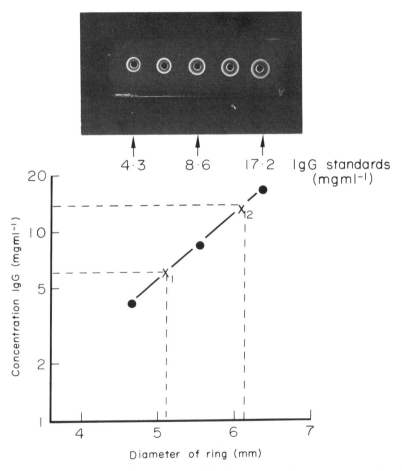

Fig. 5.9. Measurement of IgG concentration by single radial immuno-diffusion
A calibration curve is constructed from the diameter of the precipitation rings formed at equilibrium by IgG standards of known concentration. The concentration of unknown samples can then be determined with reference to the standard curve.

116

close together, are identical in terms of their antigenic determinants then the two rings of precipitation fuse completely. If the antigens are non-identical then each ring forms independently. Since the work of Ouchterlony, simpler procedures are used to test the relationships between antigens or antibodies.

5.3.3b DOUBLE DIFFUSION IN TWO DIMENSIONS

In this procedure antigen and antibody are allowed to migrate towards each other in a gel and a line of precipitation is formed where the two reactants meet. As this precipitate is soluble in excess antigen, a sharp line is produced at equivalence, its relative position being determined by the concentration of the antigen and antibody in the agar. The local concentration of each reactant depends not only on its absolute concentration in the well, but also on its molecular size and the rate at which it is able to diffuse through the gel.

Multiple lines of precipitation will be present if the antigen and antibody contain several molecular species.

This technique has the particular advantage that several antigens or antisera can be compared around a single well of antibody or antigen.

Materials and equipment

2% agar in barbitone buffer (Section 5.3.3)
Antigen and antibody solutions (see procedure for details)
Gel punch (pattern as in Fig. 5.10)

Method

1 Melt the agar in a boiling water bath.
2 Pour agar onto pre-coated slides; use a levelled surface.
3 Punch pattern required (see Fig. 5.10).

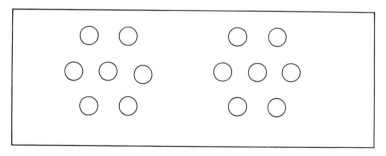

Fig. 5.10. Typical well pattern in agar for qualitative comparison of antisera or antigens
The number, size and distance between wells depends on the number and strength of the antisera and antigens.

117

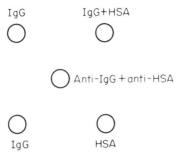

Fig. 5.11. Design of Ouchterlony plate to show reactions of identity and non-identity
IgG human or mouse IgG, HSA human serum albumin: with their respective antisera.

4   Suck out agar plugs with a Pasteur pipette connected to a water vacuum pump.
5   Fill the wells with antibody or antigen until the meniscus just disappears.
6   Place the slide in a humid chamber and incubate overnight at a constant temperature. (Diffusion and therefore precipitation is quicker at 37° and lines will be seen within 3 hours.)

Suggested antibody and antigen patterns

A straightforward demonstration of identity and non-identity can be shown using the antigen mixtures as in Fig. 5.11. In addition, this technique may be used to show the relationships between IgG molecules and their enzymic digests prepared in Chapter 7. Arrange the wells as shown in Fig. 5.12.

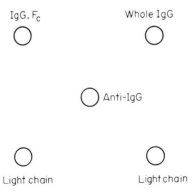

Fig. 5.12. Well arrangement to demonstrate spur formation, lines of identity and lines of non-identity
IgG.Fc: prepared by papain digestion of IgG (Section 7.7.1). Light chain: prepared by reduction and alkylation of IgG (Section 7.6.1).

Antigen concentration

Initially use 1 mg ml^{-1}. Alter concentration, if required.

Antiserum

Use whole anti-IgG, non-absorbed. Specific anti-IgG sera available commercially are absorbed with light chains to render them class-specific (see Section 7.6.2).

Interpretation of results

There are three basic patterns of precipitation as shown in Figs. 5.13 and 5.14.

1 The REACTION OF IDENTITY occurs between identical antigenic determinants, the lines of precipitation fuse to give one continuous arc.
2 REACTION OF NON-IDENTITY. Where two antigens do not contain any common antigenic determinants the two lines are formed independently and cross without any interaction.
3 REACTION OF PARTIAL IDENTITY. This has two components: (a) those antigenic determinants which are common to both antigens give a continuous line of identity, (b) the extra determinant on one of the antigens gives, in addition, a line of non-identity so that a spur is formed. Of course, there may be unique determinants in both antigens, this would give rise to two spurs.

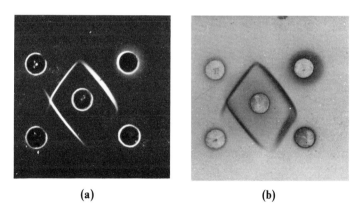

(a)   (b)

Fig. 5.13. The relationship of human IgG sub-classes
In a and b: Wells 1–4 contain human IgG1, IgG2, IgG3 and IgG4 respectively and the central well contains rabbit anti-human IgG. (Antisera prepared by immunizing rabbits with IgG obtained from normal human serum by ion-exchange chromatography, see Section 7.3.)
   Antiserum (a) recognized sub-class differences between IgG1 and IgG4, hence the double spur, but failed to recognize IgG3. Antiserum (b) recognized sub-class differences associated with IgG1 alone and so produced a single spur. Both antisera were raised against the same pool of antigen, the variation is due to the rabbits used for immunization.

119

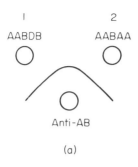

(a)

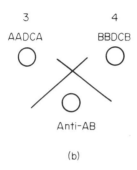

(b)

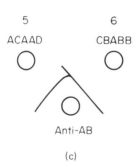

(c)

Fig. 5.14. Explanation of basic patterns of precipitation obtainable in Ouchterlony immunodiffusion

A–D represent antigenic determinants present within a series of protein molecules, 1–6, used as antigens. An antiserum has been raised against two of these determinants, A and B. (a) The precipitation lines have fused completely showing the presence of identical determinants in proteins 1 and 2. Note, however, the detection is purely qualitative and, in addition, does not give any information on the other determinants present. (b) The two precipitation lines cross without any interaction. Proteins 3 and 4 do not, therefore, share any determinants detectable by the antiserum. (c) The two precipitation lines have fused, but in addition a spur has formed towards the well containing protein 5. Hence, proteins 5 and 6 share some common determinants but protein 6 has additional unique determinants detected by the antiserum.

120

All these concepts of identity and non-identity are in terms of recognition by the antiserum. An antiserum recognizing many determinants on the antigen molecules is necessary for the demonstration of all these features.

The design of the Ouchterlony technique may be varied to obtain semi-quantitative data:

5.3.3c   RELATIVE ANTIGEN CONCENTRATION

As the position of the precipitation line is determined by the relative concentrations of the antigen and antibody, a semi-quantitative estimate of relative antigen concentration can be obtained by comparing the position of the lines using several concentrations of antigen and a constant antiserum, as shown in Fig. 5.15. Usually full

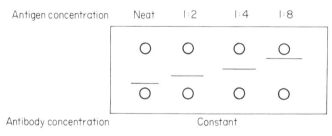

Fig. 5.15. Relative antigen concentration determined by double diffusion in agar
An unknown concentration of the same antigen can be measured by comparison with the standard dilutions to give a relative measure of antigen concentration.

Alternatively, the antiserum can be diluted to determine a relative antibody titre.

measurements are not made with this technique, instead it is used to give a rapid indication of antibody titre (especially with peaks from column chromatography, Sections 7.2 and 7.3).

5.3.3d   ESTIMATION OF MOLECULAR WEIGHT AND DIFFUSION COEFFICIENT

It is an interesting and useful feature that antigens with a molecular weight and diffusion coefficient close to IgG tend to give straight lines of precipitation with antibody. If the antigen has a rather lower molecular weight and higher diffusion coefficient than IgG, the arc of precipitation curves towards the antiserum well. Conversely, antigens with higher molecular weight and lower diffusion coefficient form arcs that bend towards the antigen well. You may demonstrate this using albumin, IgG and Keyhole Limpet Haemocyanin, with their respective antisera (See Fig. 5.16).

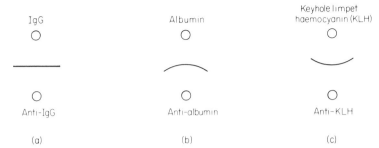

Fig. 5.16. Estimation of molecular weight by double diffusion in agar
(a): molecular weight of antigen = molecular weight of IgG in antiserum.
(b): molecular weight of antigen < molecular weight of IgG in serum.
(c): molecular weight of antigen > molecular weight of IgG in serum.

5.3.3e   NEPHELOMETRY

Although single radial immunodiffusion is a simple technique to set up it becomes rather tedious for the examination of multiple samples. For this reason many laboratories now quantitate antigen–antibody complexes by nephelometry. In this technique monochromatic light is used to illuminate a cuvette containing a suspension of the immune complex. The light is deflected by the complexes and the amount of light scattered is proportioned to the quantity of complex. The most sensitive instruments, incorporating laser light sources, are able to detect nanogram amounts of complex. Many of the machines are automated so that many hundreds of samples may be processed each day.

5.3.4   IMMUNOELECTROPHORETIC ANALYSIS

So far we have studied antibody–antigen interaction solely by simple diffusion. Increased resolution, and often quicker results, can be obtained by a combination of electrophoresis and immunodiffusion in gels. Serum proteins separate in agar gels, under the influence of an electric field into albumin, α_1-, α_2-, β- and γ-globulins. If you are not familiar with this electrophoretic separation of serum proteins, it is advisable to perform a simple agar gel electrophoresis as this will aid understanding of the patterns obtained with the later techniques.

5.3.4a   AGAR GEL ELECTROPHORESIS

Materials and equipment

2% agar in barbitone buffer (Section 5.3.3)
Barbitone buffer (Appendix I)
Precoated microscope slides (Section 5.3.3)
Normal and myeloma sera (see Appendix II for myeloma sera)

122

10% glacial acetic acid in water (v/v)
Electrophoresis tank and power pack (Appendix II)
Gel punch (pattern as in Fig. 5.17)

Method

1 Melt the agar in a boiling water bath.
2 Mark the end of the slide that will be positive during the electro-phoresis. If required, number the slides.
3 Pour 3–5 ml of agar onto the slide on a levelled surface.
4 When the agar is firm punch the pattern shown in Fig. 5.17. (Small wells are required, not as large as those used for simple immunodiffusion. A fine Pasteur pipette or a cut hypodermic needle may be used.)
5 Suck out the agar plugs.
6 Fill the wells with serum to which a small amount of bromo-phenol blue dye has been added.
7 Fill the electrophoresis tank with full-strength barbitone buffer.
8 Place the slide in the electrophoresis tank and connect each end of the slide to the buffer chambers with rayon or filter paper wicks. Close the tank.
9 Apply a current of about 8 m amps per slide. The voltage drop will be about 5–7 volts cm^{-1}.
   The bromophenol blue dye binds to the serum albumin and as this is the fastest migrating band it serves as a marker throughout the electro-phoresis. If excess dye has been added, however, a bright blue band of free dye will run in front of the albumin towards the anode.
10 When the albumin band (blue) nears the end of the slide— about 60 min—remove the slide and fix the proteins by immersing the slide in 10% glacial acetic acid.
11 Cover the slide with fine filter paper and leave to dry.
12 Dampen the paper and remove, stain the slide with Coomassie brilliant blue (Section 5.3.3a).

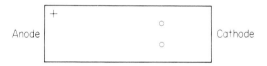

Fig. 5.17. Basic well pattern for agar gel electrophoresis

Suggested design

One well should contain normal serum and the other serum from a patient with multiple myelomatosis (a disease in which a single clone of antibody-forming cells become malignant and produce large amounts of monoclonal antibody).

Results

The main serum proteins should show clearly as oval bands. Identify each band (albumin, α_1, α_2, β and γ), and assign the abnormal monoclonal band to one of these (cf. Fig. 5.18).

Technical note

The negative charge of the agar generates an electro-osmotic flow of water through the gel. This flow, and not the potential difference, is responsible for most of the separation seen with some of the γ-globulins, which are near their isoelectric point under the conditions used. This is discussed in more detail later.

5.3.4b   IMMUNOELECTROPHORESIS

Immunoelectrophoresis is a powerful analytical technique with great resolving power as it combines prior separation of antigens by electrophoresis with immunodiffusion of these separated antigens against an antiserum (see Fig. 5.19).

Materials

As for agar gel electrophoresis, but in addition, anti-human serum.

Fig. 5.18 (opposite). Electrophoresis of serum samples
(a) Agar gel electrophoresis.
   Well 1—normal serum.
   Well 2—serum from patient with multiple myeloma.
Myeloma patients show an overproduction of antibody, often of a single clone, in this case running in the gamma-globulin region. You can see by inspection that there is an apparent decrease in the albumin content of the myeloma serum.
(b) Electrophoresis on cellulose acetate membranes.
   Sample 1—normal serum as in (a)
   Sample 2—myeloma serum as in (a), two preparations.
The principle of this separation of serum proteins is basically similar to that described for agar gel electrophoresis, except that the sample is applied onto the membrane as a band rather than via a well. The advantages of this technique are (i) it is easier to discern the individual protein bands and (ii) it is possible to clear the membrane either with glycerol or one of the commercially available clearing oils. Thus the protein content of each band can be determined by scanning photometry.
   The 'hawk-shaped' band seen in sample 3 is often observed with myeloma protein and is probably caused by overloading of this band.
(c) The traces obtained from scanning samples 1 and 2 of (b) are shown here. By integrating the area under each peak (this is usually done automatically by the scanner) it is possible to determine the total protein content of each band, and so confirm the observation made in (a), that there is indeed an albumin: gammaglobulin reversal in the myeloma serum.
   Sample 1—normal serum, above—albumin : γ-globulin ratio 4·5.
   Sample 2—myeloma serum, below—albumin : γ-globulin ration 0·7.

124

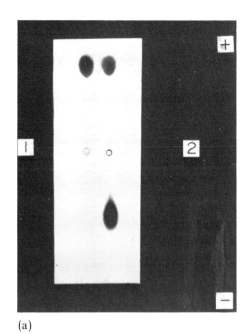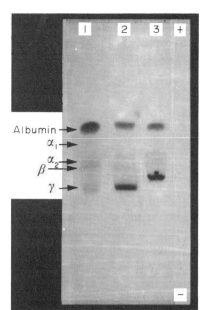

(a)

(b)

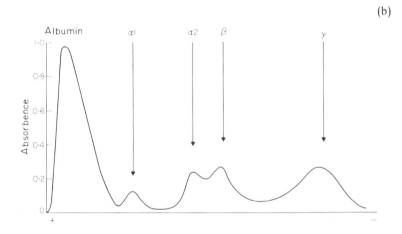

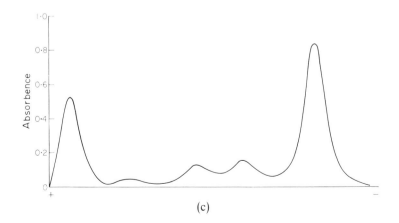

(c)

125

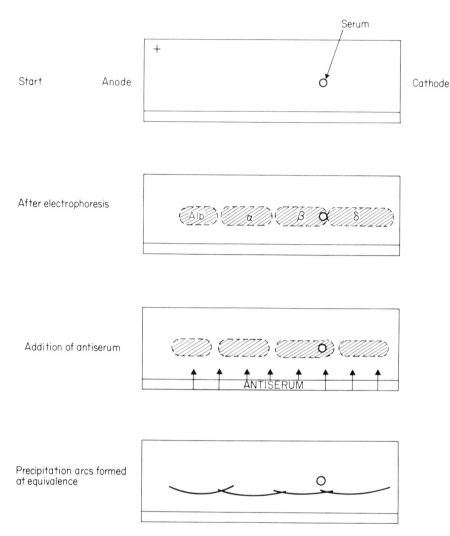

Fig. 5.19. Theoretical basis of immunoelectrophoresis
The antigen diffuses from a point source after the initial electrophoresis and interacts with the antiserum advancing on a plane front thus producing an arc of precipitation at equivalence.

Method

1 Prepare slide as for agar gel electrophoresis (Section 5.3.4a).

2 Cut the pattern shown in Fig. 5.20. (Although cutters and moulds are available commercially for many different patterns, the holes can be made with hypodermic needles (cut and sharpened) and the trough with razor blades.)

3 Suck out the agar wells but do not remove the agar from the trough as this may cause abnormalities in the banding during electrophoresis.

126

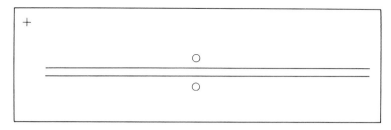

Fig. 5.20. Pattern for immunoelectrophoresis
It is convenient to mark the positive end of the slide before pouring on the agar. Alternatively mark the agar itself with a carbohydrate binding dye, for example, alcian blue (1 % solution). Do not remove the central agar trough before electrophoresis. Up to three wells and two troughs can be cut into agar on an ordinary microscope slide.

4   Fill one well with normal human serum and the other with myeloma serum.

5   Electrophorese as before (Section 5.3.4a).

6   Remove the agar trough and fill with anti-whole human serum.

7   Leave the slide to incubate overnight in a humid chamber at a constant temperature. (Again lines will appear within 2 to 3 h if the slide is incubated at 37°.)

8   Examine the lines produced and identify the IgG, IgA and IgM bands, and the bump in the precipitation arc typical of monoclonal immunoglobulin in the myeloma serum. The result obtained should be similar to that shown in Fig. 5.21 although the relative distribution of the bands will depend on the batch of agar used and the initial electrophoresis distance. At the pH of the barbitone buffer (pH 8·2) the γ-globulins are close to their isoelectric point and so would not migrate appreciably in the electric field applied. However, as mentioned earlier, the negative charge on the agar generates an electro-osmotic flow of water in the gel which sweeps

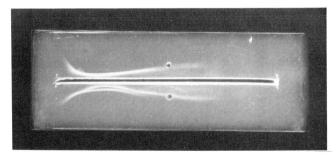

Fig. 5.21. Immunoelectrophoresis of human serum
Sample a: normal human serum showing normal IgG precipitation arc.
Sample b: serum of a patient with multiple myeloma, in this case the monoclonal protein is identified as IgG because of the 'bump' in the IgG precipitation arc towards the antiserum well.
Antiserum in central trough: rabbit anti-human immunoglobulin. (Photograph of unstained preparation.)

the β_2- and γ-globulins towards the cathode. Often agarose is used as a supporting medium. This has a lower charge and so generates a smaller electro-osmotic flow.

5.3.4c   CROSS-OVER ELECTROPHORESIS

γ-globulins are exceptional in their cathodic migration; most other proteins move to the anode. This useful property is used in cross-over electrophoresis to cause antibody and antigen to migrate towards each other in gel and form lines of precipitation. The technique is similar to a simple Ouchterlony but much faster because it is electrically driven, and more sensitive as all the antigen and antibody are moved towards each other rather than diffusing radially.

Materials and equipment

As for agar electrophoresis, but in addition, albumin and anti-albumin.

Method

1   Prepare slide as for agar gel electrophoresis (Section 5.3.4a).
2   Punch two wells as in Fig. 5.22.

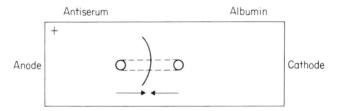

Fig. 5.22. Cross-over electrophoresis
As seen in section 5.3.4a IgG moves towards the cathode at pH 8·2 because of the electroendosmotic flow; if a negatively charged antigen is used this will move towards the anode and precipitate on contact with the antiserum IgG.

3   Place anti-albumin in the anodal well and albumin in the cathodal well.
4   Run the slide in an electrophoresis tank as before (Section 5.3.4a).
5   Examine after 10 to 15 min.

This technique lends itself to the rapid processing of many antisera or antigens and is used in many clinical screening procedures, for example, the detection of Australia Antigen.

Just as cross-over electrophoresis is related to Ouchterlony double diffusion, electrophoresis in antibody-containing media is related to the single radial immunodiffusion (SRID) test. Again the speed of cross-over electrophoresis is utilized to provide a fast quantitative assay. As in the SRID test, the antiserum is incorporated into agar and wells are cut to hold the antigen. When an electric current is applied, the antigen migrates anodally into the agar while the antibody migrates cathodally. At first soluble complexes are formed in antigen excess. As the antigen migrates further, it becomes more dilute, because antigen is held back in complexes, eventually equivalence is reached and an insoluble precipitate is formed. The precipitate redissolves and moves forward as more antigen reaches it. Finally, when no more antigen remains to enter the precipitate a stable arc is formed which becomes stationary. Rocket shapes of precipitation are usually formed and the area under the rockets is proportional to the concentration of antigen (see Figs. 5.23 and 5.24).

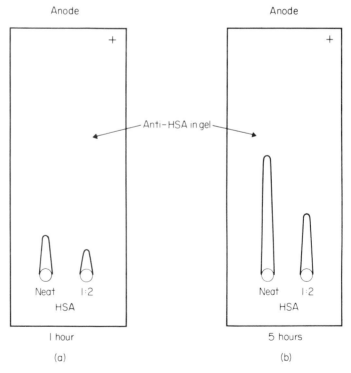

Fig. 5.23. Electrophoresis in antibody-containing media
Precipitates are formed (slide a) which redissolve in antigen excess until equivalence is reached at which point a stationary precipitate forms (slide b).

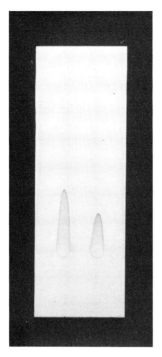

Fig. 5.24. Electrophoresis of human serum albumin (HSA) into agar containing anti-HSA
At equilibrium, the height of the precipitation arc is proportional to the antigen concentration.

Materials

2% agar in barbitone buffer (Section 5.3.3.)
Human serum albumin (HSA) (Appendix II)
Anti-HSA
Phosphate buffered saline (PBS) (Appendix I)
Pre-coated slides (Section 5.3.3)
Levelling table
Gel punch
56° water bath
Electrophoresis tank and power pack

Method

1   Melt agar in a boiling water bath and then allow to cool to 56°.
2   Add antiserum to test tube—use about 0·1 ml and add 0·9 ml PBS.
3   Mix and warm to 56°.
4   Add 2 ml agar to the diluted antiserum and mix.
5   Pour onto pre-coated slides on the levelling table.
6   Punch two wells. (If a complete standard curve is required, use a larger plate.)

7   Fill the wells with antigen solutions—250 μg ml^{-1} and 125 μg ml^{-1} respectively.

8   Electrophorese at about 8 m amps slide^{-1}, 5–10 volts cm^{-1}.

9   Run for at least two hours.

10   The peaks may be measured immediately, but this is easier after staining (Section 5.3.a).

11   Plot the height of the peaks against the antigen concentration if a full standard curve has been determined. If the slide was run until the precipitin arcs became stationary, the relationship of peak height to antigen concentration is linear.

Unfortunately this technique cannot easily be used to measure immunoglobulin levels. Obviously if IgG is used as antigen it migrates in the same direction and at the same speed as the anti-IgG antibody and therefore no rockets can form.

Further refinements of this technique using a two stage, two-dimensional process will be described later in the section on complement (Section 6.2.5).

5.4   SECONDARY INTERACTIONS—AGGLUTINATION

Antisera may be compared semi-quantitatively by determining the end point of their respective titration curve. The sera are diluted until they no longer give a visible reaction with antigen, either by precipitation or agglutination. This is a relative measure of the antigen-binding capacity of a serum and can only be used to compare antisera when they are tested in parallel with the same antigen.

Conversely, the concentration of an antigen in solution may be determined by the degree of inhibition of a standard, homologous agglutination system (cf. Section 5.4.4).

5.4.1   HAEMAGGLUTINATION

The simplest form of this test involves the agglutination of erythrocytes (as antigens) by increasing dilutions of anti-erythrocyte sera.

Materials and equipment

Anti-sheep erythrocyte sera (Anti-SRBC) (Appendix II and Section 5.4.1b)
Normal serum as control
2% v/v sheep erythrocytes (SRBC) in PBS (Appendix II and Section 1.2.1)
0·1 M 2-mercaptoethanol in PBS
Microhaemagglutination trays (V-shaped) (Appendix II)

131

Diluting loops or tulips (0·025 ml, Appendix II)
Standard dropping pipettes (0·025 ml, Appendix II)
Sealer strip (Appendix II)

Method

For each antiserum and control serum prepare two rows of dilutions as follows:

1   Add 1 drop of PBS to all the test holes with the dropping pipette. (Hold the pipette vertically to deliver 0·025 ml.)
2   Flame the diluting loops to incandescence in a Bunsen flame and quench in distilled water.
3   Blot the tips of the loops on absorbent paper.
4   Touch the meniscus of the test serum with the tip of the loop. (To collect exactly 0·025 ml of serum the loop must not be immersed in the serum.)
5   Put the loop in the first well of the tray. Repeat for a second row of the same serum.
6   Rotate the loops in the wells, lift out cleanly and rotate in the next well. Repeat to the end of the plate.
7   Add one drop of PBS to each well of the left-hand row of dilutions with the dropping pipette.
8   Add one drop of 0·1 M 2-mercaptoethanol in PBS to each well of the right-hand row of dilutions. (This reagent is toxic and so this and all subsequent steps MUST be carried out in a fume cupboard.)
9   Add 1 drop of SRBC suspension to all the wells used, and 1 drop to an empty well, as control. (Add 2 drops of PBS to this control well.)
10   Cover the tray with a sealer strip and mix the contents of the wells by shaking.
11   Leave the tray at room temperature for 1 hour. (This may be reduced to 30 min for demonstration purposes.)

Assessment of results

Read the plate either on a white surface or using a magnifying mirror (Appendix II). A typical pattern of agglutination is shown in Fig. 5.25. The 2-mercaptoethanol in each right-hand row of the duplicate dilutions causes the IgM pentamer to fall apart and so it is no longer able to agglutinate the cells. The titre of the 2-mercaptoethanol resistant antibody is roughly equivalent to that due to IgG in the serum, and so the greater titre obtained without 2-mercaptoethanol is due to the IgM. A more exact estimate of the IgG and IgM agglutination titres may be determined using indirect haemagglutination with specific anti-class sera.

132

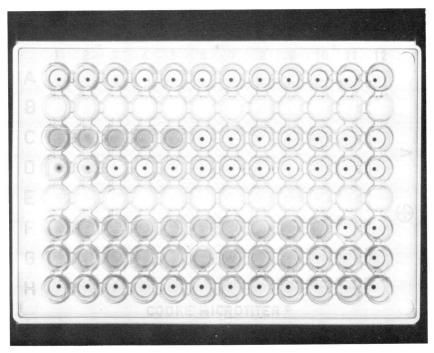

Fig. 5.25. Haemagglutination test on primary and secondary response antisera

Doubling dilutions starting at 1 : 2. Antigen: sheep-erythrocytes.

Well A: normal mouse serum, pre-immunization bleed.

Well C: mouse serum from an animal 5 days after one intraperitoneal injection of 10^8 sheep erythrocytes.

Well D: as for C but with one drop of 2 mercaptoethanol (0·1 м).

Well F: mouse serum from an animal 7 days after third injection of 10^8
sheep erythrocytes (previous injections given at 0, 10 and 20 days).

Well G: as for F but with one drop of 0·1 м 2 mercaptoethanol.

Well H: sheep erythrocytes alone.

(Note in wells not receiving 2 mercaptoethanol one drop of saline was
added to equalize the dilution effect.)

With reference to Sections 5.4.1 and 5.4.1a interpret this plate.

Technical notes

1   Many antisera or normal sera contain spontaneous anti-SRBC
antibodies (heterophile antibodies). These are usually of low titre
($< 1 : 10$) and so dilutions are usually made starting at 1 : 5 or
1 : 10, and not 1 : 2 as described here.

2   The final concentration of RBC in the trays may be varied from
0·5–1·5%. If the cells are valuable, for example, RBC coupled with
soluble antigen, then a lower concentration may be used for reasons
of economy.

3   The haemagglutination test detects IgM antibodies preferentially not only because of the multivalency of this antibody, but also
because of the relatively large size of IgM. Hence, as erythrocytes

133

are further apart when agglutinated by IgM compared to IgG, the repulsive force due to the cell's zeta potential is less.

4   You should not see any spontaneous agglutination of red cells in the control well. This is seldom a problem with fresh cells as they have a high negative zeta potential which causes the cells to repel each other. When erythrocytes are coupled to soluble antigens, however, the surface change is often reduced and so spontaneous agglutination may occur. This is discussed in Section 5.4.2b, Technical notes.

Suggested experimental protocol

5.4.1a   PRIMARY VERSUS SECONDARY ANTIBODY RESPONSE

In the primary response there is an early production of IgM antibody which soon declines and is replaced by IgG. By contrast, the IgG production is greatly accelerated in the secondary response, the peak titre is attained rapidly and it declines slowly. There appears to be no accelerated IgM production, the kinetics are essentially that of the primary response.

Compare the total and 2-mercaptoethanol resistant haemagglutination titres of sera taken from mice immunized with sheep erythrocytes as follows:

(i) 2×10^8 SRBC given i.p.—bleed 3–4 days later.
(ii) 2×10^8 SRBC given i.p. on day 0 and day 7—bleed 7 days later.

5.4.1b   CHANGE IN ANTIBODY TITRE WITH REPEATED ANTI-
GENIC CHALLENGE

You will use a hyperimmune rabbit anti-SRBC serum later in the book (Section 10.1) so test bleeds taken from the rabbit throughout the period of immunization may be used here.

Immunization schedule (per rabbit)

1   Take a 10 ml sample bleed from the central ear artery of the rabbit. Separate the serum, heat inactivate and store at $-20°$. This will serve as a control for the antiserum.
2   Homogenize 10^9 SRBC (in 1 ml of PBS) in 1 ml of Freund's complete adjuvant (Appendix II).
3   Inject the rabbit at two intramuscular sites with the homogenate.
4   At 2 weeks take another sample bleed, separate and store the serum.
5   At 4 weeks give the rabbit a second intramuscular challenge with SRBC in Freund's complete adjuvant.
6   At 6 weeks take another sample bleed for serum.

Titrate each test bleed in the haemagglutination assay described above. Boost the rabbit every 2 weeks with 10^8 SRBC given intraperitoneally until a haemagglutination titre of about 1 : 1280–2560 is obtained. At this point exsanguinate the rabbit by cardiac puncture, separate the serum and store for use in Section 10.1.3.

5.4.2 AGGLUTINATION OF ANTIGEN-COATED ERYTHROCYTES

Erythrocytes may be coupled to soluble antigens by various methods and agglutinated by antisera to the coupled antigens.

1 *Spontaneous uptake*. Erythrocytes will adsorb polysaccharides to their surface during incubation. Although this is a non-covalent binding, there is very little leaching off of the antigen during the test.

2 *Coupling to chemically modified erythrocytes*.

5.4.2a TANNED ERYTHROCYTES

This procedure is suitable for most protein antigens; in the protocol below human serum albumin is used.

Materials

Sheep erythrocytes (SRBC) in Alsever's solution (Appendix II)
Phosphate saline buffer (Appendix I)
Borate-succinate buffer (Appendix I)
Saline (Appendix I)
Tannic acid
Human-serum albumin (HSA) (Appendix II)
40% aqueous formaldehyde

Method

1 Wash SRBC 3 times with 40 volumes of saline by centrifugation (300 g for 10 min).

2 Adjust SRBC suspension to 4% v/v in phosphate saline buffer, pH 7·5.

3 Add 2·5 mg of tannic acid to 50 ml of phosphate saline buffer and mix with 50 ml of 4% SRBC suspension.

4 Incubate at 37° for 15 min.

5 Spin down cells very gently (100 g for 20 min). If the cells are pelleted too quickly they will agglutinate.

6 Divide the cells into two aliquots, and wash each with 50 ml phosphate saline buffer (100 g for 20 min). One aliquot will be used for antigen coating and the other as control cells.

7 Resuspend one aliquot of cells in 50 ml phosphate saline buffer and add 50 ml of HSA solution (2 mg ml^{-1} initial concentration).

8 Incubate at 37° for 30 min.

135

9   Wash in phosphate saline buffer by gentle centrifugation and resuspend in 100 ml of borate-succinate buffer.

10   Resuspend the second aliquot of cells in 100 ml of borate-succinate buffer. The control cells are not coated and are used both to absorb the test antisera and as control cells in the assay.

11   Add 10 ml of 40% formalin to both cell suspensions while stirring. The formalin must be added dropwise during 20–30 min.

12   Leave overnight at 4° and add a further 10 ml of formalin to both suspensions.

13   Leave the cells to settle (24 hours) and pour off the supernatant.

14   Add a large volume of borate-succinate buffer and resuspend the cells by vigorous shaking.

15   Allow cells to settle (24 hours) and repeat wash in borate-succinate buffer.

16   Adjust both cell suspensions to 1% v/v and add 0·2% formalin (final concentration) as a preservative.

The cells can be stored at 4° for up to 2 years.

5.4.2b   ASSAY PROCEDURE

Materials and equipment

As for Section 5.4.1, but use HSA-coated and control erythrocytes and rabbit anti-HSA serum (Section 1.4.6)

Method

1   Titrate the antiserum as described in Section 5.4.1, but use an initial dilution of 1 : 5 (4 drops of buffer to the first well). (OMIT the 2-mercaptoethanol from the left-hand row and the 1 drop of buffer from the right-hand row.)

2   Add one drop of the 1% suspension of HSA-coated SRBC to the right-hand row of dilutions.

3   Add one drop of 1% control (uncoated but tanned) SRBC to the left-hand row of dilutions.

4   Place one drop of coated or uncoated cells in an empty well to test for spontaneous agglutination. (Add one drop of buffer to each of these control wells.)

Again positive agglutination is seen when the cells form a continuous carpet on the base of the cup. If no agglutination has occurred the cells fall as a tight button to the bottom of the V-shaped cup (see Fig. 5.25).

Technical notes

1   If agglutination occurs with control cells the antiserum must be absorbed to remove heterophile antibodies as follows:

Add 0·1 ml of serum to 1 ml of packed control cells.
Incubate at 37° for 10 min and spin off the erythrocytes. Repeat the test.

2   If the coated or control cells agglutinate spontaneously, add 1% normal serum to the buffers used in the assay.

Antigens may also be coupled to erythrocytes using bisdiazotized benzidine, glutaraldehyde and chromic chloride. The basic principles are similar to those described above and the exact technical details may be found in the references cited at the end of this chapter.

Other particles such as bentonite or latex may be used as antigen carriers for agglutination tests. They have the advantage of not being antigenic but have a more limited range of applications than the antigen-coated erythrocyte assay described above.

5.4.3   LATEX AGGLUTINATION

Latex beads provide a convenient carrier for antigens in agglutination tests. They have not yet achieved the popularity of erythrocytes, perhaps because it is not so easy to perform quantitative assays in micro titre plates with these beads. However, sophisticated equipment has been developed (PACIA, Technicon) which quantitates the degree of agglutination of the latex beads very accurately. This apparatus has led to a whole new field of immunoassay known as Particle Counting Immunoassay which has a sensitivity approaching that of radioimmunoassay. It is, of course, simple to set up basic slide agglutination tests without any expensive equipment.

Coating the beads with antigen is not difficult especially when using IgG or albumin as antigens as these bind readily to polystyrene latex but many proteins, including the other immunoglobulin isotypes, bind less well. Fortunately it has been suggested that the simple expedient of substituting DNP groups into these proteins enables them to bind firmly to the latex. Best of all, antigens may be covalently coupled to latex particles with carbodiimide and full details of this procedure may be found in a 1974 United States Patent Number 3, 857, 931.

5.4.3a   LATEX COATING

Materials

Latex suspension 10% w/v (Appendix II)
Antigen, IgG or DNP substituted protein (Section 1.3.1a)
0·27 M and 0·054 M, Glycine-saline buffer pH 8·2 (Appendix I)

Method

1   Wash 800 μl latex suspension twice by adding 40 ml 0·054 M glycine-saline; mix and centrifuge at 12 500 *g* for 15 min.
2   Resuspend the latex in 20 ml 0·054 M glycine-saline and add 300 μl of a 10 mg ml^{-1} solution of antigen.
3   Mix the suspension for 30 min at room temperature.
4   Wash the latex twice by adding 40 ml 0·054 M glycine-saline; mix and centrifuge at 12 500 *g* for 15 min.
5   Resuspend the latex in 20 ml 0·27 M glycine-saline containing 0·1 % of an irrelevant protein to block any remaining latex protein-binding sites and store at 4°.

5.3.4b   SLIDE AGGLUTINATION

Material

Coated latex (Section 5.4.3a)
0·27 M Glycine saline buffer, pH 8·2 (Appendix I)

Method

1   Prepare doubling dilutions of test antiserum.
2   Add 25 μl of antiserum dilution to 25 μl coated latex on a glass slide.
3   Rock gently for 2 min and read agglutination visually, illuminating the slide from the side, against a dark background.

Technical note

Even in screening assays it is important to dilute the sera as pro-zones may occur, where no agglutination is seen at the highest concentrations.

Applications

Several commercial latex agglutination tests are available, one of the most widely used being for the detection of autoantibodies in rheumatoid arthritis. Patients with rheumatoid arthritis often develop antibodies to 'self IgG'. This antiglobulin antibody, known as rheumatoid factor is readily detected by its ability to agglutinate latex particles coated with IgG.

Latex particles may also be used in inhibition assays and a commonly used pregnancy test is based on this principle. Human chorionic gonadotrophin is present in the urine of pregnant women after conception and can be detected by its capacity to inhibit the agglutination of HCG-coated latex by an anti-HCG serum.

138

BLOOD GROUPING

A simple slide agglutination test may be used for blood grouping.

Materials

Standard Group A serum (Appendix II)
Standard Group B serum (Appendix II)
Human erythrocytes

Method

1 Adjust the erythrocyte suspension to approximately 4% v/v and place two separate drops on a glass slide.
2 Add one drop of either group A or B serum to each drop of erythrocytes.
3 Rock the slide and observe the agglutination over 5 min.

To avoid a transfusion reaction it is necessary to cross-match the donor and recipient blood. One drop of recipient serum is mixed with donor cells and vice versa. If no agglutination occurs in either combination then the donor and recipient are compatible.

Slide agglutination has now been largely replaced by a tube agglutination test which, among other advantages, offers greater sensitivity. (Agglutination summary table below.)

The only other blood-group antigens for which donor and recipient must be routinely typed is the rhesus or Rh system; the most important antigen of which is the Rh_0 or D antigen. Red cells are typed as positive or negative using an anti-D(Rh_0) serum.

5.4.5   RHESUS INCOMPATIBILITY

If a Rh_0 positive child is borne to a Rh_0 negative mother there is a danger of sensitization to the D antigen by the escape of fetal cells into the maternal circulation at parturition. Two classes of antibody

Agglutination reactions

	Standard antiserum*		
Blood Group	Anti-A (Group B serum)	Anti-B (Group A serum)	Saline
O	−	−	−
A	+	−	−
B	−	+	−
AB	+	+	−

* A full typing reaction would normally include anti-A B serum from an O donor to detect the rare A samples not agglutinated with anti-A.

have been detected in this situation: one which is able to induce agglutination of D positive erythrocytes and later shown to be IgM. The second type of antibody could not induce agglutination and was originally referred to as incomplete antibody (a misnomer as will be seen later). This second antibody belongs to the IgG class.

Clinically the IgG anti-D antibody is of much greater importance as this class alone is able to cross the placenta. Thus during a SECOND pregnancy with a Rh_0 positive fetus anti-D antibody may enter the fetal circulation and bring about the destruction of fetal erythrocytes by the processes described in Section 4.5.2.

Sensitization to the D antigen is now routinely suppressed by the administration of passive anti-D antibodies to the mother 36 hours after parturition. Maternal anti-D antibody production and sensitization is presumably suppressed via the 7s antibody feed-back loop. (See Uhr and Möller reference at end of chapter.)

Anti-D antibodies may be detected using rabbit anti-human immunoglobulin antibodies which cross-link IgG and anti-D in the presence of a serum-BSA mixture. (The latter mixture is used to reduce the red-cell surface charge—zeta potential—and so facilitate agglutination.)

5.5   SUMMARY AND CONCLUSIONS

Antibody molecules are capable of recognizing antigen specifically and combining with it to form a complex. When dealing with small monovalent haptens these complexes can never be larger than $hapten_2$-$antibody_1$, if the antibody is of the IgG class. With multivalent antigens, for example, proteins, we have seen that complexes of varying size can be formed depending on the concentration of antibody and antigen. The quantitative precipitin curve demonstrates the full range of complex formation from antibody to antigen excess.

The concept of the formation of complexes of varying size, some of which are soluble, is of importance not only for the interpretation of the patterns of precipitation in gels, but also for understanding the different *in vivo* pathological processes which may occur with changes in complex size. The presence of high concentrations of soluble complexes may give rise to immune complex-mediated hypersensitivity (Section 4.5.3) with all the associated immunopathological complications.

To understand all the implications of an antigen–antibody interaction it is necessary to consider the following:

(a) Amount of antigen and antibody
(b) Affinity of the combination
(c) Antibody class and sometimes sub-class
(d) Associated biological activity of antibody, antigen and complex.

FURTHER READING

BOORMAN K.E., DODD B.E. & LINCOLN P.J. (1977) *Blood Group Serology* 5e. Churchill Livingstone, Edinburgh.

CAWLEY L.P. (1969) *Electrophoresis and Immuno-Electrophoresis.* Little Brown, Boston.

CLAUSEN J. (1969) *Immunochemical Techniques for the Identification and Estimation of Macromolecules.* North-Holland, Amsterdam.

CROWLE A.J. (1969) *Immunodiffusion.* Academic Press, London.

CROWLE A.J. (1978) Immunodiffusion analyses useful in clinical chemistry. *Advances in Clinical Chemistry* **20**.

LEMIEUX S., AVRAMEAS S. & BUSSARD A.E. (1974). Local Haemolysis Plaque Assay using a New Method of Coupling Antigens on Sheep Erythrocytes by Glutaraldehyde. *Immunochem* **11** (5), 261.

LEVINSKY, R.J. & SOOTHILL J.F. (1977) A test for antigen antibody complexes in human sera using IgM of rabbit antisera to human immunoglobulins. *Clin. exp. Immunol.* **29**, 428 (This paper gives details of latex coupling)

MILFORD WARD A. & WHICKER J.T. (eds.) (1979) *Immunochemistry in Clinical Laboratory Medicine.* MTP Press, Lancaster.

MOLLISON P.L. (1979) *Blood Transfusion in Clinical Medicine* 6e. Blackwell Scientific Publications, Oxford.

NOWOTNY A. (1979) *Basic Exercises in Immunochemistry* 2e. Springer-Verlag, Berlin.

OUCHTERLONY O. (1970) *Handbook of Immunodiffusion and Immunoelectrophoresis.* Ann Arbor, Michigan.

OUCHTERLONY O. & NILSSON L.A. (1978) Immunodiffusion and immunoelectrophoresis. In D.M. Weir (ed.) *Handbook of Experimental Immunology* 3e, 19. Blackwell Scientific Publications, Oxford.

PINCKARD R.N. (1978) Equilibrium Dialysis and Preparation of Hapten Conjugates. In D.M. Weir (ed.) *Handbook of Experimental Immunology* 3e, 17. Blackwell Scientific Publications, Oxford.

STEWARD M.W. (1978) Introduction to methods used to study antibody–antigen interactions. In DM Weir (ed.) *Handbook of Experimental Immunology* 3e, 16.1. Blackwell Scientific Publications, Oxford.

6   Antibody effector systems

Antigen–antibody interaction can result in visible expressions of complex formation such as precipitation and agglutination (Sections 5.3 and 5.4). In turn this complex is capable of activating several accessory systems, for example, the complement sequence, which amplify and extend the original reaction.

6.1   COMPLEMENT

The complement pathway is a multicomponent system of serum proteins which are present in normal serum in an inactive state. When the first component is activated by combination with the immune complex it is then able to activate several molecules of the next component. So the process is repeated for components C1–9 as an amplifying cascade until the bacterium, or other foreign cell with which the original complex was formed, is lysed.

Other effector functions are activated by by-products of the complement cascade: activated C3 is chemotactic for granulocytes and promotes phagocytosis, activated C3 and C5 have anaphylatoxin activity and cause degranulation of mast cells.

We will describe techniques by which the total serum content of complement may be measured as well as the major C3 component.

6.1.1   TOTAL HAEMOLYTIC COMPLEMENT

As complement is added to antibody-coated erythrocytes an increasing proportion of the cells are lysed as shown in Fig. 6.1. The curve approaches 100% lysis asymptotically and so it is difficult to determine the total lytic unit of complement (CH_{100}) therefore one normally defines the 50% lysis point (CH_{50}).

The von Krogh equation for the sigmoid dose response curve of complement-mediated cytolysis was arrived at empirically and in its basic form may be written as:

$$x = k\left(\frac{y}{100 - y}\right)^{1/n} \tag{1}$$

where x = amount of complement (ml of undiluted serum)
y = proportion of cells lysed
k = 50% unit of complement
n is a constant.

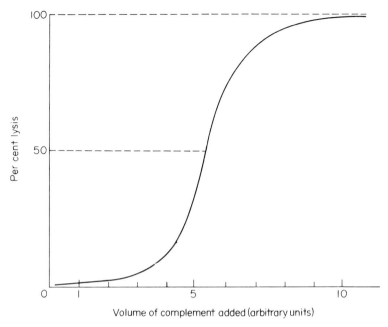

Fig. 6.1. Lysis of sheep erythrocytes, sensitized by horse anti-SRBC, in the presence of human complement
The curve of complement-mediated lysis approaches the 100% lysis value asymptotically and so accurate determinations of serum complement levels are made on the 50% lysis point as shown in the graph.

The CH_{50} unit is determined under standardized conditions which depend upon

(1) erythrocyte and antibody concentration
(2) buffering conditions of the medium
(3) temperature.

Hence the definition of the CH_{50} unit is arbitrary and depends wholly on the conditions used.

6.1.2   STANDARDIZATION OF ERYTHROCYTES

Materials and equipment

Barbitone buffered saline (Appendix I)
Sheep erythrocytes (Appendix II)
0·04% ammonia solution
Fresh or preserved guinea-pig serum
Horse haemolytic serum (Appendix II)
Spectrophotometer

Method

1   Dilute barbitone buffered saline to working strength. Check for fungal or bacterial contamination as these are anti-complementary.

143

Sensitization of sheep erythrocytes with antibody (30 ml of 3% SRBC)

Strictly, the antiserum should be titred until the highest dilution giving full complement fixation is reached. However, for most purposes it is sufficient to use a 1 : 150 dilution of the sensitizing antiserum.

2   Wash 4 ml of the erythrocyte suspension (ca. 25% in Alsever's solution) three times in barbitone saline buffer (200 *g* for 3 min).

3   Resuspend the washed erythrocytes in 15 ml of barbitone saline buffer (use a measuring cylinder).

4   Mix 1 ml of erythrocytes with 25 ml of ammonia solution to lyse the cells and read the OD at 541 nm.

For a 6% SRBC suspension, in a 1 cm cuvette, the OD should be 0·48–0·50. Adjust the suspension as required.

5   Mix 15 ml barbitone buffered saline, 0·1 ml of horse haemolytic serum and 15 ml of 6% SRBC.

6   Incubate at 37° for 15 min.

Use the sensitized cells within 24 h.

6.1.3   COMPLEMENT ASSAY—estimation of CH_{50}

1   Set up the tubes as in the protocol and remember to use fresh or preserved serum as the complement source.

2   Incubate at 37° for 60 min.

3   Place the tubes on ice and add 2 ml of buffer to each tube.

4   Centrifuge at 200 *g* for 10 min at 4°.

5   Remove a sample of each supernatant (1–7) and read OD at 541 nm.

Protocol

	1	2	3	4	5	6	7
Buffer (ml)	1·10	1·05	1·00	0·90	0·80	1·20	1·2 ml of ammonia solution
Guinea-pig serum (ml) initial dil. 1 : 30	0·10	0·15	0·20	0·30	0·40	0·00	
Sensitized erythrocytes (ml) suspension	0·3 —————————————————————→						

Calculation of results

1   Assuming that tube 7 represents total lysis, calculate the % lysis for each tube.

2   Plot the % lysis against the complement concentration (ml of undiluted serum). This will yield a sigmoid curve as in Fig. 6.1.

This dose response curve follows the von Krogh equation given earlier (1). This equation may be logarithmically transformed so

144

that the data fall on a straight line.

$$\log x = \log k + \frac{1}{n} \log\left(\frac{y}{100 - y}\right)$$

3 Plot $\log x$ against $\log\{y/(100 - y)\}$ for each dilution of complement used. The straight line has a slope of $1/n$ (the exact value depends on experimental conditions, but it should be within 20% of 0.2).

The abscissa intercept of the line, where $\log\{y/(100 - y)\} = 0$, is the log dilution resulting in 50% lysis. The complement level of a serum is normally expressed as the number of CH_{50} units ml^{-1} of serum.

Technical note

Complement components are highly labile and so fresh serum must be prepared by clotting the blood at 4°. Preserved guinea-pig serum is available commercially as a source of complement. Here the complement components are stabilized by lyophilization of serum in a hypertonic salt solution.

6.2 CLASSICAL AND ALTERNATE PATHWAY OF COMPLEMENT FIXATION

In the haemolytic system just considered the complement cascade was activated by the combination of C1 to an antigen–antibody complex. Recently several substances have been described that are able to activate C3 directly, for example, zymosan and endotoxin. Interestingly, among these by-pass activators are those classes of human and guinea-pig immunoglobulins which are not able to activate the classical pathway.

This capacity of bacterial polysaccharides to activate the complement system directly may indicate that complement was involved in a primitive form of immunity before the appearance of immunoglobulin during evolution. The activation and binding of C3 to zymosan by the alternate pathway is used to advantage by immunologists as a simple means of isolating C3 as shown in the following section.

In the classical pathway certain inorganic molecules, calcium and magnesium, are required for the initial activation step. It is thought that the trimolecular complex that forms, C1 (C_{1q}, C_{1r}, C_{1s}), may be linked together through calcium.

6.2.1 ASSAY FOR C3

C3 is the predominant component of the complement sequence (there is about 1 mg ml^{-1} in normal serum) and it is as this component is activated that the greatest amplification step of the cascade takes place.

C3 may be assayed in a simple immunodiffusion test using anti-C3 in an agarose gel (agar is not recommended because of anti-complementary effects—see haemolytic plaque technique— Section 3.1.2). Anti-C3 is available commercially but an acceptable antiserum, for routine use, can be raised quite simply.

6.2.2 ANTI-C3 SERUM

Materials

Fresh human or guinea-pig serum, as source of complement
Zymosan (Appendix II)
Saline (Appendix I)
Barbitone buffered saline (Appendix I)
Freund's incomplete adjuvant (Appendix II)
Rabbit

Method

1   Boil 500 mg of zymosan for 30 min in 50 ml saline.
2   Centrifuge and discard the supernatant.
3   When cool, mix the precipitate with 11 ml of fresh serum (see Technical note, Section 6.1.3).
4   Incubate for 1 h at 37° with mixing.
5   Centrifuge and discard supernatant.
6   Wash the zymosan–C3 complex 6 times with barbitone buffered saline.
7   Store complex at $-20°$.
8   Immunize rabbit every 10 days for 30 days with 13 mg of zymosan–C3 complex in Freund's incomplete adjuvant (Appendix II).

Zymosan binds C3 preferentially but not specifically. The antiserum therefore tends to show other specificities if immunization is prolonged.

6.2.3 SINGLE RADIAL IMMUNODIFFUSION ASSAY FOR C3

A similar assay to that described in Section 5.3.3a may be used, but substituting agarose for the agar. Anti-C3 prepared as above is incorporated into a layer of agarose on a microscope slide and serum samples and standards are placed in wells cut in the gel. Diffusion for 24 h will allow rings of precipitation to form. The size (diameter) of these rings is proportional to the C3 concentration.

146

6.2.4 ANALYSIS OF C3 ACTIVATION

The inactive and active forms of C3 share many antigenic determinants and so they are detected simultaneously in the simple immunodiffusion test described in the previous section. However, C3 in its inactive state has a β_{1C} electrophoretic mobility which changes to a β_{1A} mobility after activation. It is therefore possible to show the appearance of activated C3 and the disappearance of inactive C3 by immunoelectrophoresis.

Further, this reaction may be quantitated using two dimensional immunoelectrophoresis. The two forms of C3 are first separated by simple electrophoresis in agarose and then quantitated by the size of the rocket arcs formed during electrophoresis, in the second dimension, into a gel containing anti-C3.

6.2.5 TWO-DIMENSIONAL IMMUNOELECTROPHORESIS

Materials and equipment

Barbitone buffer (Appendix I) containing 0·01 M ethylene diamine tetra-acetic acid, di-sodium salt (EDTA)
Agarose
Anti-C3 serum (Appendix II or Section 6.2.2)
3 × 1-inch microscope slide (not precoated)
$3\frac{1}{4}$ × $3\frac{1}{4}$-inch lantern slide (precoated as in Section 5.3.3) (Appendix II)
Electrophoresis tank and power pack (Appendix II)

Method

First dimension

1   Prepare a 2% agarose solution in the barbitone buffer + EDTA, Na$_2$ (Section 5.3.3a).
2   Layer 3 ml of agarose solution onto the microscope slide and allow to set. Use a levelled surface.
3   Cut a 1 mm well in the centre of the slide, remove the agarose plug, and fill the well with the serum sample.
4   Apply a potential difference of 150 volts (constant voltage setting on power pack) for 2–3 h.
5   Cut and remove a 5 mm wide longitudinal strip of agarose from the centre of the slide. It must, of course, include the sample.

Second dimension

1   Prepare a 1 : 50–1 : 100 dilution of anti-C3 in 2% agarose solution (as in Section 5.3.3a).

147

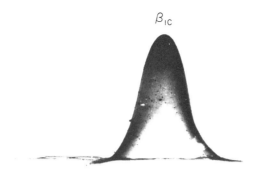

(a) Fresh human serum

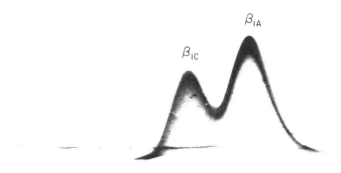

(b) Serum treated with heat aggregated IgG.

Fig. 6.2. Quantitation of C3 activation

Although the inactive and active forms of C3 share many antigenic determinants, the activation of C3 is accompanied by a change in electrophoretic
mobility from β_{1C} to β_{1A}. It is therefore possible to quantitate C3 activation
by combining electrophoresis in one dimension with 'rocket' immunoelectrophoresis in the second dimension. (Photograph courtesy Dr C.
Loveday.)

   Activation of C3: C1q, C1r and C1s are linked, probably through
calcium, to form a tri-molecular complex. The binding of C1q to the Fc of
the immune complex (in this case we have substituted heat-aggregated IgG)
initiates the esterase activity of the C1s component which activates C4 and
C2. (The complement components were numbered before their order in the
activitation sequence was known.) The resulting C1.4.2. complex has 'C3
convertase' activity and so splits C3 (β_{1C} mobility) to C3a and C3b (β_{1A}
mobility).

   The two rocket arcs of C3a and C3b are fused because of shared antigenic
determinants.

2   Place the agarose strip at one end of the $3\frac{1}{4}$-inch square glass
plate (precoated) and cover the whole slide with 12 ml of agarose
containing anti-C3.

3   Place the plate in the electrophoresis tank. The cathode must be
at the end of the plate with the agarose strip, i.e. the electric field will

cause the separated complement components to enter the antibody-containing gel at right angles to the first electrophoresis. Electro-phorese at 40–50 volts overnight.

4   Wash and stain the precipitin arcs (Section 5.3.3a).

Suggested samples for quantitation:

(i)   Fresh serum.

(ii)   Aged serum.

(iii)   Serum taken from the complement fixation test described in the next section.

(iv)   Serum treated with zymosan or endotoxin (both are by-pass activators). Use 1 mg ml^{-1} of activator for 15 min at 37°.

A specimen result is shown in Fig. 6.2.

6.3   DETECTION OF ANTIBODY OR ANTIGEN BY COMPLEMENT FIXATION

An antibody, antigen or antigen–antibody complex may be detected by estimating either complement consumption or fixation. As men-tioned earlier, because of the amplifying cascade sequence of complement, a small amount of antigen–antibody complex will cause massive complement fixation or consumption (depending on whether you assay the complex or the supernatant for complement components). Accordingly, the complement fixation reaction is a very sensitive technique for measuring very small amounts (<1 μg) of antigen or antibody. However, it has the disadvantage that (a) it is a relative and not an absolute measure, and (b) it detects only certain antibody classes. In the human, for example, IgG1, IgG2 (weakly), IgG3 and IgM activate the classical complement pathway, whereas IgG4, IgA and IgE cannot. There is, however, relatively poor complement activation via the alternative pathway by these latter 3 immunoglobulin classes if they are first heat aggregated.

6.3.1   QUANTITATIVE COMPLEMENT FIXATION ASSAY

It is possible arbitrarily to standardize complement activity using antibody sensitized erythrocytes (Section 6.1.2).

If instead of defining the CH_{50} as before, we define the minimum amount of complement required to lyse all of the standard volume of sensitized red cells (minimum haemolytic dose—MHD) we have an extremely good indicator system for complement consumption tests.

Hence in the complement fixation assay a soluble antigen is allowed to react with antibody and so fix complement. When the indicator system of sensitized erythrocytes is added the degree of

149

lysis observed will be proportional to the amount of complement remaining in the supernatant.

The assay is made semi-quantitative by titrating the test serum to determine the lowest dilution that still gives positive complement fixation.

Materials and equipment

Human serum albumin (HSA) 1 mg ml^{-1} (Appendix II)
Anti-HSA (Section 1.4.6 or Appendix II)
Sensitized erythrocytes (Section 6.1.2)
Barbitone buffered saline (Appendix I)
Complement source—guinea-pig serum (fresh or preserved—Appendix II)
Microtitre apparatus (Appendix II)
Microtitre trays—U-shaped wells (Appendix II)

6.3.1a ESTIMATION OF MINIMUM HAEMOLYTIC DOSE (MHD) OF COMPLEMENT

1   Reconstitute the guinea-pig serum if required.
2   Adjust to 1 : 10 dilution.
3   Set up the complement dilutions as in the protocol below.
4   Take 0·1 ml of each complement dilution and add 0·2 ml buffer plus 0·1 ml of sensitized erythrocytes.
5   Incubate for 30 min at 37° and centrifuge at 100 g for 15 min.

The titre of the first tube to show a button of erythrocytes is then taken as the MHD. In the assay 2MHD units are used.

Protocol

	Tube number						
	1	2	3	4	5	6	7
Barbitone buffered saline (ml)	0·1	0·2	0·3	0·4	0·5	0·6	0·7
Guinea-pig serum (ml) 1 : 10 initial dil.	0·1————————————————————→						
Final C dilution	1 : 20	1 : 30	1 : 40	1 : 50	1 : 60	1 : 70	1 : 80

6.3.1b ANTIBODY AND ANTIGEN ASSAY

The test is set up as shown in Fig. 6.3. The antiserum is diluted out down the plate (columns) and the antigen is diluted out across the plate (rows).

1   Put 1 drop (0·025 ml) of buffer in each well. (Hold the dropping pipette vertically.)
2   Dilute out the antiserum in the 8 columns as for haemagglutina-

150

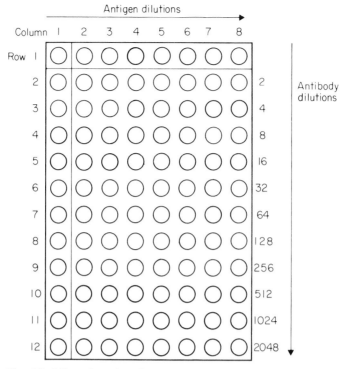

Fig. 6.3. Micro-titre plate for quantitative complement fixation assay
Row 1 contains antigen dilutions only and is a control for anti-complementary activity of the antigen.

Column 1 contains antibody alone, again this is a control for anti-complementary activity.

tion (Section 5.4.1), but start at row 2. Row 1 is used as an antigen control (see Fig. 6.3).

3 Set up antigen dilutions in tubes as in the protocol below.

4 Add 1 drop of antigen to each well in columns 2–8, tube number should correspond to column number (see Fig. 6.3). Leave column 1 free of antigen—this is the antiserum control.

Protocol

				Tube number			
	2	3	4	5	6	7	8
Barbitone buffered saline (ml)	1·0 ———————————————————————→						
HSA (ml initial conc. 1 mg ml^{-1})	1·0						
	mix ⟶ mix ⟶ mix			etc.			
		1·0	1·0				
Final HSA dilution	1 : 2	1 : 4	1 : 8	1 : 16	1 : 32	1 : 64	1 : 128

5   Add 2 MHD units of complement to each well.
6   Mix by shaking and incubate at 37° for 30 min.
7   Add 1 drop of sensitized cells to all wells.
8   Mix by shaking and incubate at 37° for 30 min.
9   Shake and stand at 4° for 60 min.

Examine the wells for the presence of unlysed erythrocytes; indicating previous complement fixation. The end-point titre of this test is usually taken as the first well showing approximately 50% lysis of indicator cells.

There should not be any complement fixation in either the antigen or antiserum controls, i.e. haemolysis should be complete.

Technical notes

1   Because IgM has a higher haemolytic efficiency (cf. Section 3.1.2), this antibody class is preferentially detected.
2   In the checkerboard design given above, both the antigen and antiserum concentrations were varied. For routine use, once the optimum level of either antigen or antibody has been established, a single concentration is usually used for the detection of unknown concentrations of antigen or antibody.
3   The final step of settling the indicator cells at 4° for 60 min may be considerably shortened by gently centrifuging the trays in special holders (Appendix II).
4   If any component is anticomplementary the test must be repeated with fresh reagents.

6.4   **DETECTION OF ANTIGEN–ANTIBODY COMPLEXES BY ANTI-C3 IMMUNOFLUORESCENCE**

Circulating immune complexes are either removed by phagocytic cells or they become deposited in blood vessels and tissues, where they may act as a focus for subsequent tissue damage. These complexes can be detected by using fluorescent antisera to immunoglobulins, but this can lead to problems with background staining. It is preferable to use anti-C3 conjugated with fluorescein. This conjugate is able to detect C3 wherever it has been bound into an immune complex. For every molecule of antibody there are usually many molecules of C3 bound around the area of the complex, and so complexes may be detected more sensitively by an anti-C3 conjugate than by an anti-Ig conjugate.

Using anti-C3, immune complexes can be demonstrated in the kidneys of patients with systemic lupus erythematosus. 'Lumpybumpy' characteristic granular deposits are seen along the glomerular basement membranes. These complexes appear to involve DNA as the antigen. Immune complex deposition can also take place after bacterial infection. In acute glomerulonephritis, following acute streptococcal infection, the same lumpy deposits may be demonstrated in the kidney, this time involving streptococcal antigen.

The $(NZB \times NZW)F_1$ mouse also exhibits a form of glomerulonephritis caused by immune complex deposition. In biopsies from the kidney deposits are found containing DNA, immunoglobulin and C3. If some of these mice can be obtained, cryostat tissue sections can be prepared from the kidney and the sections examined with rabbit anti-mouse C3 serum conjugated with fluorescein (Sections 6.2.2, 1.6.1 and 3.1.1a).

6.5 OPSONIC AND IMMUNE ADHERENCE TO PHAGOCYTIC CELLS

The ability of antibody and complement to induce lysis of invading bacteria is by no means their only rôle in combating infection. The cells which produce the specific immune response, seen here as antibody production, usually act in concert with the reticuloendothelial (RE) system. The RE system consists of many different types of phagocytic cells spread throughout the tissues of the body. As has been seen (Section 4.1.1) foreign particles are taken up fairly slowly by the cells of the RE system. In the presence of antibody and complement, however, this process of uptake is greatly accelerated by two mechanisms:

A. Opsonic adherence

Phagocytic cells have on their surfaces receptor sites for the Fc portion of immunoglobulin. Hence the coating of a bacterium by antibody could have two effects, firstly the surface charge of the organism and consequently the repulsion between bacterium and phagocyte, will be reduced, and secondly, the immunoglobulin coat will have many free Fc portions exposed which will bind to the Fc receptor sites on the phagocytes.

B. Immune adherence

Phagocytes also have sites on their surface for the binding of activated C3. As C3 is usually fixed by the antibody–bacterium complex, this will further aid the attachment of the bacterium to the phagocyte.

Not only do these two phenomena facilitate binding of the bacterium to the phagocyte, they also promote phagocytosis, or if the foreign object is too large to be engulfed they probably promote the release of lysosomal enzymes.

Not all antibody classes are able to induce immune adherence; in man this property is limited to IgG_1 and IgG_3 and in mouse it is limited to IgG_{2a} and IgG_{2b}.

153

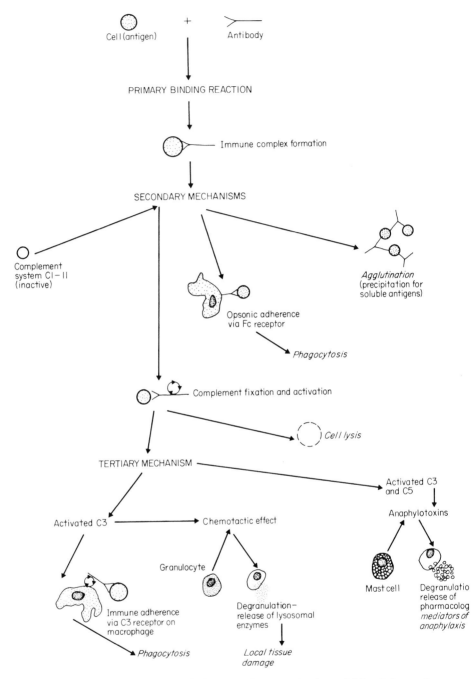

Fig. 6.4. Summary of the secondary mechanisms initiated by antigen–antibody complex formation

SUMMARY AND CONCLUSIONS

It is convenient at this point to reconsider the possible interactions resulting from the combination of an antigen with its antibody. As can be seen from Fig. 6.4 the initial event is specific, but all the other systems brought into play are non-specific, and some are mutually exclusive.

The complexity of the interaction shown in Fig. 6.4 has been greatly reduced by starting almost at the end of the specific immune response. When all the initial events of cell selection and triggering are also considered, the true complexity of the intact immune response can be envisaged.

FURTHER READING

ATTASI M.Z. (ed.) (1978) *Immunochemistry of Proteins*, Vol. 3. Plenum Press, New York.

DORRINGTON K.J. (ed.) (1978) The structure and function of the constant region: a symposium. *Molecular Immunology* **16**, 11.

EDELMAN G.M. (1970) The covalent structure of a human γG-immunoglobulin. XI. Functional implications. *Biochemistry* **9**, 3197.

FEARON D.T. & AUSTEN K.F. (1977) Immunochemistry of the classical and alternative pathways of complement. In Glynn & Steward (eds.) *Immunochemistry: an Advanced Textbook*. John Wiley, Chichester.

FEINSTEIN A. & BEALE D. (1977) Models of immunoglobulins and antigen–antibody complexes. In Glynn & Steward (eds.) *Immunochemistry: an Advanced Textbook*. John Wiley, Chichester.

LACHMAN P.J. & HOBART M.J. (1978) Complement Technology. In D.M. Weir (ed.) *Handbook of Experimental Immunology* 3e 5a. Blackwell Scientific Publications, Oxford.

METZGER H. (1974) The effect of antigen binding on the properties of antibody. *Advances in Immunology* **18**, 169.

7 Isolation and structure of immunoglobulins

The immunoglobulin classes differ from each other and from the other serum proteins by their solubility in aqueous solution, molecular size, electrostatic density and isoelectric point. These characteristics can be used to isolate immunoglobulins and to fractionate them into classes.

Recently, it has been found that certain immunoglobulin classes are bound by particular proteins. This has led to the development of affinity techniques for the isolation of immunoglobulin isotypes (Section 8.5).

7.1 SALT FRACTIONATION

The relative solubility of proteins in pure water or in various salt solutions has been used for over one hundred years as a basic fractionation technique. Serum may be separated into its euglobulin (insoluble) and pseudoglobulin (soluble) fractions by dialysis against distilled water. Although this is often used as the first step in the purification of IgM, the euglobulin fraction is always contaminated with IgG, and IgM denaturation often occurs. In addition, this method gives very low yield.

As the salt concentration of the medium is raised there is an interference with the interaction of water molecules with the charged polar groups on protein molecules, thus rendering them less hydrophilic. This allows a greater hydrophobic interaction between protein molecules and so they eventually become insoluble. The salt concentration at which each protein precipitates is different, but between closely related molecules, such as immunoglobulins, the difference is not sufficiently great to give high-grade purity of the precipitate. However, it is often useful as a first step in isolation as many unwanted serum proteins, for example albumin, will remain in solution when immunoglobulins are precipitated. Besides its use for purification, salting out is important for concentration of immunoglobulins from dilute solution.

Ammonium sulphate precipitation is the most widely used technique for the preparation of a crude immunoglobulin fraction from whole serum (see Section 1.2.2). This salt has the advantage of a high solubility which is only minimally dependent on tempera-

156

ture, varying only about 3% between $0°$ and $25°$, whereas sodium sulphate, the other salt most often used, is five times as soluble at $25°$ as at $0°$. Although relatively 'pure' IgG may be rapidly prepared by precipitation at a $33·3\%$ saturation of ammonium sulphate, if a high yield is required 50% saturation will be necessary. Smaller fragments of the molecule require much higher salt concentrations for precipitation.

7.1.1 RAPID CONCENTRATION OF LIGHT CHAINS

After column chromatography samples are often recovered in dilute solution in large volumes of buffer. It is important to concentrate these rapidly as denaturation occurs in dilute solution. Ammonium sulphate precipitation is useful for this, using the solid salt to limit the total working volume of solution. The method below is suitable for light chains (Section 7.6) Fab regions (Section 7.7) and is also applicable for preparing Bence Jones proteins from the urine of patients with multiple myeloma. (Bence Jones proteins are free light chains, identical with those combined with heavy chains in the serum myeloma protein, but at low concentration. During protein synthesis in plasma cells light chains are produced separately from the heavy chains and a pool of free light chains exists within the cell. In a plasmacytoma there is often a slight over-production of light chains and these are secreted.)

Materials

Fab or light chains from column chromatography or urine from patient with multiple myeloma or urine from mouse with a transplanted chemically induced tumour
Solid ammonium sulphate

Method

Steps 1–2 are only for urine samples, otherwise start at 3.
1   Dialyse the urine against cold, running tap water for 24 hours to remove inorganic salts and urea.
2   Filter or centrifuge to remove any insoluble material.
3   Adjust pH to 5·5 (salt precipitation is most effective at the isoelectric point of the protein required).
4   Add solid ammonium sulphate to 75% saturation. At $25°$, 575 g solid ammonium sulphate is required for 1000 ml of solution (see also nomogram, front inside cover). Add the salt slowly with stirring, otherwise it will form lumps bound up with protein which are very difficult to dissolve.
5   When all the salt has been added stir for 1 hour at room temperature to equilibrate.

157

6   Centrifuge at 1000 *g* for 15 min and discard the supernatant. (Take care to wash any salt off the rotor head or corrosion will occur.)

7   Redissolve the precipitate in PBS.

Ammonium sulphate precipitation is often used to prepare crude γ globulin fractions from whole serum (Section 1.2.2a). For many applications this is sufficient, but even if more highly purified material is required, salt precipitation provides a useful first step in the isolation procedure.

7.1.2   EFFECT OF PROTEIN CONCENTRATION ON SALT-INDUCED PRECIPITATION

The protein concentration in the medium influences the precipitation limits of the protein and also affects the co-precipitation of the other proteins. Accordingly, when precipitating serum (Section 1.2.2) ammonium sulphate is added slowly to avoid high local concentration which would decrease the specificity of the precipitation.

7.2   SIZE FRACTIONATION

Serum proteins may be isolated and fractionated on the basis of the molecular size using gel filtration.

7.2.1   PRINCIPLES OF MOLECULAR SIEVING

Using porous gels of cross-linked dextran (Sephadex), agarose (Sepharose or Biogel-A), polyacrylamide (Biogel-P) or mixtures of agarose and acrylamide (Sephacryl) proteins may be separated on the basis of their molecular dimensions. An equilibrium is maintained between the liquid phase around the gel particles and the gel phase. Depending upon the pore size of the gel, molecules may diffuse from the liquid phase into the gel phase. The rate at which a molecule moves down a column of the gel beads depends upon the number of beads that are entered. Because the solute molecules maintain a concentration equilibrium between the gel and liquid phases the sample moves down the column as a band. Large proteins, above the exclusion limit of the gel, will not enter the beads and so move with the advancing solute front while small molecules enter the beads and must traverse this space as well as the volume around the beads. All sizes of excluded proteins appear in the effluent simultaneously and so will not be separated. Molecular weight is not the only factor governing the entry of molecules into the gel; molecular shape and hydration are also important. Proteins and polysaccharides have very different exclusion limits in

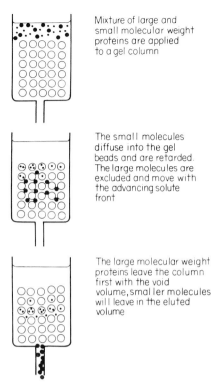

Mixture of large and small molecular weight proteins are applied to a gel column

The small molecules diffuse into the gel beads and are retarded. The large molecules are excluded and move with the advancing solute front

The large molecular weight proteins leave the column first with the void volume, smaller molecules will leave in the eluted volume

Fig. 7.1. Principles of molecular size sorting on a gel bead column
Mixture of large and small molecular weight proteins are applied to a gel column. The small molecules diffuse into the gel beads and are retarded. The large molecules are excluded and move with the advancing solute front. The large molecular weight proteins ieave the column first with the void volume, smaller molecules will leave in the eluted volume.

terms of molecular weight. However, within a related group of molecules, for example immunoglobulins, the molecules will leave the column in order of decreasing size (Fig. 7.1). Some molecules such as nucleotides have a tendency to bind to dextran columns and this will alter their behaviour during separation.

Many gels are available for exclusion chromatography, each differing in their chemical composition, physical form and pore size. The following basic requirements should be considered in selecting a gel for separation of any protein mixture.

Basic requirements

1   Correct pore size—the proteins must be able to diffuse into the gel for molecular sieving to occur. The exclusion limits of the different grades and types of gel are available from the manufacturers. (See Appendix III for Sephadex.)
2   The gel must be inert—any charged groups on the gel or affinity for the material to be separated will interfere with size separation.

159

3   Bead size—the gel must be finely dispersed to allow rapid diffusion and effective separation, but this must be balanced against optimum flow rate as very fine particles tend to slow the flow of solute molecules. The presentation of the gel in bead form gives good flow characteristics.

Sephadex (Appendix II). This is the most widely used material for gel filtration. It is prepared by cross-linking alkaline dextran with epichlorohydrin and is swollen in phosphate buffered saline or water for use.

Sepharose and Biogel-A (Appendix II). These consist of small spheres of agarose, a linear polysaccharide of D-galactose and 3,6-anhydro-L-galactose. It contains no ionizable groups but has the unfortunate characteristic of congealing at elevated temperatures or in the presence of solutes capable of breaking hydrogen bonds, for example urea, this problem has now been overcome by the introduction of cross-linked Sepharose. Unlike Sephadex it can be used to separate very large molecules, even in the range of viruses.

Biogel-P (Appendix II). This gel is a copolymer of acrylamide and methylenebis-acrylamide. Its fractional range corresponds roughly to that of agarose, but as it is a plastic it has the enormous advantage of not being susceptible to attack by micro-organisms.

Sephacryl. This is becoming very popular for gel filtration. Each bead consists of a mixture of agarose and acrylamide. It is a rigid gel capable of good resolution at comparatively high flow rates, S300 is especially useful for fractionating large serum proteins including immune complexes.

PARAMETERS OF GEL FILTRATION (see also Section 1.2.3).

Large molecules, above the exclusion limit, cannot enter the gel pores and remain in the solute around the beads, i.e. in the VOID VOLUME V_o. Small buffer molecules are able to pass into the gel freely and so enter the INCLUDED VOLUME V_i, as well as the space around the beads and so traverse the volume $V_i + V_o = V_t$, the TOTAL SOLVENT VOLUME.

Molecules of intermediate size may enter the gel, but less freely than buffer molecules, and so they are eluted from the column at an intermediate volume between V_o and V_t, known as the ELUTION VOLUME V_e.

7.2.2   APPLICATIONS OF GEL CHROMATOGRAPHY

1 Desalting or rapid 'dialysis'

Sephadex G-25 excludes all molecules over 5000 molecular weight. Its use in desalting and rapid 'dialysis' of protein solutions has been described in detail in Section 1.2.3.

2 Protein fractionation

From the previous sections it is obvious that the major use of gel chromatography is the isolation and purification of molecules of different molecular size. It is possible, however, to separate molecules of the same size if they have different affinities for the gel material.

3 Molecular weight determinations of proteins

Molecular weight determinations may be made on protein samples equilibrated against and run in guanidine, in which case the protein adopts a random coil configuration. Proteins of known molecular weight are used as standards. (Pharmacia supplies sets of dyed proteins as size standards.)

7.2.3   BASIC COLUMN TECHNIQUE

Fig. 7.2 shows the ideal equipment for gel filtration. This equipment is available commercially and is invaluable for serious fractionation work.

Equipment

Columns. Many different types of column are available each with their own minor advantages and disadvantages. The column must have a small dead space (see Fig. 7.2) to minimize mixing of the sample eluting from the column. We have found Pharmacia columns of 2·5 cm and 1·5 cm internal diameter and 100 cm height to be satisfactory (Appendix II). (The same columns with water jackets have internal diameters of 2·6 and 1·6 cm, respectively.) Also, the new 'generation' of Wright columns are easy to use (Appendix II). For reasons discussed later (Section 7.2.4) it is an advantage to have columns fitted with a flow adaptor (see Fig. 7.2).

Pump. Peristaltic pumps provide an even flow rate with little solvent turbulence. Alternatively, a simple reservoir such as a Marriotte flask can be used. It is important to maintain a constant pressure on the column.

Monitoring and collection of fractions. For most runs a fraction collector is vital. The LKB Ultrorac (see Appendix II) is widely used and reliable. A flow-through UV analyser (e.g. Uvicord, Appendix II) and chart recorder can be connected to this. If an analyser is not available the fractions must be processed in a UV spectrophotometer after collection.

161

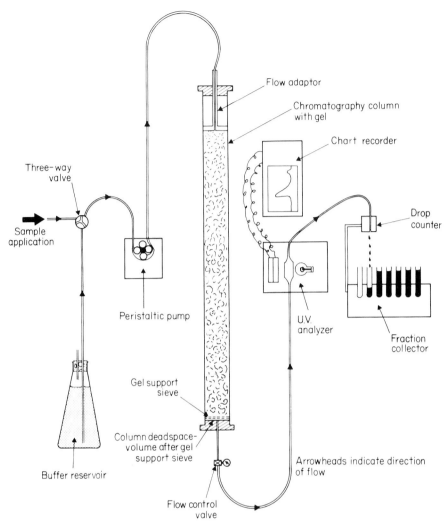

Flow adaptor

Chromatography column
with gel

Chart recorder

Drop
counter

Three-way
valve

Sample
application

Peristaltic pump

U.V.
analyzer

Fraction
collector

Gel support
sieve

Column deadspace-
volume after gel
support sieve

Buffer reservoir

Arrowheads indicate direction
of flow

Flow control
valve

Fig. 7.2. Equipment for column chromatography
The equipment shown above allows efficient chromatographic separation
of protein mixtures. Although, as described in the text, some items of equipment are not essential they save greatly in time and effort.

7.2.4   FRACTIONATION OF SERUM ON G-200
         SEPHADEX

Sephadex G-200 excludes proteins over 800,000 molecular weight
and so is extremely useful for the isolation of IgM. Sephacryl, S200,
which is preswollen is also very useful for fractionation in this
molecule weight range (Section 8.5.1, gel filtration). Although
Sephacryl gives better resolution at higher flow rates, it is significantly more expensive than Sephadex.

162

Materials and equipment

Sephadex G-200 (Appendix II)

Phosphate buffered saline (PBS) (Appendix I)

Column chromatography equipment (Fig. 7.2, Section 7.2.3, Appendix II)

Mouse serum, preferably use an immune serum, e.g. mouse serum 4–5 days after injecting with 2×10^8 sheep erythrocytes (SRBC)

Method

1   Heat 17 g (dry weight) Sephadex G-200 in about 750 ml PBS in a boiling water bath for 5 h. This will provide sufficient swollen gel for a 100×2.5 cm column. *Swelling the gel by boiling is more rapid than at room temperature and expels the air from the gel.*

2   Cool the gel to the operating temperature. *Generally room temperature is suitable but with labile materials 4° must be used. The gel must be poured and the column run at the same temperature. As gases are more soluble at lower temperatures, bubbles will form in a column poured at 4° and run at room temperature.*

3   De-gas the gel under a vacuum. Air bubbles in the gel will distort the protein bands during the run.

4   Pour the gel into the column along a glass rod to avoid air bubbles. Take great care that the column is vertical. All the gel must be poured into the column at one time. Use an extension tube or reservoir (Appendix II). Leave the column outlet open during packing. A column of 100 cm $\times$ 2.5 cm generally takes about 5 hours to settle.

5   Once the gel has settled, fit the flow adapter.

6   Pack the column by running through at least two column volumes of buffer. The flow rate should be about 20 ml h^{-1}. After packing, lower the flow adapter if required.

If the column tends to pack down after several runs you are probably running the column too fast. If a flow adapter is used, packing after extended use may be avoided by using descending and ascending flow chromatography alternatively.

8   When the column is not in use add thiomersal to a concentration of 0.005% to stop microbial growth. This must be completely flushed out of the column before adding a sample as it absorbs at the same wavelength as protein. Alternatively columns may be run with buffer containing sodium azide 0.01 M. Azide gives less absorption at 280 nm.

Sample application

The gel surface must not be disturbed during sample application as this would cause distortion of the bands. The simplest procedure is to feed the sample through the pump and then through the flow adapter.

163

If an adapter is not available place a nylon net or a layer of G-25 Sephadex (about 5 mm) on top of the gel to protect the surface. Add a little sucrose to the sample to increase its density and layer it gently onto the gel surface below the free buffer, with a long Pasteur pipette.

1   Apply a sample volume of up to 8 ml of serum.
2   Run the column at 20 ml h^{-1}.
3   Collect samples of 2–5 ml.

Distribution of serum proteins in eluted volume

Three major peaks should be eluted as shown in Fig. 7.3.

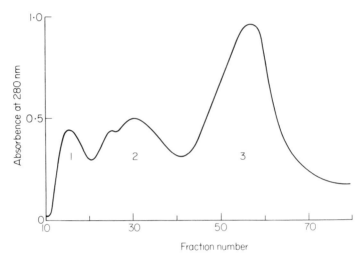

Fig. 7.3. Elution profile of serum proteins from a column of G-200 Sephadex A 5 ml sample of mouse serum was applied to a column of bed volume 100 × 2·5 cm, and the proteins eluted with phosphate buffered saline.

PEAK 1

The first peak contains the macroglobulins, IgM and α2 macro-globulin, plus some lipoproteins. Also on some occasions large haemoglobin–haptoglobin complexes are present. These are easily distinguishable by their reddish brown colour. Some IgA may be found towards the end of the elution of this peak.

PEAK 2

Most of the IgG is in this peak, together with IgA in the first fractions.

PEAK 3

This contains mainly albumin and other small globulins.

Occasionally the first two peaks are not resolved satisfactorily. This is due to weak non-covalent interactions between the IgG molecules causing them to aggregate and so contaminate the first peak. In these cases, run the column in 0·1 M acetate buffer, pH 5·0. Lowering the pH increases the positive charges on the IgG molecules increasing the repulsive forces between them and so preventing aggregation.

Examination of fractions

After concentration each fraction should be examined by agar gel electrophoresis and immunoelectrophoresis with anti-mouse immunoglobulins or anti-mouse serum. Compare your patterns with those in Fig. 7.4.

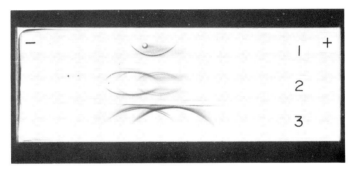

Fig. 7.4. Immunoelectrophoretic analysis of protein peaks eluted from G-200 Sephadex
Sample wells 1–3 contain the eluted peaks 1–3 from Fig. 7.3. The electrophoresed proteins were visualized by precipitation with a rabbit anti-mouse immunoglobulin serum. Identify the proteins in each sample with reference to the figures in Appendix III. (A more detailed analysis would require a longer initial electrophoresis.)

7.2.5   ULTRACENTRIFUGATION

The techniques of analytical and preparative ultracentrifugation have been widely applied in immunochemistry, both for molecular-weight determinations and isolation procedures.

Preparative ultracentrifugation in sucrose density gradients is particularly useful for the isolation of chicken IgM. Chicken IgM cannot be isolated by gel filtration as the IgG forms soluble aggregates very readily and so appears within the excluded fraction of Sephadex G-200 as a major contaminant of the IgM. The difference in size between the IgG dimers and the IgM is still sufficiently great, however, to allow good resolution in the ultracentrifuge.

A detailed treatment of the basic techniques available, for example, rate separation and isopycnic separation, both with and without a density gradient, is beyond the range of this book. (See reference McCall and Potter, 1973 at end of chapter.)

7.2.6   POLYACRYLAMIDE GEL ELECTROPHORESIS IN SDS

In electrophoresis the migration of proteins is dependent on the charge, size and shape of the molecules. However, in the presence of sodium dodecyl sulphate (SDS) proteins all become negatively charged and have similar charge to weight ratios, owing to their binding the negatively charged detergent molecules. When these SDS coated proteins are placed in an electric field, the separation of the proteins will now depend only on their size and shape. By varying the concentration of the polyacrylamide gel, used as the medium for the electrophoresis, different molecular weight ranges may be set up. Proteins may be fractionated in the native state but better resolution is usually obtained if the disulphide bonds are first reduced, allowing separation of the individual peptide chains. After reduction most proteins will take up similar shapes and the resulting separation will be on size alone. There are two exceptions to this behaviour: (a) heavily glycosylated proteins bind less SDS than unglycosylated molecules of similar molecular weight; (b) some proteins such as J chains do not unfold completely and retain some of their native configuration.

Materials and equipment

STOCK SOLUTIONS

(A) 4x Separation gel buffer Tris-HCl buffer, 1·5 M pH 8·8 (Appendix I).
(B) 4x Stacking gel buffer Tris-HCl buffer 0·5 M pH 6·8 (Appendix I).
(C) 10x Electrode buffer Tris-glycine pH 8·3 (Appendix I).
(D) Acrylamide solution; Acrylamide 30 g; NN' methylenebis acrylamide 0·8 g.

Sodium dodecyl sulphate
N,N,N'N'-tetramethylethylene diamine
Aqueous isobutanol
Ammonium persulphate
Methanol
Acetic acid
Coomassie blue
Periodic acid
Schiffs reagent
Sodium metabisulphite
Slab gel apparatus (Appendix II)

166

Method

1   Assemble the slab gel mould with spacer bars and stand vertically in narrow tray.

2   Add 12·5 ml solution A to 13·3 ml solution D and make up to 50 ml with distilled water.

3   Degas the solution under vacuum.

4   Prepare blocking gel by taking 10 ml of this solution and add 3 mg ammonium persulphate and 10 μl TEMED.

5   Use this to block the bottom of the gel mould.

6   After polymerization of the blocking gel, take the remaining 40 ml solution and polymerize with 12 mg ammonium persulphate and 40 μl TEMED.

7   Run into mould to within 3 cm of the top. Seal the top of this separation gel by applying 1 ml of aqueous isobutanol (isobutanol saturated with distilled water). *This ensures that the polymerized gel will have a flat surface.*

8   After polymerization wash off the isobutanol with distilled water.

9   To prepare the stacking gel, add 2·5 ml solution B to 1 ml solution D, make up to 10 ml with distilled water and de-gas under vacuum.

10   Polymerize the gel with 3·0 mg ammonium persulphate and 10 μl TEMED and run onto the top of the separation gel.

11   Insert the plastic comb for forming the sample wells and leave to polymerize for about 15 min.

12   Remove comb and run the gel within 30 minutes.

SAMPLE PREPARATION

Reduced sample—

1   Dialyse the sample into 1 : 4 dilution of solution B. Only 25 μl of sample will be loaded onto the gel but it is convenient to work with larger volumes at the dialysis and reduction stage. To obtain an optimum loading you should aim for 2–20 μg per band.

2   To 100 μl dialysed sample add 40 μl of 10% SDS plus 10 μl 2-mercaptoethanol plus 20 μl glycerol and a trace of bromophenol blue. Make up to 200 μl with distilled water and boil for 3 min.

Unreduced sample—

This is prepared as for the reduced sample but the 2-mercapto-ethanol is replaced with 20 μl of 100 mM iodoacetamide.

167

1   Set up gel apparatus and apply electrode buffer C (diluted 1 to 10) to top and bottom of the plates.
2   Run the samples into the well, 25 μl per well, the samples will sink through the buffer.
3   Turn on the current with the anode at the bottom. Run at 3 W until the bromophenol marker reaches the bottom of the separation gel. (If the gel apparatus has a cooling plate a current of up to 6 W may be used.)

Staining and molecular weight estimation

Proteins (minimum detection limit 1 μg ml^{-1})

1   Fix the gel in a mixture of 40% methanol, 10% acetic acid for 4 h.
2   Stain in 0·1% Coomassie blue in methanol-acetic for 5 h.
3   Destain in 30% methanol, 10% acetic acid for 2 h.
4   Complete the destaining in 10% methanol, 10% acetic acid.
5   Reswell and store in 7% acetic acid.

Carbohydrates (minimum detection limit 5 μg ml^{-1})

1   Fix gel in 40% methanol, 10% acetic acid for 4 h.
2   Reswell in 7% acetic acid.
3   Oxidise in 1% periodic acid in 7% acetic acid for 1 h in the dark.
4   Wash in 7% acetic acid for 24 h, changing the wash several times.
5   Stain with Schiff's reagent at 4° for 1 h in the dark.
6   Differentiate in 1% sodium metabisulphite in 0·1 M hydrochloric acid.

Molecular weight determination

Marker substances must be run to calibrate the gel. Suitable molecules are:
IgG: 150 000
Phosphorylase a: 94 000
Bovine serum albumin: 68 000
IgG heavy chain: 52 000
Aldolase: 40 000
DNAase: 31 000
Chymotrypsinogen: 25 000
RNAase: 14 000
Cytochrome C: 12 500

Plot the mobility of the marker substances relative to the solvent front on a scale of 0 to 1 against the log of the molecular weight.

Unknown substances may then have their molecular weights read off this standard curve.

7.3   **ION EXCHANGE CHROMATOGRAPHY**

Ion exchange chromatography has become one of the most popular methods for the separation of serum proteins and the isolation of immunoglobulin. Proteins are bound electrostatically onto an ion exchange matrix bearing an opposite charge to the proteins. The degree to which a protein binds depends upon its charge density. Proteins are then eluted differentially by:

(a) Increasing the ionic strength of the medium. As the concentration of buffer ions is increased they compete with the proteins for the charged groups on the ion exchanger.

(b) Alteration of the pH. As the pH of the buffer approaches the isoelectric point of each protein, the net charge becomes zero and so the protein no longer binds to the ion exchanger.

Both cation, for example carboxymethyl (CM) cellulose, and anion exchangers, for example diethylaminoethyl (DEAE) cellulose, are available but the latter is used more widely for the fractionation of serum proteins.

Cellulose remains the favoured support for the diethylamino-ethyl group but the physical form of some of the cellulose supports are not ideal for column chromatography. Recently a beaded form of cellulose has been introduced (DEAE-Sephacel). It has good flow characteristics and is supplied pre-swollen and ready for use.

7.3.1   BATCH PREPARATION OF RABBIT IgG WITH
            DEAE CELLULOSE

For preparing IgG alone a batch technique based on the method of Reif, 1969, may be used. The DEAE cellulose is equilibrated under conditions of pH and ionic strength which allow all the serum proteins to bind *except* IgG. The pre-equilibrated serum is simply stirred with the cellulose and the supernatant containing IgG removed. This method, although suitable for rabbit IgG, is not nearly as efficient for human IgG and so a gradient separation will be described for the latter.

Materials

DEAE cellulose—DE52 Whatman (Appendix II)
0·01 M Phosphate buffer, pH 8·0 (Appendix I)
1·0 M HCl

169

Method

EQUILIBRATION OF DEAE CELLULOSE

1   Place 100 g DE52 in a 1 l flask and add 550 ml 0·01 M phosphate buffer, pH 8·0.

2   Titrate the mixture back to pH 8·0 by adding 1·0 M HCl.

3   Leave the slurry to settle for 30 min, then remove the supernatant with any fines it may contain. Resuspend the cellulose in enough phosphate buffer to fill the flask. Repeat this cycle of settling, decantation and resuspension twice more.

4   Pour the slurry into a Buchner funnel containing 2 layers of Whatman No. 1 filter paper. Suck the cellulose 'dry' for 30 sec to leave a damp cake of cellulose.

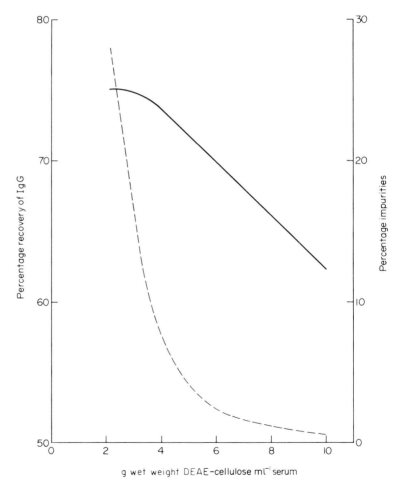

Fig. 7.5. Relationship of purity and yield of IgG to the amount of ion-exchanger used per ml of serum

———— curve of percentage recovery of IgG.

– – – – curve of percentage of impurities.

(After Reif (1969) *Immunochemistry*, **6,** 723.)

170

The degree of purity of the IgG is governed by the ratio of ion exchanger to serum. Fig. 7.5 illustrates the problems involved. For high purity more cellulose is added but this leads to losses of IgG through binding to the ion exchanger. The precise proportions used depends on the purpose for which the IgG is intended. Reasonable purity (about 96%) and good yield (about 70%) are obtained using 5 g (wet weight) cellulose for every ml of serum.

1   Weigh the cellulose into a beaker; for 10 ml serum use 50 g wet weight. Mix the 10 ml serum with 30 ml distilled water, to lower its ionic strength, and add to the cellulose at 4°.
2   To equilibrate stir thoroughly every 10 min for 1 h at 4°.
3   Pour the slurry onto a Buchner funnel and suck through the supernatant containing IgG. Wash the cellulose quickly with three volumes of 20 ml of 0·01 M phosphate buffer, pH 8·0.

The combined effluents contain the IgG.

7.3.2   EXAMINATION OF IgG PREPARATION

1   Determine IgG content of effluent and of original serum by single radial immunodiffusion (Section 5.3.3a) and calculate the yield of IgG.
2   Measure total protein and calculate the percentage purity of IgG.
3   Run immunoelectrophoresis against anti-whole rabbit serum and identify main contaminants.
4   Compare purity and yield with other techniques, e.g. salt fractionation, ionic strength gradient elution from DEAE-cellulose and use of specific anti-IgG immunoadsorbent column (Section 8.1).

7.3.3   COLUMN PREPARATION OF IgG WITH AN IONIC STRENGTH GRADIENT

For maximum yield and purity a column technique using gradient elution is preferred for the preparation of IgG of any species. For human and mouse IgG gradient elution is essential. Initially, buffering conditions are adjusted such that virtually all the serum proteins bind to the ion exchanger. The proteins are then eluted sequentially by gradually raising the ionic strength of the buffer running through the column.

Materials and equipment

Serum sample
DEAE cellulose—DE52 Whatman (Appendix II)

171

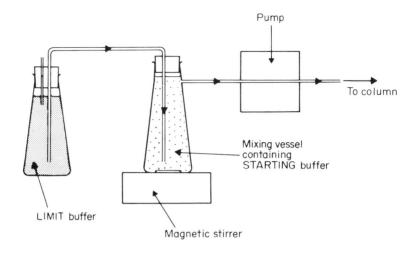

Pump

To column

Mixing vessel
containing
STARTING buffer

LIMIT buffer

Magnetic stirrer

Arrowheads indicate direction of flow

Fig. 7.6. Apparatus for the production of an exponential gradient
When the buffer concentration in the limit vessel is greater than the initial
concentration in the mixing vessel a convex gradient is produced.

Column and fraction collection apparatus (as in Section 7.2.3,
    Fig. 7.2 and Appendix II)
Gradient device (Fig. 7.6 or 7.7)
Conductivity meter
Phosphate buffers, pH 8·0, 0·005 M and 0·3 M (Appendix I)

Method

EQUILIBRATION OF ION EXCHANGER

1   Place the ion exchanger in a beaker—use 2–5 g DE52 for every
1 ml of serum. *This is wet weight as DE52 is pre-swollen.*
2   Add the basic component of the phosphate buffer (0·5 M di-
sodium hydrogen phosphate) until the pH reaches 8·0.
3   Add 0·005 M phosphate buffer, pH 8·0. There should be 6 ml
buffer for every 1 g of wet ion exchanger.
4   Disperse the cellulose and pour into a measuring cylinder and
allow to settle (settling time (min) = 2 × height of the slurry (cm)).
Remove the supernatant which contains cellulose 'fines'; these may
block the column.
5   Add a volume of 0·005 M buffer equal to half the volume of
settled cellulose and disperse.
6   Pour the slurry into the column with the flow control valve
open. (A short wide column is preferable, for example, 25 × 2·5 cm.)
7   Pack the column by pumping 0·005 M, pH 8·0, phosphate buffer
through at 45 ml h^{-1} for each cm^2 internal cross section.

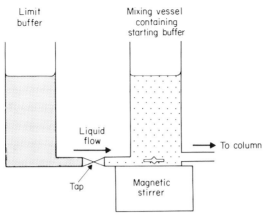

Fig. 7.7a. Formation of a linear gradient using an open mixing vessel
The effective volume of the mixing chamber reduces as the gradient is formed.

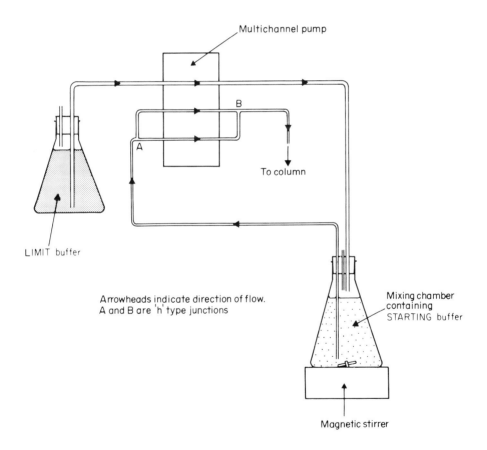

Fig. 7.7b. The production of a linear gradient by means of a multichannel pump
Tubing from B to the column must be of a sufficient internal diameter to take twice the flow rate in the rest of the system.

173

8   Monitor the buffer effluent with a conductivity meter. When the ionic strength of the effluent is that of the original buffer, the ion exchanger is equilibrated. If a meter is not available, pass 2–3 litres of buffer through the column.

RUNNING THE COLUMN

1   Dialyse the sample against the starting buffer (0·005 M, pH 8·0 phosphate buffer) (Section 1.2.3).
2   Centrifuge the sample. (Some protein will precipitate at this low ionic strength.)
3   Apply the serum to the column and pump through the starting buffer (about 60–100 ml h^{-1}). Monitor the effluent for protein.
   Most of the proteins should bind to the ion exchanger. If a high concentration of protein is detected in the effluent:
(a) *the ion exchanger or serum was not fully equilibrated or*
(b) *the absorbing capacity of the cellulose has been exceeded.*
4   Elute the proteins with a gradient of increasing ionic strength (see below). Collect fractions of approximately 5 ml.

IONIC STRENGTH GRADIENT

Gradients of varying shapes are used for different purposes. Devices such as the LKB Ultrograd are capable of forming gradients to the user's specifications (see Figs. 1.1 and 7.8). A simple exponential gradient may be produced as shown in Fig. 7.6. The limit buffer enters the mixing vessel at the same rate as the buffer is pumped onto the column. The gradient is established according to the following equation:

$$C_m = C_1 - (C_1 - C_0)e^{-v/v_m}$$

where C_m = concentration in mixing vessel
       C_1 = concentration in limit vessel
       C_0 = initial concentration in mixing vessel
        v = volume removed from mixing vessel
       v_m = volume of the mixing vessel.

For ease of calculation this equation may be rewritten as:

$$2·303 \log \frac{C_1 - C_m}{C_1 - C_0} = \frac{-v}{v_m}$$

When $C_1 > C_0$ the gradient is convex; when $C_1 < C_0$ the gradient is concave. (Latter used for density gradient centrifugation, NOT ion exchange chromatography.)

   Linear gradients may be established using an open mixing vessel (Fig. 7.7a) or by means of a multichannel pump as shown in Fig. 7.7b. In this case the equation for the gradient is:

$$C_m = C_0 + (C_1 - C_0) \cdot \frac{v}{2v_0}$$

174

where $v_0 =$ initial volume of buffer in the mixing vessel. Other symbols as in equation for exponential gradient.

Distribution of serum proteins (Fig. 7.8)

Assuming that the ion exchanger has not been overloaded with protein, the first peak should contain only IgG. This is the only pure protein that can be isolated under these conditions of pH and buffer molarity, the remaining peaks contain several proteins. Beta lipoproteins, haptoglobin and $\alpha 2$ macroglobulin will contaminate the IgA and IgM fractions.

Experiments on fractionated proteins

Carry out a similar examination of the fractions to that in Section 7.3.1. Use the purified IgG in the examination of the structure of the molecule given later in this chapter (Section 7.6). Compare the purity of protein obtained from column versus batch techniques.

7.3.4   CLASS EXPERIMENTS WITH ION EXCHANGERS

A. The conditions described for batch elution may be used in a simple experiment for class preparation of IgG.

Materials and equipment

DEAE cellulose, DE52 Whatman (Appendix II)
2 ml rabbit anti-HSA (Sections 1.2.2d and 1.4.6)
Phosphate buffer, 0.01 M, pH 8.0 (Appendix I)
10 ml plastic syringe barrels
Sintered plastic discs (Appendix II) or glass wool
10% trichloracetic acid (TCA) in water
G-25 Sephadex column (Section 1.2.3)

Preparation required

Equilibrate the ion exchanger against 0.01 M, pH 8.0 phosphate buffer (Section 7.3.1) and pack in 10 ml syringe barrels (up to the 10 ml mark), fitted with a sintered plastic disc or glass wool.

Protocol

1   Equilibrate the Sephadex G-25 column with the 0.01 M, pH 8.0 phosphate buffer.
2   Equilibrate the serum sample by passing it down the Sephadex column (Section 1.2.3).

175

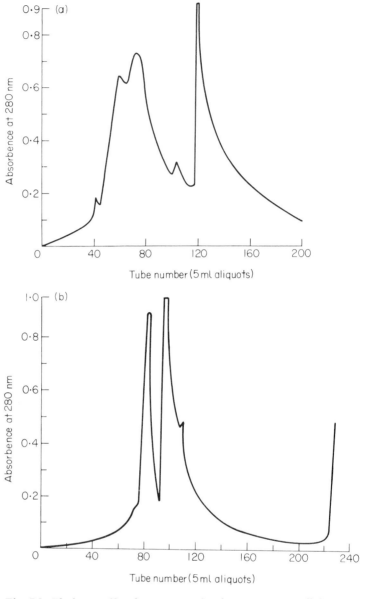

Fig. 7.8. Elution profile of serum proteins from a DEAE cellulose column using a gradient of increasing ionic strength

a) A sample of 30 ml of mouse serum, equilibrated with 0·005 M, pH 8·0 phosphate buffer, was applied to a column of DEAE cellulose (bed volume 25 × 3·3 cm) equilibrated in the same buffer. Elution was by means of a convex gradient, limit buffer 0·18 M, pH 8·0 phosphate buffer, volume of mixing vessel 110 ml.

b) Using a device to establish discontinuous gradients, such as the Ultrograd (see Fig. 1.1) it is possible to resolve the first major peak into its two major components. The first is IgG_1 alone and the second contains the other IgG sub-classes.

176

3 Add the equilibrated serum sample to the DEAE-cellulose and wash through with phosphate buffer.

4 Monitor every 5th drop of effluent for protein by collecting it into 0·5 ml TCA solution.

5 Collect the effluent as soon as a white precipitate forms in the TCA test.

6 Continue to monitor the effluent during collection, until no more precipitation occurs.

The IgG may be tested for purity and compared to the original serum as suggested in Section 7.3.1.

B. Determine the conditions for batch preparations of an unknown IgG molecule (e.g. rabbit).

Materials

DEAE-cellulose—DE52 Whatman (Appendix II)
Phosphate buffers as details in table below
Serum sample

Phosphate buffer:	1	2	3	4	5
pH	4·0	6·5	8·0	8·0	8·0
molarity	0·01	0·01	0·01	0·1	0·5

Preparation required

Equilibrate aliquots of DEAE cellulose and of serum with the buffers of different pH and ionic strength. (Table above.)

Protocol

1 Add 1 ml of equilibrated serum to 3 ml packed DEAE-cellulose equilibrated with the same buffer.

2 Mix for 10 min.

3 Centrifuge and test supernatant for IgG and for impurities by immunoelectrophoresis (Section 5.3.4b). Also check the yield of IgG by single radial immunodiffusion (Section 5.3.3a).

7.3.5   QAE-SEPHADEX ISOLATION OF IgG

Quaternary aminoethyl Sephadex is a strongly basic anion exchanger which is particularly suitable for the column separation of proteins using pH gradient elution as the swelling of QAE-Sephadex is not affected by changes in pH. IgG may be prepared and freeze dried directly using a volatile buffer which enables freeze drying to be performed without prior salt removal. It is advisable to remove β-lipoproteins from the serum before chromatography, otherwise they may break through and contaminate the IgG.

Materials

Human serum
Aerosil (Appendix II)
Diamino ethane-acetic acid buffer, ionic strength 0·1, pH 7·0 (Appendix I)
Acetic acid-sodium acetate buffer, ionic strength 0·1, pH 4·0 (Appendix I)
QAE-Sephadex A50 (Appendix II)
Column and fraction collection apparatus (as in Section 7.2.3, Fig. 7.2 and Appendix II)
Sodium hydroxide 1 M
Aquacide (Appendix II)
Dialysis tubing (Appendix II)
Centrifuge capable of 12 000 g

Method

1 Swell QAE-Sephadex A50 in the diamino ethane-acetic acid buffer. A bed volume of 20 ml of swollen gel is required per 10 ml serum.
2 Pack the gel into a suitable chromatography column and equilibrate with the diamino ethane-acetic acid buffer.
3 Remove β-lipoprotein from the serum by adding 0·2 g Aerosil to 10 ml serum and stir at room temperature for 4 h.
4 Centrifuge the serum at 12 000 g for 30 min and remove the lipid layer.
5 Equilibrate the serum with the diamino ethane-acetic acid buffer by dialysis.
6 Dilute the equilibrated serum with an equal volume of diamino ethane-acetic acid buffer.
7 Apply the sample to the column at a flow rate of 8 ml cm^{-2} h^{-1} and continue the elution with the diamino ethane-acetic acid buffer. *IgG will come straight through the column while other proteins will be retained.*
8 Elute the other proteins with the acetate buffer pH 4·0.
9 Regenerate the column by running through two bed volumes of diamino ethane-acetic acid buffer.
10 Concentrate the IgG in the first peak 10 fold as quickly as possible by placing in a dialysis bag and covering with Aquacide.
11 The concentrated sample may now be freeze dried without removing salt as the buffer is volatile.

178

Technical notes

1   It is important to concentrate the sample prior to lyophilization otherwise an insoluble precipitate may form.
2   The yield of IgG should be about 70% of the serum IgG.

7.4   PREPARATIVE ELECTROPHORESIS

A 'scaled-up' version of the analytical electrophoresis technique (Section 5.3.4a) may be used preparatively. It is especially useful for resolving molecules of similar size, but different charge, for example IgM and α-2 macroglobulin, which elute together from Sephadex G-200 (Section 7.2.4). In cases of multiple myeloma there is often so much of the single monoclonal immunoglobulin that preparative electrophoresis alone will give an isolation of high purity.

The serum proteins separate into bands as shown in the analytical electrophoresis technique, Section 5.3.4a.

7.4.1   PEVIKON BLOCK ELECTROPHORESIS

The support matrix for electrophoresis must be inert. In the past starch gels were used but they produced a carbohydrate contamination of the proteins and so have been replaced by the plastic Pevikon (copolymer of polyvinyl chloride and polyvinyl acetate).

Avoid inhalation of the dry resin, some batches may contain the highly carcinogenic vinyl chloride monomer.

Materials and equipment

Pevikon C870 (Appendix II)
Bromophenol blue dye (Appendix II)
Serum sample—either peak 1 from G-200 (Section 7.2.4) or a myeloma serum (Appendix II)
Barbitone buffer, pH 8·2, ionic strength 0·08 (Appendix I)
Phosphate buffered saline (PBS) (Appendix I)
Electrophoresis tray—plastic, approximately 22 cm × 11 cm × 1 cm.
Electrophoresis tank and power pack (Appendix II)
Sintered glass funnel and Buchner flask
Filter paper, Whatman 3 MM (Appendix II)

Method

1   Soak the Pevikon in several changes of half strength barbitone buffer and remove the finely dispersed Pevikon from the supernatant.

2   Place the filter paper wicks at either end of the electrophoresis tray and place the tray on several sheets of absorbent paper.

3   Allow the Pevikon to settle for the last time and remove the supernatant.

4   Pour the thick slurry into the tray. The surplus buffer will flow into the absorbent paper.

5   Blot the surface of the gel with filter paper to remove the excess buffer and then smooth the gel surface with a spatula.

6   Cut a trough (about 8 cm long) for the sample, about one-third the distance from the cathodal end of the gel. Use the long edge of a microscope slide.

7   Add a trace of bromophenol blue dye to a 3·0 ml sample of the serum. *This will bind to the albumin and act as a marker (Section 5.3.4a). If no albumin is present the free dye will move anodically at a greater rate.*

8   Mix the sample with a little dry Pevikon to absorb the serum and prevent the sample spreading excessively during application.

9   Apply the sample to the trough with a wide Pasteur pipette.

10   Push together the edges of the trough if required.

11   Electrophorese the block for approximately 20 hours at 4° (the lower temperature reduces the heating effect in the gel). Use a voltage drop of 3–4 volts cm^{-1}.

12   When the stained albumin band approaches the edge of the tray, stop the electrophoresis. If the free dye is used as a marker, apply the current until the dye has left the tray.

7.4.2   ELUTION OF PROTEIN BANDS

Slice the resin into 1 cm wide blocks and elute in one of the following ways:

(a) Place each block in turn on the sintered glass funnel and wash with 2 aliquots of 3 ml PBS. Suck the buffer into a test tube standing in a Buchner flask.

(b) Place each block in a centrifuge tube and mix with 6 ml of PBS. Centrifuge and remove the supernatant.

Fig. 7.9 (facing). Pevikon block electrophoresis of serum proteins
(a) Preparative electrophoresis of human IgM myeloma serum. The IgM is at a much greater concentration than in normal serum and so this single electrophoretic isolation yields reasonably pure IgM. The high background is due to UV absorption by the barbitone buffer.
(b) Separation of IgM and α2 macroglobulin. These two proteins are of similar molecular size and shape and so elute together from G-200 Sephadex. It is therefore necessary to separate the two proteins on the basis of their charge difference. In this case the samples have been dialysed against three changes of phosphate buffered saline before determining the protein content spectrophotometrically. Fractions 7–9 were combined and were found to contain only IgM on immunoelectrophoresis. Fractions 12–15 contained α2 macroglobulin.
Sample (b) derived from Fig. 7.3, peak 1.

180

7.4.3   ESTIMATION OF PROTEIN YIELD

Barbitone absorbs at the same UV wavelength as protein (280 nm) so each sample must be dialysed against PBS before the protein content can be determined.

Plot a graph of the protein content against the fraction number. A typical separation of an IgM myeloma serum is shown in Fig. 7.9a. Fig. 7.9b shows the separation of IgM and α-2 macroglobulin from the Sephadex G-200 elution peak 1 (Section 7.2.4). It should be

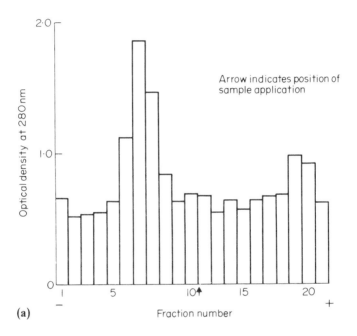

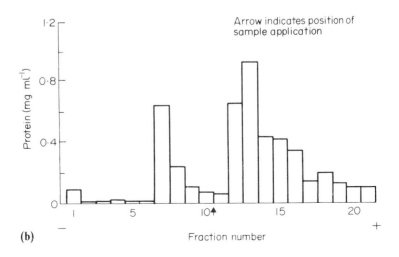

181

noted that the electroendosmotic flow is lower with Pevikon compared to agar and so the banding more closely resembles the separation in agarose.

7.5   ISOELECTRIC FOCUSING

A mixture of proteins may be resolved into fractions of differing charge by their differential migration in an electric field (Section 5.3.4a). If this electric field is applied across a continuous pH gradient, then the proteins will move to, and concentrate at their isoelectric point, i.e. the pH at which their net charge is zero. Unlike ordinary electrophoresis at a single pH, the protein is concentrated to a very narrow band while the electric current is applied.

In isoelectric focusing a protein purified to a single peak by molecular sieving and ion-exchange chromatography may be resolved into several bands. Indeed, the product of a single lymphocyte clone, e.g. a myeloma protein, usually separates into 2–5 bands because of post-synthetic changes in the molecule (see Fig. 7.10). The major post-synthetic change involves the hydrolysis of amide residues by serum enzymes to carboxyl groups, thus gaining one negative charge for each deamidation.

7.5.1   pH GRADIENT

The pH gradient is established using a mixture of carrier ampholytes. These molecules have a 'backbone' on which varying numbers of NH_3^+ and COO^- groups are attached. Under an electric field the ampholyte molecules migrate to their various isoelectric points and produce an ascending pH gradient from the anode to the cathode. Different mixtures of ampholytes are available commercially for different ranges of pH gradient (see Appendix II).

7.5.2   PREPARATIVE ISOELECTRIC FOCUSING

On a preparative scale the pH gradient can be established in a column containing a sucrose density gradient. For general, low resolution fractionation, a pH gradient of 3·0–10·0 is used, whereas for high resolution of immunoglobulin a narrower pH gradient of 5·0–8·0 or 7·0–10·0 is preferable. Because of the danger of protein denaturation by anodic oxidation or cathodic reduction, it is an advantage to apply the protein sample at the centre of the column.

Fig. 7.10a (facing). Serum isoelectric spectra: thin-layer polyacrylamide gel electrofocusing (5% gel, pH range 5–10) (Courtesy of Jan Obel)

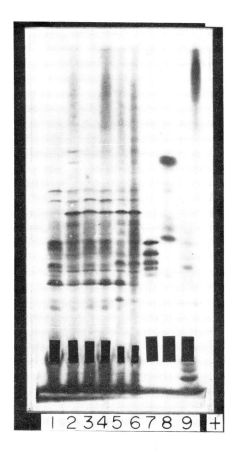

Fig. 7.10a (cont.) Samples were loaded on filter paper strips of various size depending on the loading volume. After focusing, the plate was stained with Coomassie brilliant blue dye.

Samples 1–6: Serum samples from individual mice challenged with an antigen of very few antigenic determinants. Under these conditions, it is possible to limit the number of different lymphocyte clones stimulated and so an analysis of the resulting antibody is possible in terms of its isoelectric spectrum. The migration of two antibodies from two different mice to the same position in the same pH gradient may be used as a criterion of clonal identity. This has been used, for example, to determine the frequency with which a single clone repeats within a population of mice.

It should be noted in this case we are comparing proteins alone as no method has been used to demonstrate antibody activity in any of the observed bands (cf. section on identification of antibody, Section 7.5.3).

Samples 7–9: Myeloma proteins isolated by DEAE-cellulose chromatography. Each sample was eluted as a single peak.

Sample 7: IgG_{2a} myeloma. The five bands probably result from a single clone of plasma cells and so the sample is probably of a single antibody specificity. The spectrum of pI values results from the post-synthetic changes after secretion into the serum.

Sample 8: IgG_{2b} myeloma. This preparation has at least three major contaminants.

Sample 9: IgA myeloma, partially purified. This protein is more basic and so has migrated towards the anode. To resolve this sample satisfactorily it would be necessary to use a lower pH range.

183

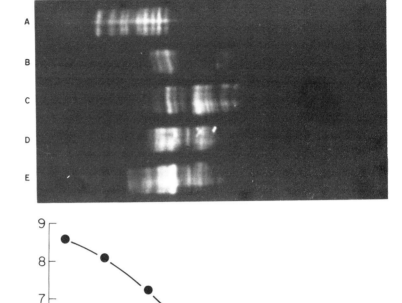

Fig. 7.10b. Isoelectric spectrum of anti-DNP antibodies from CBA/J mice
Sera from X-irradiated CBA/J mice receiving column fractionated spleen
cells (as in Section 8.2.4) were focused (Section 7.5.3) and then treated with
[125]I labelled DNP-HOP-lysine. Antigen binding bands were detected by
autoradiography with X-ray film. (Courtesy of Andrew Brown.)

After focusing the fractions are recovered by running the sucrose
out of the bottom of the column through a UV cell. This must be
done immediately the electric field has been turned off to prevent
diffusion of the bands.

7.5.3 ANALYTICAL ISOELECTRIC FOCUSING

For the resolution of small samples of protein the pH gradient may
be stabilized by polyacrylamide or Sephadex gel. Although we will
describe the usual technique using a polyacrylamide gel, it is often
an advantage to use Sephadex gel for small-scale preparative
isoelectric focusing. Sufficient quantities of purified protein may be
eluted from slices of the gel for immunization (see Radola, 1969.
Reference at end of chapter).

Materials and equipment

Sample: IgG isolated by ion exchange chromatography (Section 7.3.3) and Bence Jones proteins (Section 7.1.1).

Stock solutions for gel:

(1) N,N,N′,N′–tetramethylethylene diamine 5% v/v

(2) Acrylamide 100 g ⎫
    N,N′–bismethylacrylamide 3 g ⎭ to 300 ml with water

(3) Riboflavin 2 mg in 100 ml water

Stock subbing solutions:

Ilford No. 1 gelatine powder 5% w/v

Potassium chromium sulphate 1% w/v

Ampholine, pH range 3–10 (Appendix II)

Ethylene diamine 5% v/v.

Phosphoric acid 5% v/v.

Staining and destaining solutions as in Section 5.3.3a.

Glass plates 7.5×15 cm (as in Fig. 7.11) (Appendix II)

Electrophoresis tank (described below)

Power pack (500 volts)

Filter paper, Whatman 3 MM (Appendix II)

Method

CONSTRUCTION OF ELECTROPHORESIS TANK

This may be built from a plastic box with an airtight lid. The type sold for refrigerator storage is suitable. Mount carbon rod electrodes in this box, either attaching them to one side or resting them on perspex supports. Platinum wire should connect these electrodes to terminals on the box. To maintain humid conditions, plastic sponge is attached to the lid and base.

Well designed apparatus for this technique is now available from commercial sources (Appendix II).

PREPARATION OF THE GEL

The gel may be prepared by chemical polymerization using ammonium persulphate but photopolymerization with riboflavin is preferable as this avoids the risk of artifacts resulting from the action of persulphate on the sample.

For a 7.5×15 cm gel about 10 ml of solution is required:

1 Mix 0.05 ml stock solution (1) with 1.5 ml solution (2) plus 0.5 ml of 40% Ampholine carrier ampholytes and make up to 10 ml with water.

2 De-gas the mixture with a vacuum pump until bubbling ceases.

3 Add 1 ml of solution (3). Briefly gas solution with CO_2 until pH is 6.5. *This is required because of the instability of riboflavin at a higher pH.*

4 Cast the gel immediately.

1   Dip the isoelectrofocusing plate in the 0·1% gelatine 'subbing' solution with potassium chromium sulphate 0·01% and air dry.
2   Siliconize the second plate and attach the polythene tubing.
3   Assemble the mould as in Fig. 7.11.
4   Pipette 10 ml of gel mixture into the mould and expose to UV light for 2–3 h to polymerize the gel. (This must be done in a humid atmosphere.)
5   Prise away the siliconized plate and store the gel in a humid box at 4° until use. (Cast gels may be stored in this way for 2–3 weeks.)

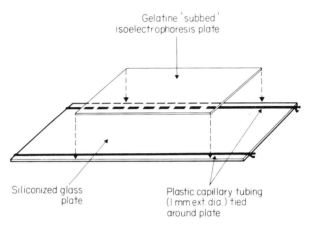

Gelatine 'subbed' isoelectrophoresis plate

Siliconized glass plate

Plastic capillary tubing (1 mm ext. dia.) tied around plate

Fig. 7.11. Mould for casting thin-layer polyacrylamide gels
Run the 'gel solution' between the glass plates and after photopolymerization remove the siliconized plate with a scapel blade.

SAMPLE APPLICATION

1   Pipette about 10 μl of sample (10–20 mg ml^{-1}) onto Whatman 3 MM paper, 10 mm × 5 mm.
2   Place the paper on the gel surface towards the anodal end. Leave the paper in place during the electrofocusing. Several samples may be placed on the gel at the same time (as in Fig. 7.10a).

E. ELECTROFOCUSING

1   Wet the cathode rod with 5% v/v solution of ethylene diamine and the anode rod with 5% v/v phosphoric acid. Remember to maintain the same polarity in all future runs. (The strong acid and base prevent the ampholytes from approaching the electrodes.)
2   Turn the gel plate upside down (gel underneath) and place onto the electrodes.
3   Moisten the plastic sponges to maintain humidity, close the lid and place the box at 4°.

186

4 Apply the current. The maximum power per plate must not exceed 500 mW to avoid excessive heating and distortion of the gel. As the pH gradient is established the current will fall and so the voltage may be increased.

Running voltages for above plate (use constant voltage setting on power pack) (see Table below)

Time (hours)	Voltage (Volts)	Corresponding Current (m Amps)
0–4	150	3
4–overnight	250–300	1·5–2
last 3 hours	500	< 1

Examination of the gel

Measurement of pH gradient:

1 Remove 5 mm discs of gel with a sharp cork borer at close intervals along the plate.
2 Disperse each disc in 1 ml freshly distilled water for 2 hours.
3 Measure the pH with a microelectrode.
Flat membrane electrodes are available for pH determination directly on the gel (Radiometer, Copenhagen).

Staining the protein bands

Most protein stains are unsuitable as they bind to the ampholytes as well as the proteins. The following procedure is suitable without ampholyte removal.

1 Immerse the gel in the Coomassie brilliant blue staining solution for 30 min (see Section 5.3.3a).
2 Differentiate in the destaining solution until the background is clear.
3 For a permanent record the gel may be dried onto the glass plate with a hair drier.

Interpretation of results

The major difficulty with this technique is the embarrassing number of protein bands resolved, even with so-called 'purified' proteins. The IgG from normal serum will give so many lines that any real interpretation is impossible, except to give some idea of the heterogeneity of immunoglobulins.

The Bence Jones proteins should be more restricted. If the previous isolation has been thorough about 3 or 4 bands should be seen. When myeloma proteins or free light chains are isolated from within the tumour cells a single molecular species can be seen. After

187

contact with serum for just 1 hour, post synthetic modifications occur, as mentioned earlier, producing the multiple bands resolved by isoelectric focusing (see Fig. 7.10a).

Identification of antibody

Haptens may be presented to animals so as to stimulate only a small number of lymphocyte clones and elicit a more homogeneous antibody response than 'normal' antigens. If the haptens are radio-actively labelled it is possible to detect individual species of anti-body molecules by autoradiography combined with isoelectric focusing. When sera are focused on the same plate it is possible to identify common clonal products between individual mouse sera (Figure 7.10b).

Note

Because of their size, IgM molecules are not included in the polyacrylamide gels and so cannot be analysed by the system described. This is not, however, a problem with preparative isoelectric focusing using a sucrose density gradient. The tendency for these large molecules to precipitate at their isoelectric point may be overcome by using 6 M urea in the medium. LKB have now introduced a new agarose isoelectrofocusing gel which may be used for intact IgM.

7.6   **STRUCTURE OF IMMUNOGLOBULIN MOLECULES**

Although the techniques described in this section provide valuable research tools, historically they were used to elucidate the basic structure of immunoglobulin molecules.

7.6.1   REDUCTION OF IgG TO HEAVY AND LIGHT CHAINS

Use the IgG prepared by ion-exchange chromatography (Section 7.3.1 or 7.3.3).

Materials and equipment

IgG
Tris-hydrochloric acid buffer, 0·15 M, pH 8·2 (Appendix I)
2-mercaptoethanol
Iodoacetamide
Propionic acid, 1 M

Sodium hydroxide 0·1 M
Nitrogen cylinder
Methyl cellulose or polyethylene glycol 40 000
G-100 Sephadex column, equilibrated with 1 M propionic acid at 4°
Dialysis tubing

Method

1   Dialyse the IgG sample against Tris-HCl buffer (Section 1.2.3) and adjust the protein concentration to 30 mg ml^{-1}.

2   De-gas the IgG solution with a water vacuum pump and then bubble in nitrogen.

3   Add 2-mercaptoethanol to a final concentration of 0·1 M. 2-mercaptoethanol is toxic and so this procedure must be carried out in a fume cupboard. *The solution is de-gassed and the reduction carried out in the presence of nitrogen as 2-mercaptoethanol is oxidized by atmospheric oxygen. Alternatively, reduction may be carried out with 0·02 M dithiothreitol which is less susceptible to oxidation. Again this agent is dangerous and will cause a severe headache if inhaled.*

4   Incubate at room temperature for 1 hour.

To prevent reassociation of the reduced interchain S–S bonds when the reducing agent is removed, they are alkylated with iodoacetamide.

5   Add iodoacetamide to a final concentration of 0·12 M and maintain the pH at 8·0 for 1 h by the dropwise addition of sodium hydroxide.

6   Concentrate the sample in dialysis tubing against methyl cellulose or polyethylene glycol 40 000, to the original protein concentration.

7   Apply the sample to the G-100 Sephadex column equilibrated with 1 M propionic acid at 4° (see Section 1.2.3) and collect fractions of 5 ml.

A typical elution profile is shown in Fig. 7.12.

Identification of peaks

1   Collect both peaks and calculate recovery.

2   Concentrate the recovered samples to 1 mg ml^{-1} and dialyse overnight against phosphate buffered saline.

3   Analyse each peak by Ouchterlony immunodiffusion (Section 5.3.3b) using anti-light chain and anti-IgG Fc antisera. (Commercial antisera—Appendix II.)

Expected results

If the reduction, alkylation and column fractionation are successful the first peak eluted should react with the anti-IgG serum alone, and the second peak with the anti-light chain serum alone. Thus the

189

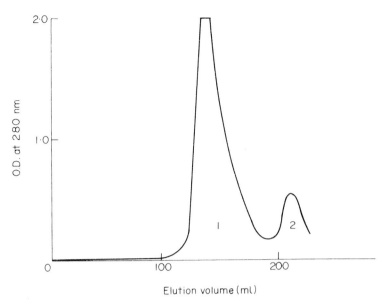

Fig. 7.12. Elution profile of reduced and alkylated IgG from a Sephadex G-100 column

The reduction of the molecule achieved under the conditions described is only partial, i.e. not all of the S–S bonds are broken. The intrachain S–S bonds in each V and C region domain can only be reduced after unfolding the IgG molecule in 8 M urea or 5 M guanidine.

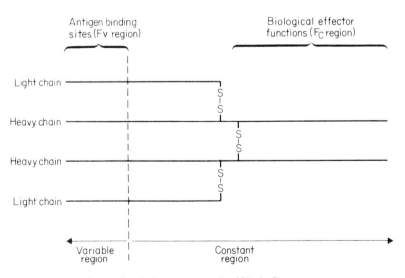

Fig. 7.13. Polypeptide chain structure of rabbit IgG

The interchain disulphide bonds are broken by reduction in 2-mercapto-ethanol yielding two heavy (H) and two light (L) chains per IgG molecule.

The variable region consists of three hypervariable stretches of amino acids interspersed with more conservative sequences, and is responsible for antigen binding. The biological effector functions controlled by the Fc region include complement fixation, placental passage and skin and cell fixation.

190

protein peaks may be identified as heavy (H) and light (L) immuno-globulin chains respectively. However, separation of the two chains may not be complete and the eluted sample may be contaminated with H–L chain intermediates.

The two types of chains obtained by reduction of IgG are called heavy and light simply on the basis of their molecular weight; rabbit heavy and light chains have values of 50 000 to 53 000 and 22 000 to 25 000 respectively. The molecular weight of rabbit IgG is 150 000 and it is composed of two heavy and two light chains as shown in Fig. 7.13.

The heavy- and light-chain preparations may be used to immun-ize rabbits as in Section 1.4. The properties of these antisera will be discussed in Section 7.6.2.

Technical note

Store the heavy- and light-chain fractions at physiological pH and ionic strength, preferably at $-20°$. The light chains should be com-pletely soluble but the heavy chains may precipitate.

7.6.2   DETECTION OF LIGHT- AND HEAVY-CHAIN DETERMINANTS ON IMMUNOGLOBULINS

Reduction of the IgG molecule resulted in the production of heavy and light chains. The antisera made against each chain should be absorbed with the other type of chain to render it specific.

If the other immunoglobulin classes are similarly treated with sulphydryl reducing reagents they are also split into heavy and light chains. Using specific antisera or by amino acid sequencing it can be shown that all the classes share similar light chains but have unique heavy chains.

Materials

Anti-light chain
Anti-γ heavy chain
IgG, IgA, IgM (each at 1 mg ml^{-1}) (Appendix II, if required)
IgG heavy and light chains (1 mg ml^{-1})
Ouchterlony immunodiffusion equipment (Section 5.3.3b)

Method

1   Pour an agar slide and punch the pattern in Fig. 7.14.
2   Fill the wells as in Fig. 7.14.
3   After incubating overnight at room temperature wash and stain the slide (Section 5.3.3a) to detect any weak reactions.

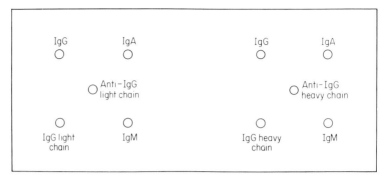

Fig. 7.14. Design of immunodiffusion slide to demonstrate the relationship of the heavy and light chains of the major immunoglobulin classes

Interpretation of results

The anti-light chain serum should react with all classes showing that the light chains are similar. But the anti-γ heavy chains will react solely with the IgG and the type of heavy chain against which it was made. This demonstrates that each class of immunoglobulin has a specific type of heavy chain. There are, in fact, two types of light chain, κ and λ, but either type may be associated with each H chain class.

7.7 CLEAVAGE OF IgG BY PROTEOLYTIC ENZYMES

For half a century it was known that antibody may be cleaved into active and inactive fragments by digestion with pepsin and papain. The significance of these observations for antibody structure was realized by Porter in 1958 in experiments similar to those described below using rabbit IgG.

7.7.1 PAPAIN DIGESTION

Materials and equipment

IgG fraction of rabbit or mouse anti-HSA (prepared in Section 7.3.4 by ion-exchange chromatography)
Papain (Appendix II)
Cysteine
Ethylene diamine tetra-acetic acid, Na$_2$ salt (EDTA)
0·5 M, pH 8·0 phosphate buffer (Appendix 1)
DEAE-cellulose column equilibrated with 0·005 M, pH 8·0 phosphate buffer

Method

A. MOUSE IgG

1   Adjust the concentration of the IgG to 20 mg ml^{-1} in phosphate buffer. Add cysteine and EDTA to a final concentration of 0·01 M and 0·002 M respectively.
2   Add 1 mg of papain for every 100 mg IgG used.
3   Incubate at 37° for 4 hours.
4   Dialyse the digest against 0·005 M, pH 8·0 phosphate buffer.

When the cysteine and EDTA are removed by dialysis, the enzyme is inactivated. At this stage crystals might be formed. Spin these off and keep for later examination.

5   Apply the dialysate to the DEAE-cellulose column and fraction-ate with a gradient of increasing ionic strength (starting buffer 0·005 M, pH 8·0 phosphate; limit buffer 0·3 M, pH 8·0 phosphate) as in Section 7.3.3. Collect and concentrate each peak.

A typical elution profile is shown in Fig. 7.15.

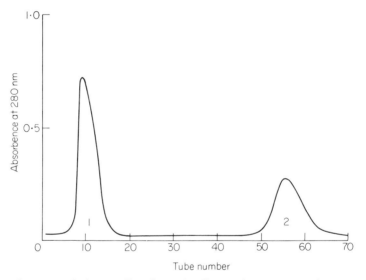

Fig. 7.15. Elution profile of papain digest of mouse IgG from DEAE-cellulose
Sample equilibrated in 0·005 M, pH 8·0 phosphate buffer and applied to a DEAE-cellulose column equilibrated in the same buffer. Elution with linear gradient, limit buffer 0·2 M, pH 8·0 phosphate buffer.

B. RABBIT IgG

Rabbit IgG is digested under the same conditions as mouse IgG but a different separation technique is required.

1   Following digestion for 4 hours, dialyse the sample against 0·01 M sodium acetate buffer pH 5·5. Spin off any crystals which form.

193

2   Apply the dialysate to a carboxymethyl-cellulose (CM-cellulose) column. *This column is prepared as for DEAE-cellulose (Section 7.3) but the cellulose is pre-equilibrated with 0·01 M sodium acetate buffer.*
3   Run the column with 200 ml of 0·01 M sodium acetate buffer, pH 5·5.
4   Apply a gradient of increasing ionic strength (starting buffer 0·01 M sodium acetate, pH 5·5; limit buffer 0·9 M sodium acetate, pH 5·5), as in Section 7.3.3. Collect and concentrate each peak. *The first two peaks contain Fab, while the third smaller peak contains the Fc. On dialysing the concentrated samples against phosphate buffered saline, crystals of the Fc fragment will appear.*

C. HUMAN IgG

Human IgG is also digested under the same conditions as mouse IgG but purification of the Fab and Fc is relatively more complex using ion-exchange techniques. It is much easier to take advantage of the IgG binding property of staphylococcal protein A. Protein A binds to IgG molecules through their Fc regions and has no affinity for Fab. As protein A does not bind IgG3, the IgG preparation should be protein A purified before digestion (Section 8.5.2).

Materials

Sephadex G150 (Appendix II)
Chromatography column and fraction collection apparatus (as in Section 7.2.3, Fig. 7.2 and Appendix II).
Aquacide (Appendix II)
Protein A-Sepharose CL 4B (Appendix II)
Phosphate buffered saline (PBS) (Appendix I)
1·0 M Sodium hydroxide
0·1 M Glycine-HCl buffer, pH 2·8 (Appendix I)

Method

1   Prepare a G150 Sephadex column equilibrated with PBS (Section 7.2.3).
2   Pass the dialysed digest through the column and collect fractions.
3   Any undigested IgG will come through in the breakthrough volume. The Fab and Fc will come later in one peak.
4   Concentrate the Fab/Fc peak to the pre gel filtration volume by placing in a dialysis bag and covering with Aquacide.
5   Set up a protein A-Sepharose 4B column as in Section 7.6.2.
6   Apply the Fab/Fc peak to this column and wash through with PBS. *The capacity of the column for binding Fc is 8 mg ml^{-1} of swollen gel.*
7   Collect the Fab which comes straight through the column.
8   Elute the bound Fc with glycine-HCl buffer pH 2·8.

9   Titrate the pH of the purified Fc to near neutrality with NaOH and then dialyse against PBS.

10   Regenerate the column by running through 2 column volumes of PBS. Store the column at 4°.

Technical note

The binding of IgG to protein A involves tyrosine residues on the protein A. Therefore the Fc may be eluted by passing glycosyl tyrosine down the column (Section 7.6.2).

Examination of fragments

1 CRYSTALS FORMED DURING DIGESTION

Porter identified a fragment of rabbit IgG which crystallized but had no antibody activity. This was called the Fc fragment. However, using mouse IgG it is likely that the crystals will be formed by cystine.

Dissolve the crystals in a minimum volume of PBS and check for the presence of Fc by Ouchterlony immunodiffusion (Section 5.3.3.b) using an antiserum to rabbit immunoglobulin. If Fc is present retain the original sample for examination in next section.

2 ELUATE FROM DEAE-CELLULOSE

If enzyme digestion has not gone to completion the second peak from DEAE-cellulose will be contaminated with the whole IgG molecules. You may quantitate this undigested IgG by a precipitin curve using HSA as described in Section 5.3.1.

If IgG is present in the second DEAE-cellulose peak, as shown by precipitation, it can be removed by fractionation on G-100 Sephadex equilibrated with phosphate buffered saline. The whole IgG will leave the column first, followed by a protein peak which is able to combine with antigen but will not cause precipitation. This is known as the Fab fragment.

Immunological analysis of the fragments

Compare the undigested IgG, Fab and Fc by immunoelectrophoresis using an antiserum raised to rabbit total immunoglobulin. (IgG-specific antisera sold commercially usually react only with the Fc fragment.)

The IgG molecule and fragments will be observed in the order Fab, IgG, Fc, cathode to anode (Fig. 7.16).

195

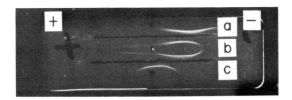

Fig. 7.16. Immunoelectrophoresis of fractions from DEAE-cellulose chromatography of papain digest of mouse IgG
Sample a. Peak 1, DEAE-cellulose. Fab.
Sample b. Original IgG.
Sample c. Peak 2, DEAE-cellulose. Fc.
The proteins were visualized by precipitation with rabbit anti-mouse whole IgG. (Photograph of unstained preparation.)

Antibody activity of the fragments

The ability of the IgG fragments to bind antigen may be tested by inhibition of precipitation of HSA by the original IgG fraction of the anti-HSA serum.

1   Determine the equivalence precipitation of IgG anti-HSA with HSA (Section 5.3.1).

2   Attempt to inhibit the precipitation at equivalence by adding an equal concentration of either fragment before addition of the whole IgG. This will test the antigen-binding capacity of the fragments independently of their ability to cause precipitation (cf. Section 5.3.2).

Additional class experiments

1   Small quantities of Fab and Fc can be separated by Pevikon block electrophoresis (Section 7.4.1) and so a large-scale digestion and fractionation may be avoided.

2   The progress of digestion may be monitored by electrophoresis, showing the disappearance of the IgG molecule and the appearance of the Fab and Fc fragments. Remove samples from the digestion mixture at 0, 10, 30 min and at 4 h and electrophorese as described in Section 5.3.4a. (Keep samples on ice and electrophorese after 4 h sample collected.)

7.7.2   PEPSIN DIGESTION

Historically, pepsin digestion of IgG was found to yield a molecule with two-thirds the molecular weight of the original molecule and with intact antigen-binding activity. This is the $F(ab')_2$ fragment. The other one-third of the IgG molecule was digested into smaller polypeptide chains, without antibody activity.

Materials and equipment

IgG fraction of rabbit anti-HSA (prepared in Section 7.3.4 by ion-exchange chromatography)
Pepsin (Appendix II)
0·1 M sodium acetate
Phosphate buffered saline (PBS) (Appendix I)
Acetic acid glacial
G-100 Sephadex column equilibrated with PBS

Method

1　Adjust the IgG solution to 20 mg ml^{-1} and dialyse 10 ml against 0·1 M sodium acetate for 3 hours.
2　Adjust the pH of the dialysate to 4·5 with acetic acid.
3　Add 2 mg of pepsin for each 100 mg of IgG used.
4　Incubate at 37° overnight.
5　Centrifuge and discard any precipitate that may form. Adjust the pH of the supernatant to 7·4 and dialyse against PBS. This inactivates the enzyme.

Analysis and isolation of fragments

1　ISOLATION OF F(ab')$_2$

Apply the digest to a G-100 Sephadex column equilibrated with PBS. A typical elution profile is shown in Fig. 7.17.

Examine activity of peaks 1 and 2 only. Peak 3 contains Fab', peak 4 pFc' (see below) and peak 5 contains small polypeptides.
(a) Investigate the ability of proteins in peaks 1 and 2 to precipitate HSA. Use the equivalence conditions determined in Section 5.3.1.
(b) Resuspend an equivalence precipitate (2 mg approximately) of each precipitating peak with albumin in 1·0 ml of 0·15 M Tris-HCl,

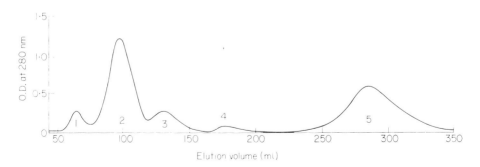

Fig. 7.17. Elution profile of IgG pepsin digest from G-100 Sephadex
A 2 ml sample of digest (20 mg ml^{-1}) was applied to a column of Sephadex G-100 (Bed volume 90 × 2·5 cm) equilibrated with phosphate buffered saline.

pH 8·2 (Appendix I) and add 10 μl of 2-mercaptoethanol. Observe the dissolution of the precipitate.

(c) Perform immunoelectrophoresis on the protein in peak 2 and on the precipitate dissociated with 2-mercaptoethanol (in (b) above) using an antiserum to rabbit immunoglobulin (Fig. 7.18).

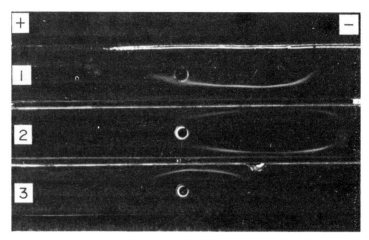

Fig. 7.18. Immunoelectrophoresis of G-100 Sephadex fractions of IgG pepsin digest
Well 1: Human IgG before digestion.
Well 2: G-100 Sephadex fraction 2—$F(ab')_2$.
Well 3: G-100 Sephadex fraction 4—pFc′.
Samples were visualized after electrophoresis by precipitation with rabbit anti-human immunoglobulin. (Photograph of unstained preparation.)

In Section 10.1.3 we will investigate the ability of a peptic digest of an anti-sheep erythrocyte preparation to agglutinate erythrocytes and to fix complement. In addition, you should test the ability of the $F(ab')_2$ to form cytophilic rosettes with macrophages, as in Section 6.5.1.

As well as producing $F(ab')_2$, pepsin digestion of IgG gives a small polypeptide, of 27 000 molecule weight, called pFc′. This corresponds to the last homology region, C_H3, at the C-terminal end of the molecule. The fragment includes the C_H3 regions from both heavy chains, held together with non-covalent forces. The intra-chain disulphide bond is intact and the molecule appears to maintain its normal tertiary structure as the biological property of binding to macrophages can be demonstrated with isolated pFc′.

Conclusion from analysis of peptic fragments

Peak 1 (Fig. 7.17) contains undigested IgG with intact antibody activity (see also Section 7.7.1). Peak 2 contains the $F(ab')_2$ fragment which retains the ability to bind antigen to form insoluble precipitates. Accordingly, the $F(ab')_2$ molecule must be divalent, i.e.

it has two combining sites. On reduction with 2-mercaptoethanol (Section 7.6.1), the $F(ab')_2$ is split into 2 Fab′ molecules by reduction of the interchain disulphide bonds.

7.8   SUMMARY AND CONCLUSIONS

7.8.1   ISOLATION OF IMMUNOGLOBULINS

In this chapter we have described the basic techniques available for fractionating immunoglobulin molecules. Many refinements of these techniques are possible, for example in the mouse and human, subclasses of the IgA and IgG classes have been recognized and isolated, particularly in cases of multiple myelomatosis. Further, using isoelectric focusing, it is now possible to solve the age-old problem of heterogeneity of antibody; here the products of single antibody-producing cell clones may be identified and isolated.

Although very high sample purity may be obtained, it is important to remember that the degree of protein denaturation increases with the number of manipulations. Thus many properties may be attributed to the final purified sample that are simply artifacts induced by denaturation during preparation.

When isolating immunoglobulins it is advantageous to combine several different fractionation methods rather than recycling the sample. For example, IgM may be prepared by gel filtration followed by electrophoresis, and IgG may be prepared by combining salt fractionation with ion exchange chromatography. It is obvious that a 'two dimensional' separation on charge and size has a greater resolving power than either technique alone.

7.8.2   STRUCTURE OF IgG

The structure of the IgG molecule and its digest fragments is shown in Fig. 7.19.

7.8.3   STRUCTURE OF IgM

Mammalian IgM has a pentameric structure and each of the five sub-units consists of two heavy and two light chains (see Fig. 7.20). The μ heavy chains are rather longer than the γ heavy chains having one extra homology region. The subunits are linked together covalently through disulphide bonds between the heavy chains. J chain is involved in the polymer formation. This chain has a molecular weight of about 25 000 and is rich in cysteine. It is always found associated with polymeric inmunoglobulins, both IgM and IgA, but never with monomeric immunoglobulins.

199

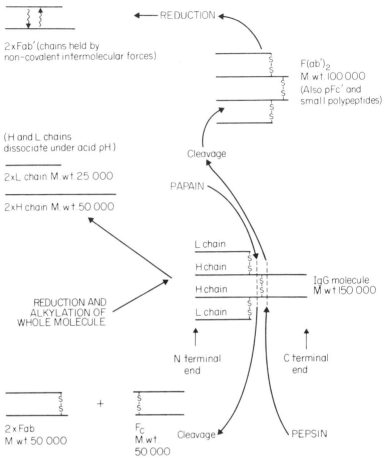

Fig. 7.19. Summary diagram of the structure of rabbit IgG and its reduction and enzymic cleavage products
Depending on the conditions under which cleavage takes place, it is possible to obtain similar fragments with trypsin, chymotrypsin and thermolysin.

7.8.4   STRUCTURE OF IgA

7S IgA molecules are found in serum but it is in secretions that IgA predominates. This secretory IgA is predominantly a dimer of 7S subunits (Fig. 7.21). J chain is associated with this dimer. A further chain, the secretory component (M.W. 58 000) is also present attached by both covalent and non-covalent forces. This secretory component is produced in a separate cell from the plasma cell producing the IgA and is added later during secretion. The function of secretory component is to transport IgA across the epithelial cells layer at external or internal body surfaces. It may also protect IgA from proteolytic enzymes in the gut.

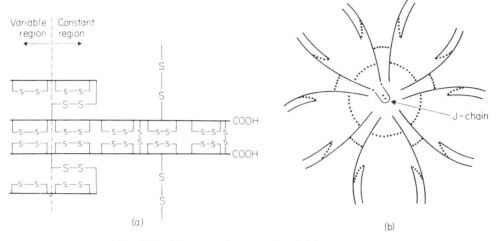

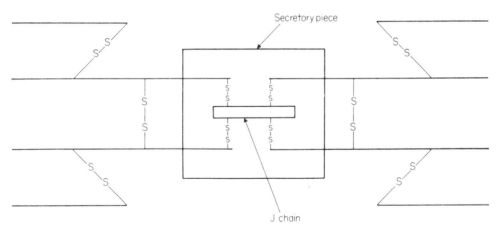

Fig. 7.20. Diagram of mammalian IgM

(a) Monomer—showing S–S bonds between monomers and H and L chains, as well as the intrachain S–S bonds associated with the V and C region domains.

(b) IgM pentamer—although it would appear from the diagram that the full IgM molecule should have 10 antigen-combining sites, in fact one of each pair is often blocked by steric hindrance when combining with large antigens.

...... di-sulphide bonds.

Fig. 7.21. Polypeptide chain structure of mammalian IgA (Dimer)

FURTHER READING

ALLEN R.C. & MAURER H.R. (1974) *Electrophoresis and Isoelectric Focusing in Polyacrylamide Gel.* W. de Gruyter, Berlin.

DETERMAN H. (1969) *Gel Chromatography* 2e. Springer-Verlag, Berlin.

FISCHER L. (1971) *An Introduction to Gel Chromatography.* North-Holland, Amsterdam.

KABAT E.A. (1976) Structural concepts in immunology and immuno-chemistry, 2e. Holt, Rinehart & Winston, New York.

McCALL J.S. & POTTER B.J. (1973) *Ultracentrifugation.* Bailliere Tindall, London.

MILSTEIN C. & PINK J.R.L. (1970) Structure and evolution of immuno-globulins. *Progr. Biophys. Mol. Biol.* **21,** 211.

Pharmacia Fine Chemicals (1978) *Gel filtration theory and practice.* Pharmacia Fine Chemicals, Uppsala.

RADOLA B.J. (1969) Thin-layer Isoelectric Focusing of Proteins. *Biochim. biophys. Acta* **24,** 61.

RIGHETTI P.G. & DRYSDALE J.W. (1974) Isoelectric focusing in gels. *J. Chromatogr.* **98,** 271.

STANWORTH D.R. (1973) Ultracentrifugation of Immunoglobulins. In D.M. Weir (ed.) *Handbook of Experimental Immunology,* 2e. Blackwell Scientific Publications, Oxford.

STANWORTH D.R. & TURNER M.W. (1978) Immunochemical analysis of immunoglobulins and their subunits. In D.M. Weir (ed.) *Handbook of Experimental Immunology* 3e, 6. Blackwell Scientific Publications, Oxford.

202

8 Affinity chromatography

PURIFICATION OF ANTIBODIES

As we know from Chapter 5 an antibody reacts specifically with its own *antigenic determinant* to form an antigen–antibody complex.

If an animal is immunized with an antigen it will respond with antibodies all reacting with the antigen to some degree. Serum from this animal will have the usual range of immunoglobulins but those reacting with this antigen will be at a relatively higher concentration, compared to normal serum.

To study a particular antibody in detail it is of great advantage to be able to separate it from the surrounding, non-specific antibody molecules. The precipitated antigen–antibody complex has already done this for us! Unfortunately, the antibody in combination with its antigen has already completed the interesting reactions before we could follow them.

We must separate the complex, remove the antigen and we will then have purified antibody in a reactive state.

The forces binding antibody to antigen are those involved in any protein–protein interaction:

1   Coulombic
2   Dipole
3   Hydrogen bonding
4   van der Waals
5   Hydrophobic bonding

All these forces depend on the charge of the molecules taking part in the reaction; the net charge of the molecules in turn depends on the pH of the medium. If the pH of the medium is lowered sufficiently the protein molecules change conformation, gain H^+ ions and so repel each other. We are now faced with the problem of physically removing the antigen or the antibody, because when the pH is returned to neutrality the complexes would re-form.

If the antigen is *insoluble* it can be removed easily.

There are many methods available for rendering either the antigen or antibody insoluble, some of which are described in the following sections. The antigen in its insoluble form is known as the IMMUNOADSORBENT and the whole purification process is AFFINITY CHROMATOGRAPHY.

PREPARATION OF IMMUNOADSORBENT

In this experiment antibodies to mouse immunoglobulin are purified but the identical method can be used for other proteins.

Materials and equipment

Sepharose 4B (Appendix II)
Cyanogen bromide (THIS CHEMICAL IS VERY TOXIC AND **MUST** BE HANDLED IN A FUME CUPBOARD)
2·0 M sodium hydroxide
Phosphate buffered saline (PBS) (Appendix I)
Borate saline buffer, pH 8·3, ionic strength 0·1 (Appendix I)
Mouse immunoglobulin (Section 1.2.2c)

Method

1   Pipette 14 ml of Sepharose (about 200 mg) into a 50 ml glass beaker and add 10 ml of distilled water.

ALL PROCEDURES MUST NOW BE CARRIED OUT IN A FUME CUPBOARD

2   Weigh a stoppered tube, add some solid cyanogen bromide, replace the stopper and re-weigh the tube.
3   Dissolve the cyanogen bromide in distilled water to a final concentration of 50 mg ml^{-1}.
4   Place the Sepharose beads on a magnetic stirrer and titrate the pH to 11·0–11·5 with 2·0 M NaOH.
5   Add 10 ml of the cyanogen bromide solution (USE A PIPETTE SAFETY BULB).
6   Maintain the pH at 11·0–11·5 by dropwise addition of sodium hydroxide for 5–10 min until the pH becomes stable.
7   Wash the activated beads on a sintered glass funnel with 100 ml of water, and then 100 ml of borate buffered saline.
8   Wash the beads into a glass beaker, allow them to settle and remove the supernatant.
9   Add 100 mg of mouse immunoglobulin at 5–10 mg ml^{-1} (initial concentration).
10   Leave the beads stirring with the protein overnight at 4° (*most of the uptake occurs within the first 4 hours and so this stage can be abbreviated*).
11   Wash the beads on a sintered glass funnel with 10 ml PBS and collect the washings. (Use negative pressure and collect washings in a tube standing in a side arm flask.)
12   Wash the beads thoroughly with PBS to remove the rest of the unbound immunoglobulin.

13   A UV spectrophotometer reading of the washings will give the amount of unbound protein and so the approximate quantity of protein bound to the column can be calculated.

The immunoadsorbent is now ready. Store in PBS containing azide (0·1 M)

Technical note

In step 6, wash the gel with borate saline buffer as soon as the pH becomes stable. The rate of inactivation by hydrolysis is highly pH dependent.

8.1.2   USE OF IMMUNOADSORBENT FOR ANTIBODY PURIFICATION

Materials and equipment

Rabbit anti-mouse immunoglobulin (Section 1.4.2)
Immunoadsorbent—mouse Ig on Sepharose 4B (Section 8.1.1)
Glycine-HCl buffer, 0·1 M, pH 2·5 (Appendix I)
Trichloracetic acid, 10% aqueous solution (TCA)
Tris (hydroxymethyl) aminomethane
Phosphate buffered saline (PBS) (Appendix I)
Chromatography column (Appendix II)

Method

1   Pour the immunoadsorbent into the column and equilibrate with 20 ml PBS. Close the column.
2   Run 20 ml of antiserum through the column—do not use positive pressure—allow it to run under 1 *g*.
3   Wash the unbound protein from the column. If a Uvicord or similar flow-through UV cell is available, wash the column until the absorbance is <0·1 (see Fig. 8.1), otherwise wash with 200 ml PBS. Close the column.

We now have the antigen–antibody complex.

Dissociation of complex

1   Pipette out twenty 0·5 ml aliquots of TCA into small glass tubes. (*Use this to sample the effluent for protein during elution if a flow-through UV cell is not available.*)
2   Add glycine-HCl buffer to the top of the column and collect the effluent when protein is first detected.
3   Stop collecting the effluent when protein is no longer detectable.

The first stage of the elution is now complete and part of the anti-body has been recovered. The low pH will, however, eventually denature the antibody so we must raise the pH.

205

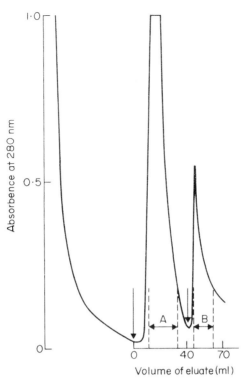

Fig. 8.1. Elution of antibody from an immunoadsorbent with glycine–HCl buffer

The unbound protein was washed away with phosphate buffered saline until the absorbance at 280 nm was below 0·1%. A first population of antibody molecules was eluted with 0·1 M, pH 2·5 glycine–HCl buffer (first arrow). When elution was complete a second population of antibody was eluted off with the same buffer containing 10% dioxane (this second elution was started at the second arrow). To reduce the total sample volume only the volumes A and B were collected.

4   Titrate the protein solution to pH 8·5 with solid Tris. Mix thoroughly and monitor with a pH meter or indicator papers.

We are now going to alter the elution conditions to recover a second batch of antibody.

5   Add glycine-HCl + 10% dioxane to the column. Monitor the effluent and collect the second batch of antibody.

6   Adjust the pH to 8·5 with solid Tris.

7   Read the absorbance of each protein solution at 280 nm and calculate the recovered protein. (*Remember to use the correct reference solution for the spectrophotometer!*)

8   Concentrate the samples in dialysis tubing against either sucrose or polyethylene glycol 40000 or by negative pressure dialysis (Fig. 8.2).

9   When the sample volume has been reduced to 3–5 ml, dialyse against 5×1 l PBS.

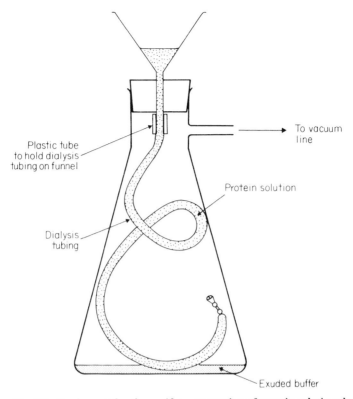

To vacuum line

Plastic tube to hold dialysis tubing on funnel

Protein solution

Dialysis tubing

Exuded buffer

Fig. 8.2. Equipment for the rapid concentration of protein solutions by negative pressure dialysis
It is advisable to test the system for leaks using phosphate buffered saline before adding the protein solution to the dialysis tubing.

10   Spin off the precipitate and determine the protein content of each sample.

This method of antibody purification is highly reproducible and so it is not necessary to calculate the antibody content of the sample routinely. However, a specimen calculation is given below.

8.1.3   CALCULATION OF RECOVERY FROM IMMUNOADSORBENT

Total weight of immunoglobulin on column = 92·0 mg on 200 mg of Sepharose 4B.

Volume of antiserum for antibody purification = 10 ml.
Antibody content of serum calculated from Fig. 8.3, at equivalence conditions as in Section 5.3.1:
Antibody content of serum = 5·2 mg ml^{-1}.

% yield of antibody from serum:
immediately 81·5%
after concentration and dialysis 47·8%

| | Total protein concentration in eluate | |
Eluant	immediately	after concentration and dialysis
Glycine-HCl	36·4 mg ⎱ 42·4 mg	23·0 mg ⎱ 25·0 mg
Glycine-HCl + 10% dioxane	6·0 mg ⎰	2·0 mg ⎰

Calculation of antibody content of eluate

From Fig. 8.3: Weight of antibody in 200 μg of eluted protein
= 490 – 160
= 230 μg.

Hence all the recovered protein has retained antibody activity. (In general, at least 90% of the recovered protein should be antibody.)

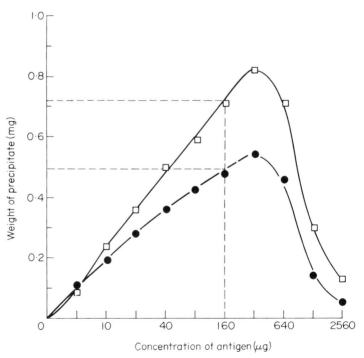

Fig. 8.3. Precipitin curves of anti-immunoglobulin antiserum and antibody
□———□ 0·1 ml of original serum.
●———● 200 μg of purified antibody.

208

Antibodies with high affinity antigen binding sites are the essential constituents of a 'strong', high titre antiserum. However, when these antibodies are linked to Sepharose and used as solid phase immunoadsorbents they give virtually irreversible binding to antigen.

It is rarely possible, therefore, to isolate antigen or antibody by true affinity methods, simply because a sufficiently high concentration of free competitor cannot be obtained to compete effectively with the solid phase reagents.

Most techniques for the release of material from antibody affinity columns rely on deforming agents to alter the shape of the reacting molecules and so lower their net binding affinity. Acid buffers are usually sufficient to release an acceptable proportion of bound material, most of which will regain full activity when a near neutral pH is restored. The addition of dioxan to an acid buffer will increase yield from an affinity column (by reducing hydrophobic interactions) with little additional loss of recovered material due to irreversible denaturation.

Other, more effective eluting buffers may be used. These are more effective because they deform (and denature) to a greater extent. In order of increasing harshness they are:

1   3·5 M potassium thiocyanate in 0·1 M, phosphate buffer, pH 6·6 (Appendix I).
2   8·0 M urea.
3   7·0 M guanidine hydrochloride.

Although these reagents will release bound material more effectively, they may produce an unacceptably high proportion of denatured material.

When using anti-immunoglobulin affinity columns to isolate a particularly valuable antibody, for example, a monoclonal antibody produced by a hybridoma cell line (Chapter 11), it is usual to saturate high affinity anti-immunoglobulin sites by a cycle of pretreatment with normal mouse immunoglobulin and acid elution (Section 11.8.3).

Technical notes

1   Under the conditions described, the Sepharose should bind 90–100 mg of mouse immunoglobulin. Approximately the same uptake can be expected with other common protein antigens, with the notable exception of bovine serum albumin where only 20–30 mg are bound.

2   Although the proportion of antibody in the final sample is fairly constant, the actual yield of antibody relative to the serum concentration varies with serum pool and species. The greatest loss of antibody occurs due to denaturation and precipitation after elution, concentration and dialysis. (See also Section 8.1.4.)

3   In this experiment the immunoadsorbent has been used below its maximal capacity; in general it should be able to deplete 1 ml of antiserum for each mg of antigen on the column.

4   Pre-activated Sepharose is available commercially (Appendix II) this avoids the use of cyanogen bromide. For large-scale preparations, however, it is relatively expensive.

8.1.5   PRACTICAL APPLICATIONS OF IMMUNOADSORBENTS

Besides their use for isolation of pure antibodies, immunoadsorbents are widely used to render antisera specific by depletion of cross-reacting antibodies (Section 1.6.6), and for quantitative adsorption (Section 9.1).

Although the method described used an antigen immunoadsorbent to isolate antibody, it is possible to prepare antigen or immunoglobulin by the same procedure using an antibody immunoadsorbent column (Section 11.8.3) or a cellular immunoadsorbent column (Section 11.8.2).

8.2   **AFFINITY CHROMATOGRAPHY OF LYMPHOID CELLS**

Cells can be isolated on the basis of any reactive molecules expressed on their surface membrane. These molecules can either be (a) specific receptors, for example antigen receptors, or (b) antigens, for example immunoglobulin molecules (which are also receptors), histocompatibility or blood-group antigens, etc.

In the first, and simplest, system we will describe cells are adsorbed to the immunoadsorbent on the basis of their membrane content of immunoglobulin, however, these cells cannot be recovered and so we must work with the normal versus the depleted population. In the second system these cells may be recovered but in a slightly altered form; this is explained in Section 8.2.2.

8.2.1   B CELL DEPLETION FOR T CELL ENRICHMENT

A. Anti-immunoglobulin columns

Materials and equipment

5 g Degalan V_{26} plastic beads (Appendix II)
0·1 M phosphate buffer, pH 6·4 (Appendix I)
Phosphate buffered saline (PBS) (Appendix I)
10 mg purified rabbit anti-mouse immunoglobulin antibodies (Section 8.1)

Method

1   Wash 5 g of Degalan beads with distilled water, and then equilibrate with 30 ml phosphate buffer. Suck beads dry.

2   Add 10 mg purified antibody (initial concentration 5 mg ml^{-1}).

3   Incubate at 45° for 2 h then at 4° overnight.

4   Recover unbound antibody and calculate amount adsorbed to beads as in Section 8.1.1.

Control column

Many cells passing down a column of protein coated onto plastic beads will stick non-specifically because of the strong non-covalent intermolecular forces at the surface of the bead. Hence retention of the cells will not only be related to the antiserum on the column. As a control for non-specific retention of cells a column of an irrelevant antibody, for example, anti-Keyhole Limpet haemocyanin must be prepared and used in an identical manner to that described for the anti-immunoglobulin column.

Cell fractionation

Materials and equipment

Mouse spleen or lymph-node cells
Two 20 ml plastic syringe barrels
Sintered plastic discs for columns (Appendix II)
Tissue culture medium containing 5% fetal bovine serum and
    EDTA, 5 mM (All components are required)
Degalan beads coated with (a) anti-Ig and (b) an unrelated antibody

Method

1   Pour the coated plastic beads into the syringe barrels fitted with sintered plastic discs and equilibrate each with 30 ml of medium.

2   Seal off the column with a needle and rubber bung.

3   Incubate the column at 37° for 30 min.

4   Incubate at 4° for 30 min before use.

5   Prepare a single-cell suspension of mouse spleen or lymph-node cells (Section 2.4.1) and deplete of phagocytic cells (Section 1.7.4). Wash in medium and adjust to 10^7 lymphocytes ml^{-1}.

6   Pipette 1 ml of lymphocytes onto each column.

7   Allow the cells to enter and re-seal column.

8   Add 1 ml of medium to the column, allow it to enter the column.

Under the conditions described the anti-Ig column will be able to deplete 10 aliquots of lymphocytes. The depleted population may be collected either as individual aliquots or as a pool.

211

9   After the last aliquot of cells, wash the column through with 15 ml of medium. Collect effluent.

10   Concentrate the effluent cells by centrifugation and count in a haemocytometer.

This is the basic fractionation procedure. To determine the change in fractionated cells perform some or all of the following experiments:

1   Calculate percentage recoveries from anti-Ig and control columns.

2   Stain an aliquot of original and anti-Ig and control column effluent cells with anti-immunoglobulin (Section 2.5.1). Calculate the % of B cells in the original population and also calculate the % recovery of B cells in the anti-Ig and control column effluent populations.

3   Fractionate rat or mouse lymphocytes and inject original and fractionated cells into F_1 or neonatal recipients respectively for 'g.v.h.' assay (Section 3.2.3).

Technical notes

1   The high non-specific retention by these columns can be minimized by a high-flow rate. At a flow rate of 2–3 ml min^{-1} about 20–30% non-specific loss may be expected.

2   All cell fractionation procedures must be carried out at 4°.

3   T-lymphocytes prepared by this technique may be contaminated by a variable proportion of null cells (see Fig. 2.1).

B.   Nylon wool columns

Spleen cell suspensions may be fractionated on the basis of their differential adherence to nylon fibres. At 37° and in the presence of serum, B lymphocytes will bind avidly to nylon wool columns, giving an effluent population of virtually pure T-lymphocytes and 'null' cells.

The technique has the obvious advantages of speed, convenience and low cost.

Materials and equipment

Nylon wool, sterile (Appendix II)
Tissue culture medium (Appendix I)
   containing 5% fetal bovine serum (FBS)
Syringe, 20 ml, plastic, sterile.

212

Method

1   Pack 600 mg of sterile nylon wool (approximately 6 ml) into a 20 ml syringe barrel and wash with tissue culture medium containing 5% FBS.

2   Seal the column and incubate at 37° for 1 h.

3   Prepare cells (as in Section 2.4.1), deplete of phagocytic cells (Section 1.7.4) and adjust to 5×10^7 lymphocytes ml^{-1}.

4   Flush column with 5 ml of warm tissue culture medium. (*This will correct any change in pH during incubation.*)

5   Add 2 ml of cell suspension dropwise to the top of the column. After it has all entered, add 1 ml of warm tissue culture medium.

6   Seal the column and incubate at 37° for 45 min.

7   Wash the column with 25 ml of warm tissue culture medium and collect the unbound cells in the effluent. Concentrate by centrifugation (150 *g* for 10 min at 4°) and determine the number of viable lymphocytes.

The effluent population should be depleted of B-lymphocytes, as evidenced by anti-immunoglobulin immunofluorescence (Section 2.5.1), and will consist of T lymphocytes and 'null' cells (see Fig. 2.1).

A proportion of the bound cells may be recovered by mechanical elution as follows:

1   Wash the column with 100 ml of warm tissue culture medium and discard the effluent.

2   Seal the column with a needle and rubber bung.

3   Add 2 ml of warm tissue culture medium and squeeze the nylon wool with blunt stainless steel forceps.

4   Unseal the column and wash with 10 ml of warm tissue culture medium. Finally replace the syringe piston and expel all the tissue culture medium.

5   Collect the effluent cells and concentrate by centrifugation (150 *g* for 10 min at 4°).

6   Count number of viable lymphocytes ml^{-1} (Section 2.4).

The cells recovered by mechanical elution will consist of B lymphocytes (as evidenced by anti-immunoglobulin immunofluorescence—Section 2.5.1) contaminated with a variable number of T lymphocytes and 'null' cells.

8.2.2   ANTIGEN-SPECIFIC CELL DEPLETION AND ENRICHMENT

In the previous section cells were fractioned on the basis of their membrane content of immunoglobulin, i.e. into T and B cells. Because of the nature of the immunoadsorbent, the enriched B cells cannot be recovered in a viable state.

In this section we will describe a technique by which the column matrix may be solubilized and the cells released. The technique as

213

described is used for the fractionation of antigen reactive lymphocytes, however, an identical technique may be used for the preparation of T and B cells. (Though, of course, anti-Ig antibodies must be substituted for antigen.)

8.2.3   PREPARATION OF ANTIGEN
IMMUNOADSORBENT

Materials

Sephadex G-200 (Appendix II)
Cyanogen bromide
0·2 M sodium hydroxide
Phosphate buffered saline (PBS) (Appendix I)
Borate saline buffer, pH 8·3, ionic strength 0·1 (Appendix 1)
DNP-human serum albumin (HSA) (Section 1.3.1)

Method

1   Swell the Sephadex G-200 in water containing sodium azide or in PBS and remove the 'fines' by settling six times in 2 litres of water.
2   Pipette 40 ml of packed Sephadex G-200 into a 150 ml beaker and add 8 ml of water.

ALL FURTHER STEPS MUST BE CARRIED OUT IN
A FUME CUPBOARD

3   Prepare a 50 mg ml^{-1} solution of cyanogen bromide (see Section 8.1.1).
4   Adjust the pH of the Sephadex to 10·5 with 0·2 M sodium hydroxide and add 2 ml of cyanogen bromide solution. (USE A PIPETTE BULB.)
5   Maintain the pH of the Sephadex at 10·5 for 7 min by dropwise addition of sodium hydroxide.
6   Wash the activated Sephadex with 100 ml of water and then 100 ml of borate saline buffer. (Use sintered glass funnel. DO NOT use negative pressure.)
7   Allow the Sephadex to settle and remove the supernatant.
8   Add 20 mg of DNP–HSA (in solution at 2·5 mg ml^{-1}) and mix for 4 h at room temperature.
9   Wash away the unbound protein with PBS and store immunoadsorbent at 4° with 0·1 M sodium azide.

Use of immunoadsorbent

Previous preparation
    Prime 5 inbred mice with 400 μg DNP–FγG on alum with *B. pertussis* (Section 10.1) 2–3 months before use.

Materials and equipment

DNP–FγG primed mice
DNP–HSA immunoadsorbent (Section 8.2.3)
Tissue culture medium (Appendix I) containing 5% fetal bovine serum and EDTA (5 mM).
Dextranase enzyme (Appendix II)
20 ml plastic syringe barrel
Sintered plastic disc for column (Appendix II)

Method

1   Pour 10 ml (packed volume) of immunoadsorbent into syringe barrel fitted with a sintered plastic disc.

2   Equilibrate the immunoadsorbent with 20 ml of medium and incubate at 37° for 30 min.

3   Transfer immunoadsorbent to a 4° cold room for 30 min before use.

4   Prepare a spleen-cell suspension from the immunized mice (Sections 1.7.3 and 2.4), remove active phagocytic cells (Section 1.7.4) and wash 3 times in medium.

5   Count and adjust the cell suspension to 10^7 viable lymphocytes ml^{-1}.

6   Add 10 aliquots of 10^7 lymphocytes to the column as in Section 8.2.1; collect the effluent as a pool (DNP depleted cells).

7   Add a further 10 aliquots of 10^7 lymphocytes to the column. Do not collect the effluent cells.

8   Finally wash the column with 20 ml of medium and seal the column.

9   Add 500 IU dextranase enzyme to the immunoadsorbent and incubate at 37° for 30 min, with shaking.

The immunoadsorbent should digest completely in this time, however, digestion may be extended for a further 30 min if required.

10   Unseal the column and collect the digest. (DNP 'enriched' cells.)

11   Wash all the cells in tissue culture medium (WITHOUT fetal bovine serum or EDTA) and count in a haemocytometer.

12   Calculate the percentage cell recovery for depleted (effluent) and enriched (digest) fractions.

8.2.4   DETERMINATION OF ANTIGEN REACTIVE CELLS IN DEPLETED AND ENRICHED POPULATIONS

We will assay the number of DNP plaque-forming cells in each population to estimate the approximate number of DNP reactive precursor lymphocytes.

215

Materials

X-irradiated mice (Section 1.8.3)
Cells from previous experiment
Mice primed to KLH (Section 1.5)
DNP on FγG and KLH (Section 1.3)

Method

1 X-irradiate the recipient mice (850 R) and reconstitute them according to the protocol below.

Protocol

Group no.	Cells primed to	Fractionation	Number of cells transferred per X-irradiated recipient	Antigen challenge (10 μg soluble antigen)
1	DNP–FγG	none	5 × 10⁶	DNP–FγG
2 (a)	DNP–FγG	none	(a) 5 × 10⁶	
	+		+	DNP–KLH
(b)	KLH	none	(b) 5 × 10⁶	
3	DNP–FγG	DNP depleted	5 × 10⁶	DNP–FγG
4	DNP–FγG	DNP enriched	*	DNP–FγG
5 (a)	DNP–FγG	DNP enriched	(a) *	
	+			DNP–KLH
(b)	KLH	none	(b) 5 × 10⁶	
6	KLH	none	5 × 10⁶	DNP–KLH

$$* \text{ The number of cells per recipient} = \frac{\text{total number recovered from digest.}}{\text{total number of recipients}}$$

Notes on protocol

1 The design of the protocol has been abbreviated from our own experience. Normally groups 1 and 2 would be replaced by a titration curve of transferred cells e.g. 2×10^5, 2×10^6, 2×10^7 and 2×10^8, to determine the dose response curve.

2 Group 4 may be omitted. T cells are not bound by these columns and so the B cells alone will not respond (cf. Section 10.1).

The design of the protocol will be appreciated more fully when Section 10.1 has been covered.

3 Challenge each group with 10 μg soluble antigen intraperitoneally as shown in protocol.

4 Assay each group of mice 7 days later for DNP plaque-forming cells as in Section 10.1.

5 Calculate the percentage depletion and enrichment for each group relative to the original population of spleen cells.

Note

It is very important, in any technique of cell separation, to consider and record cell recovery data, especially when dealing with antigen-specific cell purification. One would not expect, for example, to recover 10% of even a primed lymphocyte population on an antigen-coated column, without being aware of a large non-specific element in the isolation procedure. It is therefore essential, in experimental work, to include another, non-cross reactive antigen as an internal control for non-specific adsorption.

In addition, the calculation of the factor of enrichment of purified cells can be made, strictly, only against a full titration curve of the original population, as the pfc response curve of antigen-stimulated, transferred cells is not linear. Accordingly, the total number of pfc detected in the depleted and enriched populations may exceed the number present in the unfractionated population.

8.3 GENERAL TECHNIQUE FOR SPECIFIC CELL FRACTIONATION

The various techniques described for affinity fractionation of cells have required the preparation of an immunoadsorbent for each antigen or antibody used. In 1976, Scott described a very elegant technique, with wide application, for the fractionation of cells using antigen or antibody derivatised with fluorescein isothiocyanate.

Lymphocytes are treated in suspension with fluorescenated antigen (or antibody) and antigen binding cells isolated by anti-fluorescein immunoadsorbent columns. Column bound cells may then be released by mechanical shear (gentle stirring) in the presence of fluorescein on an heterologous carrier (this prevents reassociation of cells after mechanical release).

Initial preparations

1   Treat keyhole limpet haemocyanin (KLH) with fluorescein isothiocyanate to obtain 5 moles of fluorescein per KLH molecule (per 100 000 daltons) (Section 1.6).
2   Immunize a goat with the fluorescein-KLH conjugate (Section 1.4.7). Test for anti-fluorescein (Fl) activity (using Fl conjugated to an unrelated carrier, for example, goat gammaglobulin) by precipitation in agar (Section 5.3.3).
3   Isolate anti-Fl antibodies using a Fl-goat gammaglobulin immunoadsorbent (Section 8.1) and link to Sepharose 6B (Appendix II) using cyanogen bromide (conditions of activation as in Section 8.2.3).
4   Fluoresceinate antigen or antibody to be used for the fractionation of lymphocytes (Section 1.6).

217

Technique

Materials and equipment

As in Section 8.2.3, but in addition:

Sepharose conjugated with anti-fluorescein (anti-Fl) antibodies

Antigen (or antibody) for cell fractionation, conjugated with fluorescein (as in Section 1.6)

Bovine serum albumin, conjugated with 5 moles mol^{-1} fluorescein (as in Section 1.6)

Tissue culture medium (Appendix I) containing 5% v/v foetal bovine serum (FBS).

Method

1 Pour 3 ml (packed volume) of anti-Fl derivatized beads into a 10 ml syringe barrel. Equilibrate and incubate column (as in Section 8.2.3: use of immunoadsorbent).

2 Prepare cell suspension for fractionation (as in Section 8.2.3: use of immunoadsorbent).

3 Treat cells with Fl-antigen (or antibody) at 100 μg ml^{-1} for 30 min on melting ice.

4 Wash cells three times by centrifugation (150 g for 10 min at 4°) in tissue culture medium containing 5% FBS.

5 Adjust cells to 1×10^8 ml^{-1} and load dropwise onto the top of the anti-Fl column. *Experience has shown that a 3 ml anti-Fl column, prepared as above, will retain $1-3 \times 10^7$ Fl-labelled lymphocytes.*

6 Wash the cells into the column with 0·5 ml tissue culture medium and seal column.

7 Incubate for 5 min at 4°. Unseal the column and wash with 20 ml of cold tissue culture medium. Collect the depleted population (*cells not binding the Fl-labelled reagent*) in the effluent and concentrate by centrifugation (150 g for 10 min at 4°).

8 Add 3 ml Fl_5BSA (initial concentration 5 mg ml^{-1} protein) and stir the column gently with a fine stainless steel rod. Collect the eluted cells.

9 Wash the column with 10 ml of Fl_5BSA (initial concentration 500 μg ml^{-1} protein) and then 20 ml of tissue culture medium. Collect the eluted population.

10 Pool eluted populations from 9 to 10, and wash three times by centrifugation (150 g for 10 min at 4°) in tissue culture medium.

11 Assay the depleted (effluent), enriched (eluted) and original cell suspensions for activity as in Section 8.2.4.

8.4 **FLUORESCENCE ACTIVATED CELL SORTER**

The fluorescence activated cell sorter (FACS) undoubtedly provides the most powerful and effective means of fractionating cell populations. Its position at the end of this section is not intended to reflect

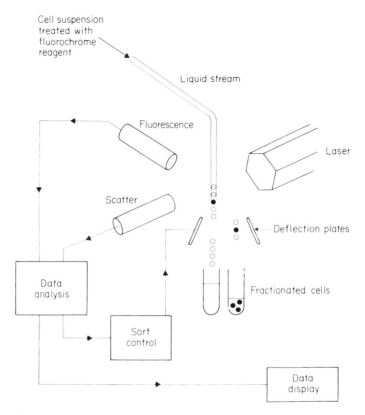

Fig. 8.4. Principle of fluorescence activated cell sorter.
● Fluorochrome labelled cell.
○ Unlabelled cell.

its importance but merely its relative rarity; the brief description is
due to our recognition that any laboratory rich enough to buy one
will certainly know how to use it.

Cell suspensions are treated with an antigen or antibody labelled
with a fluorochrome reagent. In the FACS (Fig. 8.4), a liquid stream
containing the dilute suspension of fluorochrome-labelled cells
passes through a small orifice which is vibrated to break up the
liquid into regularly spaced droplets of uniform size. Cells are irradiated with a high intensity beam of monochromatic light from a
laser. The degree of light scatter (related to cell size) and intensity of
light emitted by the laser-activated fluorochrome is measured by a
pair of photodetectors and the information processed by a
computer.

In this way, cells may be examined individually and, if required,
may be extracted from the main droplet stream by electrically
charging the appropriate droplet which is then deflected as it passes
between charged plates. Potentially, the FACS is capable of
3-channel sorting, i.e. uncharged and positively or negatively
charged droplets.

219

Although the sorting rate of the FACS is relatively low, about 10^4 cells sec^{-1}, this is offset by a prodigious increase in the frequency of positively selected cells, for example, cells at an original frequency of 1 in 10^3 or 10^4 may be purified up to a relative purity of 80–90%. Viable cells are not harmed by the separation process and can be used for *in vitro* culture or *in vivo* transfer experiments.

The degree of precision and reproducibility obtainable with the FACS is well suited to the analysis of monoclonal anti-cell surface antibodies produced by hybridization techniques (Chapter 11). If the FACS had not pre-existed, hybridoma antibodies would have required its invention.

8.5 **ISOLATION OF IgG AND IgM**

Some of the immunoglobulin isotypes may be isolated on the basis of their binding affinity to certain other proteins. For instance IgG is known to bind strongly to protein A, a cell wall protein derived from *Staphylococcus aureus*, while IgM binds strongly to protamine.

8.5.1 PREPARATION OF IgM ON PROTAMINE-SEPHAROSE

Protamine, covalently coupled to Sepharose, may be used to adsorb IgM from normal serum. After washing away free serum proteins, the IgM is eluted with NaCl. It is thought that the binding is mainly through electrostatic forces; the probable interaction being between special negatively charged areas on the IgM molecule (where there are clusters of carbonyl groups) and suitable collections of positive groups on the protamine. Only the whole 19S IgM or the fragment composed of five Fc regions are able to bind, single IgM subunits are not retained by protamine.

Materials and equipment

Normal serum
Protamine sulphate (Appendix II)
Sepharose 4B (Appendix II)
Cyanogen bromide (Appendix II)
2·0 M NaOH
0·08 M Phosphate buffer pH 7·4 containing 1·1 M or 0·007 M sodium chloride (Appendix I)
Borate saline buffer pH 8·3, ionic strength 0·1 (Appendix I)
Tris buffered saline (Appendix I)
0·1 M $NaHCO_3$ bicarbonate buffer, pH 8·9 (Appendix I)

220

Sephacryl S300 superfine (Appendix II)

Column and fraction collection apparatus (as in Section 7.2.3, Fig. 7.2 and Appendix II).

Method

PREPARATION OF IMMUNOADSORBENT

1   Couple protamine to Sepharose 4B using cyanogen bromide, Section 8.1.1 steps 1–8.

2   At step 9, add 112 mg protamine sulphate in 22 ml 0.1 M $NaHCO_3$ pH 8.9. Continue with steps 10–13.

USE OF IMMUNOADSORBENT

1   Wash the adsorbent with 0.08 M phosphate saline buffer pH 7.4 containing 0.077 M NaCl.

2   Add 28 ml normal serum and then 28 ml distilled water.

3   Stir slowly at 4° for 3 h.

4   Wash the gel, on a sintered glass filter funnel, with dilute phosphate saline buffer (one volume 0.08 M phosphate containing 0.077 M NaCl plus two volumes distilled water). *At this stage the gel may appear blue owing to adsorbed ceruloplasmin.*

5   Pack the washed gel into a chromatography column and wash through with further dilute phosphate saline buffer.

6   Elute the IgM with 0.08 M phosphate buffer containing 1.1 M NaCl.

7   Concentrate the eluate to 2–4 ml by placing in a dialysis bag covered with Aquacide.

This preparation still contains some other proteins of lower molecular weight than IgM. These can be removed by gel filtration, use either Sephacryl S300 superfine or Sepharose 6B.

GEL FILTRATION

1   Take 200 ml of Sephacryl S300 and dilute with 40 ml Tris buffered saline.

2   De-gas the gel under a vacuum.

3   Attach a gel reservoir to the column (100 cm × 16 cm) and pour the gel into the column along a glass rod to avoid air bubbles.

4   Pack and equilibrate the column with Tris-buffered saline. *As Sephacryl has a rigid structure it may be packed using fast flow rates. For best results a flow rate of 30 ml cm^{-2} h^{-1} should be used. This is equivalent to 1.0 ml min^{-1} in the 16 mm diameter column.*

5   Fit a flow adaptor to the column and apply the sample.

6   Run the column at a flow rate of less than 25 ml cm^{-2} h^{-1}. *There is greater resolution at lower flow rates.*

The IgM will be found in the first major peak. The descending arm of this peak may contain some IgA, while the other large peak contains ceruloplasmin.

Note: This technique may also be used for the isolation of mouse IgM.

8.5.2   PREPARATION OF IgG ON PROTEIN A-SEPHAROSE

The IgG binding properties of protein A make affinity chromatography with protein A-Sepharose CL-4B a very simple method for preparing IgG. The only problem is that there is some selectivity for the subclasses (Section 8.5.3). With human IgG subclasses: 1, 2 and 4 bind to the protein A but IgG3 does not.

Materials

Human serum
Protein A-Sepharose CL-4B (Appendix II)
Phosphate buffered saline (PBS) (Appendix I)
0·1 M, Glycine-hydrochloric acid buffer, pH 2·8 (Appendix I)
Sodium hydroxide

Method

1   Swell 1·5 g protein A-Sepharose CL-4B in 10 ml PBS for 1 h at room temperature and then pack it into a small chromatography column.
2   Dilute 10 ml human serum with an equal volume of PBS.
3   Filter the serum through the column at a flow rate of 30 ml h^{-1}.
4   Wash through unbound proteins with PBS until no more protein leaves the column (*monitor the protein with a UV flow cell*).
5   Elute the bound IgG with glycine-HCl buffer pH 2·8.
6   Titrate the pH of the purified IgG solution to near neutrality with NaOH, and dialyse against PBS.
7   Regenerate the column by washing with 2 column bed volumes of PBS. Store the column at 4°.

Technical notes

1   The protein A content of the swollen gel is 2 mg ml^{-1} and the binding capacity for human IgG is approximately 25 mg ml^{-1} of packed gel.
2   As the binding of protein A to IgG involves tyrosine residues on the protein A, glycosyl tyrosine (0·1 M in 2% NaCl) may be used to elute the IgG rather than the glycine-HCl buffer.

222

8.5.3   ISOLATION OF IgG SUBCLASSES USING
          PROTEIN A-SEPHAROSE

Although the subclasses of both human and mouse IgG differ
markedly from each other in their biological properties, they are
structurally very similar. This similarity has made it almost impossible to isolate single subclasses from normal serum. Therefore most
studies on the biological functions of immunoglobulin subclasses
have been made on paraproteins derived from individuals with multiple myeloma. Unfortunately, as the antigens with which these
monoclonal immunoglobulins react are rarely known, their effector
functions can only be elicited after aggregating the proteins
artificially.

Fortunately recent developments have made possible the isolation of antibodies comprising a single subclass. One technique, the
production of hybridoma antibodies (Chapter 11), results in monoclonal antibodies, whereas the other, fractionation of the IgG subclasses using staphylococcal protein A, gives polyclonal antibodies.
Already, studies using antibody prepared by the second technique
has revealed that mouse IgG1 can be complement fixing when
bound to antigen, whereas evidence from studies using myeloma
IgG1 had suggested that IgG1 did not fix complement. It has been
proposed that in certain immunoglobulins, particularly those with
shortened hinge regions, the Fab arms may sterically hinder the C1
molecules and prevent their access to the Fc region. Movement of
the Fab arms, after interaction with antigen, might alter the acces-
sibility of the Fc region to effector molecules such as C1. This ability
to prepare single subclass antibodies is likely to enhance our understanding of how antibodies work, both in controlling infections and
in producing hypersensitivity states.

A. Isolation of mouse subclasses

Mouse serum may be fractionated on protein A-Sepharose by
allowing all the IgG to bind to the adsorbent and then eluting the
separate subclasses with a stepped gradient of increasing acidity.

Materials and equipment

Mouse serum
Protein A-Sepharose CL-4B (Appendix II)
Phosphate buffered saline, PBS (Appendix I)
0·1 M Phosphate buffer pH 8·0 (Appendix I)
0·1 M Citrate buffers pH 6·0, 5·5, 4·5, 3·5 (Appendix I)
1·0 M Tris-HCl buffers, pH 8·5, 9·0 (Appendix I)
Chromatography column
Antisera to the mouse IgG subclasses (Appendix II)

223

Method

1   Swell 1·5 *g* protein A-Sepharose in 10 ml PBS for 1 h at room temperature and then pack it into a small chromatography column. Store and use this column at 4°.

2   Equilibrate the column with 0·1 M phosphate buffer pH 8·0.

3   Add 2 ml of 0·1 M phosphate buffer pH 8·0 to 4 ml mouse serum and adjust pH to 8·1 with 1 M Tris-HCl buffer pH 9·0.

4   Apply the diluted serum to the column and wash through with 30 ml of 0·1 M phosphate buffer pH 8·0 *(flow rate 0·4–0·5 ml min⁻¹ throughout)*.

5   Elute the IgG1 with 30 ml of 0·1 M citrate buffer, pH 6·0.

6   Wash the column with 25 ml of 0·1 M citrate buffer pH 5·5.

To minimize the denaturation of the IgG2a and -b antibodies, 1·0 M tris-HCl buffer, pH 8·5 should be added to the tubes prior to collecting the fractions.

7   Elute the IgG2a with 30 ml of 0·1 M citrate buffer pH 4·5.

8   Elute the IgG2b with 25 ml of 0·1 M citrate buffer pH 3·5.

9   Re-equilibrate the column to pH 8·0.

10   Determine the composition of each fraction with specific antisera preferably using radioimmunoassay (Section 9.3) or alternatively single radial immunodiffusion (Section 5.3.3a).

B. Isolation of human IgG subclasses

Recently protein A-Sepharose has also been used to separate the subclasses of human IgG. IgG3 does not bind to protein A and so IgG, prepared by ion exchange chromatography (Section 7.3) is filtered through a column of protein A-Sepharose. IgG1, IgG2 and IgG4 will bind to the adsorbent but IgG3 will come straight through. The IgG1 and IgG2 may then be differentially eluted from the adsorbent with a pH gradient of increasing acidity. Although IgG4 is a slight contaminant in the IgG2 fractions, this problem may be reduced by starting with IgG prepared using DEAE-cellulose, this is deficient in IgG4.

Materials and equipment

Protein A-Sepharose CL-4B (Appendix II)
Human IgG (Section 7.3.5) or human serum
0·15 M Citrate-phosphate buffers pH 7·0, 5·0, 4·5 (Appendix I)
0·1 M Citric acid pH 2·2
Antisera to human IgG subclasses
Chromatography column
UV flow cell

Method

1   Swell 1 g protein A-Sepharose with 10 ml citrate-phosphate buffer pH 7·0.

2 Pack into a small chromatography column and equilibrate with citrate-phosphate buffer pH 7·0.

3 Load either 5 mg human IgG or 0·5 ml human serum (in 0·5 ml pH 7·0 buffer) onto the column.

4 Wash the column through with pH 7·0 buffer. *If purified IgG was used on the column, pure IgG3 will come out with the washing buffer.*

5 Elute the IgG2 and IgG1 with a pH gradient of citrate-phosphate buffer. *This is constructed by using a gradient maker of 3 equivolume chambers connected in series. The first chamber contains 6 ml of 0·1 M citric acid (pH 2·2), the middle chamber 6 ml of citrate-phosphate buffer pH 4·5 and the final chamber, which is connected to the column, has 6 ml of citrate-phosphate buffer pH 5·0.* Use a flow rate of 12 ml h^{-1}. Monitor the eluate with a UV flow cell. Two overlapping peaks are obtained, the first being enriched for IgG2 the second for IgG1. Each of these peaks should be concentrated and recycled on the protein A column to increase resolution.

6 Wash the column with 6 ml 0·1 M citric acid and 30 ml citrate phosphate buffer to re-equilibrate the column.

7 Check the purity of the IgG subclasses with specific antisera preferably using radioimmunoassay (Section 9.3) or alternatively single radial immunodiffusion (Section 5.3.3a).

8.6   SUMMARY AND CONCLUSIONS

Much of our present knowledge on the functional relations between lymphocytes has been gained by the study of fractionated populations, either alone or after deliberate recombination. In this section, we have described only a small number of the wide variety of physical and biochemical techniques that have been used for cell fractionation.

Indeed, so many markers are now available for the delineation of lymphocyte subpopulations that they greatly exceed the number of functional attributes available.

Clearly, immunology is once again at a stage analogous to the discovery of T and B lymphocytes; we know there are lots of different types of lymphocytes, but we are not sure what they all do in the cellular complexities that underlie the control of the immune response.

FURTHER READING

Hudson L. (1978) Lymphocytes, receptors and affinity chromatography. *J. Chromatography* **159,** 123.

Hulett H.R., Bonner W.A., Sweet R.G. & Herzenberg L.A. (1973) Development and application of a rapid cell sorter. *Clin. Chem.* **19,** 813.

9 Immunochemical methods

Most of the methods described in this section were initially developed for particular applications, but they can easily be adapted for more general use.

9.1 QUANTITATION OF IMMUNE COMPLEXES

Normally immune complexes, resulting from the combination of antibody with antigen within the body, are very quickly removed by cells of the mononuclear phagocyte system. Little, if any, harm results to the individual, which is fortunate as we appear to form immune complexes, composed of antibody and food antigens, after every meal. In certain circumstances the complexes tend to persist in the circulation where they may eventually fix complement, leading to the release of anaphylotoxins and chemotactic factors. The anaphylotoxins mediate histamine release and consequently produce increased vascular permeability. Polymorphonuclear leucocytes are attracted to the site of complement fixation where they release proteolytic enzymes while engulfing the complexes, thus causing local tissue damage.

The fate of complexes formed in the circulation depends largely on their size. Large complexes are rapidly cleared by the Kupffer cells, although this system may become overloaded if too many complexes are present. Small complexes are cleared far more slowly and in some instances can be trapped in vessel walls or in filtering membranes, such as renal glomeruli or the choroid plexus. Recently there has been an enormous increase in interest in immune complex diseases resulting in numerous publications. However, recent blind trials arranged by the World Health Organisation have revealed that some of the assay systems used to detect immune complexes are, in fact, incapable of doing so. Also many of the tests which do detect complexes are extremely irreproducible, which must lead one to doubt the validity of some of the published experimental data on immune complexes.

Immune complexes may be detected by methods depending on either physical or their biological properties. We shall detail one method from each group which is well established and robust in performance. The ability of each test to detect immune complexes often varies in different diseases or even at different stages of the same disease, thus it is important to use more than one technique.

226

PRECIPITATION OF IMMUNE COMPLEXES
BY POLYETHYLENE GLYCOL

Polyethylene glycol (PEG) precipitates proteins in proportion to their molecular size and concentration. Thus, free IgG is soluble in 2% w/v PEG, but it is insoluble when part of an immune complex. Although a screening test for complexes could simply involve the measurement of the total protein precipitated from serum by PEG more accurate information can be obtained by further analysis of the precipitated proteins. For instance IgG may be quantitated in the precipitate and used as a measure of the complexed IgG in the serum. The measurement of complement components, particularly C1q and C4 also can give useful information.

Materials and equipment

Test serum samples
Veronal buffered saline (VBS) (Appendix I)
Polyethylene glycol 6000 (PEG) 20% w/v in VBS (Appendix II)
0·2 M, ethylene diamine tetra acid (EDTA), Na_2 salt titrate to pH 7·6 with 0·1 M NaOH
Plastic test tubes, 3 ml (Appendix II)
Single radial immunodiffusion plate for quantitating IgG (Section 5.3.3a)

Method

1   Adjust PEG solution to the working concentration by mixing 6 ml of 20% PEG with 3 ml 0·2 M EDTA and 1 ml VBS.
2   Add 30 μl PEG working solution to 150 μl of each test serum. (in duplicate).
3   Mix and leave overnight at 4°.
4   Centrifuge at 2000 g for 20 min at 4°.
5   Place the tubes in ice and carefully remove the supernatants.
6   Resuspend each precipitate with 2 ml of 2% PEG in 0·01 M EDTA in VBS.
7   Centrifuge at 2000 g for 20 min at 4°.
8   Remove the supernatants and redissolve the precipitates in 150 μl VBS. Incubate at 37° for 1 h to ensure that the precipitated complexes have redissolved.
9   Quantitate the precipitated IgG by single radial immuno-diffusion (Section 5.3.3a) or nephelometry (Section 5.3.3e).
10   Express the results as μg of IgG precipitated per ml of serum.
  Generally up to 100 μg of IgG will be precipitated from the serum of healthy people. Amounts above this are indicative of circulating complexes which may reach mg levels in severe cases.

Care must be taken in the collection and preparation of serum samples to avoid the loss of immune complexes by cryoprecipitation and to prevent denaturation of the sample resulting in the formation of immunoglobulin aggregates. A World Health Organization Scientific Group has recommended the following procedure: serum is prepared by allowing blood, obtained by venepuncture, to clot at 37° in glass tubes for at least 2 h. The retracted clot is removed by centrifugation at room temperature.

9.1.2   C1q SOLID PHASE ASSAY FOR IMMUNE COMPLEXES

C1q is frequently used for the detection of circulating complexes. The simple binding of C1q to immune complex may be determined, but this has the disadvantage that certain molecules, such as DNA, may also bind the C1q. We favour solid phase C1q for the assay of immune complexes because the complexes are identified by two, rather than one, marker molecules. Human C1q is first bound to the surface of plastic tubes followed by the addition of patients' sera. Complexes bound to the C1q are then revealed with radiolabelled anti-human IgG.

9.1.2a   PREPARATION OF HUMAN C1q

Materials and equipment

Fresh human serum
C1q buffers 1 to 6 (Appendix I)
Dialysis tubing (Appendix II)
Refrigerated centrifuge capable of 10 000 g.

Method

Note—the samples and buffers must be kept at 4° at all times during this preparation.

1   Dialyse 127 ml fresh human serum against 1 l of buffer 1 for 4 h.

2   Transfer the dialysis bag to a second 1 l of buffer 1 and dialyse for a further 11 h.

3   Centrifuge each sample at 10 000 g for 15 min at 4°.

4   Discard the supernatants and resuspend the precipitates in buffer 1.

5   Centrifuge at 10 000 g for 15 min at 4°.

6   Discard the supernatants. Loosen the precipitate with a glass rod and add 32 ml of buffer 2. Dissolve the precipitate by mixing on a slow roller for 10 min.

7   Centrifuge at 5000 g for 5 min at 4° to remove undissolved material.

8   Dialyse the supernatant against 4 l of buffer 3 for 4 h.

9   Centrifuge at 10 000 g for 15 min at 4°.

10   Discard the supernatant and resuspend the precipitate in buffer 3.

11   Centrifuge at 10 000 g for 15 min at 4°.

12   Discard the supernatant and redissolve the precipitate in 32 ml of buffer 4 as in step 6.

13   Centrifuge at 5000 g for 5 min at 4° to remove undissolved material.

14   Dialyse the supernatant against 4 l of buffer 5 for 5 h.

15   Centrifuge at 10 000 g for 15 min at 4°.

16   Discard supernatant and resuspend precipitate in buffer 5.

17   Centrifuge at 10 000 g for 15 min at 4°.

18   Discard the supernatant and redissolve the precipitate in 16 ml of buffer 6.

19   Measure the absorbance at 280 nm and calculate the C1q concentration. (The absorbance of C1q at 280 nm in a 1 cm cell is 1·0 for a 1156 μg ml^{-1} solution.) Aliquot the C1q and store at $-70°$.

Technical notes

1   Some authors use animal, rather than human, C1q in immune complex assays. If required, this method may be used to prepare C1q from the serum of small laboratory animals, such as rabbits and guinea pigs.

2   Do not extend the time for re-solution of the precipitates. Although more protein will go into solution, the eventual product is less pure.

3   The degree of purity may be determined by immuno-electrophoresis (Section 5.3.4b) against anti-human serum and anti-C1q or by SDS polyacrylamide gel electrophoresis (Section 7.2.6).

9.1.2b   IMMUNE COMPLEX ASSAY

Materials

Human C1q (as above)

Test sera

Gelatin (Appendix II)

Antibody against human IgG, immunoadsorbent purified and radiolabelled (Sections 8.1 and 5.2.2a).

Phosphate buffered saline (PBS) (Appendix I)

Tween 20

0.2 M ethylene diamine tetra acetic acid (Na_2) (EDTA) adjust to pH
7·5 with 0.1 M NaOH
γ-ray spectrometer (gamma counter)
Polystyrene tubes (LP3) (Appendix II)

Method

1   Dilute the human C1q to 10 μg ml^{-1} in **PBS**.
2   Place 1 ml volumes of C1q solution in polystyrene tubes and
leave for 3 days at 4°.
3   Empty the tubes and wash 3 times with **PBS**.
4   Fill the tubes with 0.01% w/v gelatin solution in **PBS** *to block
any free sites on the tubes*, and incubate at room temperature for 2 h.
5   While the tubes are being blocked, mix 50 μl of each test serum
with 100 μl EDTA solution and incubate at 37° for 30 min. Transfer
the samples to an ice bath.
6   Empty the C1q tubes and wash 3 times with **PBS**.
7   Place duplicate 50 μl samples in the C1q coated tubes together
with 950 μl of PBS containing 0.05% v/v Tween 20 (PBS-Tween).
8   Coated tubes containing 1 ml PBS-Tween (background controls) are processed in the same way as the sample tubes.
9   Incubate the tubes at 37° for 1 h and at 4° for 30 min.
10   Remove free serum proteins by washing 3 times with cold **PBS**.
11   Detect the bound complexes by adding 1 μg radiolabelled anti-
IgG antibody in 1 ml PBS-Tween to each tube and incubate at 37°
for 1 h and then 4° for 30 min.
12   Remove free radiolabelled reagent by washing 3 times with
cold **PBS**.
13   Count the tubes in a γ-ray spectrometer.

The amount of radiolabelled antibody bound is a measure of the
concentration of immune complexes in the patients serum. Generally sera from normal subjects bind less than 20 ng of radiolabelled
antibody, while patients may bind as much as 200 ng.

Technical notes

1   Enzyme labelled antibodies may be used for the detection of
complexes bound to the C1q (Section 9.4).
2   The use of antibody can be avoided altogether by using labelled
protein A. Staphylococcal protein A binds specifically to IgG,
especially subclasses IgG1, IgG2 and IgG4. It is difficult to label by
conventional techniques but this can easily be done by the following
method.

Materials and equipment—

Staphylococcus aureus protein A, 5 mg ml^{-1} in water (Appendix II)
0.12 M, carbonate-bicarbonate buffer, pH 9.0 (Appendix I)

230

Dioxane containing 10 mg ml^{-1} hydroxyphenol succinimide
Phosphate buffered saline (PBS) (Appendix I)

Method—

1   Add 0·8 ml carbonate-bicarbonate buffer and 10 μl hydroxyphenol solution to 0·2 ml protein A solution (5 mg ml^{-1}, initial concentration).
2   Incubate at room temperature for 25–30 min with occasional mixing.
3   Dialyse overnight against 1 l of PBS.
4   Iodinate as in Section 9.5.1 or Section 9.5.2.

3   A positive control should be included in all assays for immune complexes. International reference preparations will soon be available but a simple standard can be prepared from heat aggregated IgG, as below.

Materials and equipment—

Human IgG (Section 8.5.2).
Phosphate buffered saline (PBS) (Appendix I)
Water bath

Method—

1   Prepare 1 ml of a 27 mg ml^{-1} solution of IgG in PBS.
2   Place in a glass test tube and incubate at 63° for 10 min. *This aggregates approximately 10% of the IgG.*
3   Immediately cool in ice.
4   Make dilutions, from 100 to 1000 μg ml^{-1} in normal serum.
5   Include these dilutions in each immune complex assay.

9.2   AVIDITY DETERMINATION

Often it is not necessary to undertake a full affinity measurement to obtain useful information. Where antisera are being compared it is often enough to have an index which rates their binding strengths in relation to each other. Methods which do this are generally less cumbersome and use less materials than required for a Scatchard or Sips plot (Section 5.2.3).

Celada has devised a useful technique based on the ammonium sulphate precipitation test of Farr. The antiserum is reacted against different antigen concentrations over a range of antiserum dilutions. The average avidity is given by 'the slope of the regression of the amount of antiserum in the reaction mixture on the antigen concentration'.

231

Materials

As for the Farr ammonium sulphate precipitation test (Section 5.2.1)

Method

1   Dilute out anti-albumin antibody. Using 0·1 ml aliquots make 10 doubling dilutions in triplicate.

2   Similarly dilute out control normal serum not containing antibody.

3   Add albumin to each tube: to each tube of the first set add 0·2 μg, the second 2 μg and the third 20 μg (each in 0·1 ml).

4   Incubate for 30 min at 37°.

5   Add an equal volume of saturated ammonium sulphate and mix immediately.

6   After 30 min spin down the precipitate and wash twice with 50% saturated ammonium sulphate.

7   Count the radioactivity in the precipitates and calculate the μg of albumin bound.

Calculations

1   Plot the percentage of the added antigen bound against the dilution of antiserum (Fig. 9.1).

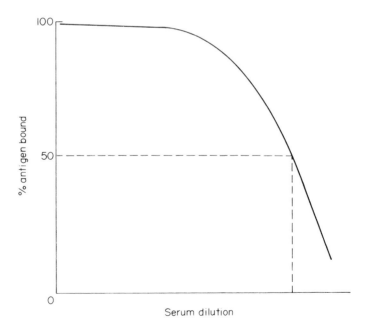

Fig. 9.1. Typical curve for the percentage of antigen bound by increasing dilutions of antiserum
The 50% binding point shown on the graph is used in all calculations.

232

2   Calculate the μl of undiluted serum which would be necessary to bind 50% of the antigen at each concentration.

If, for example, a 1/100 dilution of 100 μl of antiserum bound 50% of 20 μg, then 1 μl of undiluted antiserum would bind 50% of 20 μg.

3   Having calculated this for each antigen concentration, plot the number of μl antiserum required against the amount of albumin in the reaction mixture, on a log/log scale (see Fig. 9.2).

4   The slope of the line is a measure of the avidity. A slope approaching 0 indicates that the efficiency of binding is decreased when the antigen concentration is decreased: while high values, nearing 1, mean that dilution has little effect on the binding, as the antibody is highly avid.

Different antisera should be compared and their slopes examined. It would be interesting to examine, for example, the avidity at different times during the immune response.

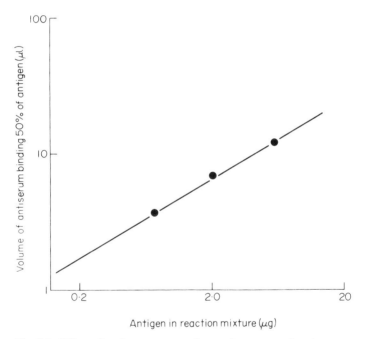

Fig. 9.2. Effect of antigen concentration on the amount of antiserum required to bind 50% of the added antigen
The slope of the graph line gives an estimate of the avidity of the antibody.

9.3   **RADIOIMMUNOASSAY**

Radioimmunoassay is a highly specialized technique with an enormous diversity of applications. It is rapid, sensitive and precise. The range of applications and degree of precision will undoubtedly increase with a wider use of monoclonal antibodies (Chapter 11).

The concentration of an unknown antigen is determined by measuring its ability to compete with a fixed amount of radiolabelled antigen for a limiting quantity of antibody. The antibody may either be immobilized on an insoluble support (Section 11.5.1) or in solution (as below). In the latter case, the assay is performed in a microtitre plate, and the precipitates collected and washed using a multiple sample harvesting machine.

9.3.1 RADIOIMMUNOASSAY OF HUMAN IgG

Preparation of ^{125}I-Fab

Materials and equipment

Human IgG (either Section 7.3.5 or Appendix II)
Sodium ^{125}iodide, carrier free (Appendix II)
Bovine serum albumin, RIA grade
Tris-buffered saline, pH 8·0 (Appendix I)
Chicken serum

1   Obtain human IgG (either Section 7.3.5 or commercially, Appendix II) and prepare the Fab fragment (Section 7.7.1c).
2   Label 10 μg of protein with 0·5 mCi^{125}I (Section 9.5) and store in 5 ml TBS containing 1% BSA.
3   Immediately before use dilute as required with TBS containing 10% chicken serum and filter under gentle pressure through a Whatman GF/B glass fibre filter.

Determination of binding curve

Materials and equipment

Anti-human IgG serum (Appendix II)
^{125}I-Fab (as above)
Bovine serum albumin, RIA grade

Fig. 9.3. Binding and inhibition curves for radioimmunoassay
(a) Various dilutions of a goat anti-human IgG serum (●——●) were added to a fixed amount of ^{125}I labelled human IgG Fab. Treatment of the same amount of ^{125}I-Fab with 10% w/v TCA gave a precipitate containing 80×10^3 cpm. A standard antiserum dilution of 1 : 5000 was used for the construction of the inhibition curve. (*The quantitative nature of this assay is evidenced by the additivity of cpm precipitated by an anti-κ, ○——○, and anti-λ, △——△, serum compared to the anti-IgG ●——● serum, PEG precipitable counts in the absence of antibody shown by broken line.*)
(b) Competition between a fixed amount of ^{125}I-Fab and increasing amounts of unlabelled IgG for a 1 : 5000 dilution of anti-IgG serum. This calibration curve may then be used for the quantitation of unknown samples within the concentration range defined by the steepest part of the curve. (Courtesy of Dr Jens C. Jensenius and Dr Hans C. Sierstad.)

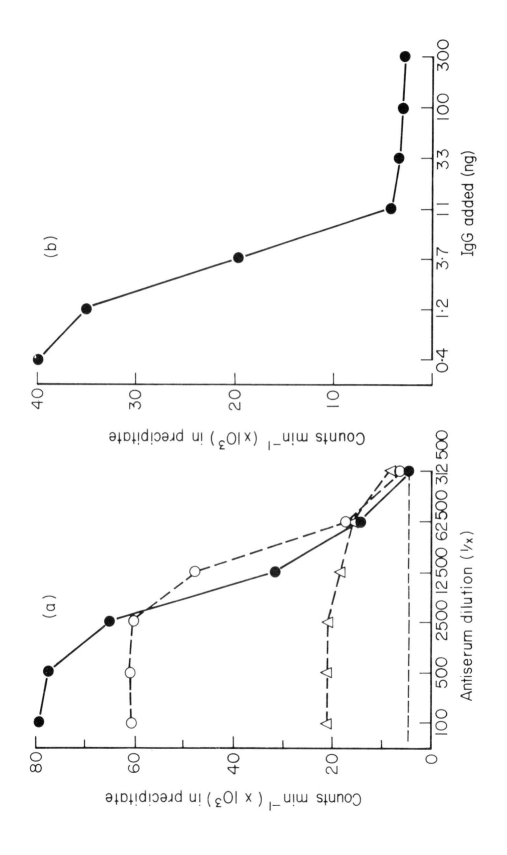

Tris-buffered saline pH 8·0 (Appendix I)

Polyethylene glycol, 6000

Microtitre plates (Appendix II)

Cell culture harvesting machine (Appendix II) Whatman GF/B glass fibre filter strips, for above machine

Method

1   Dilute the anti-IgG serum 1 : 100 and then prepare a range of 2–3 fold dilutions in TBS containing 0·1% BSA.

2   Add 100 μl of ^{125}I-Fab (dilute to yield 10^5 cpm in TCA precipitable material per well, as in 3 above) to each well of the microtitre tray. (Sufficient wells for triplicates of each antibody dilution.)

3   Add 50 μl aliquots of the diluted anti-IgG serum to appropriate wells, mix thoroughly and incubate at room temperature for 16 h.

4   Add 200 μl of 23% w/v PEG solution to each well and incubate at room temperature for 2 h.

5   Collect contents of each well onto Whatman GF/B glass fibre filter strips using a cell culture harvester.

6   Wash each precipitate with 1·5 ml of PEG, 15% w/v in TBS.

7   Determine number of cpm per sample using a gamma counter and plot a curve of cpm against antiserum dilution.

In all future assays, use the dilution of antiserum binding 50–80% of the added radioactivity.

Construction of inhibition curve

Materials and equipment

Human IgG (Appendix II)

Anti-human IgG serum (standardized as above)

^{125}I-Fab (diluted in chicken serum to half dilution used above)

Tris-buffered saline pH 8·0 (Appendix I)

Bovine serum albumin, RIA grade

Polyethylene glycol, 6000

Cell culture harvesting machine (Appendix II)

Whatman GF/B glass fibre filter strips, for above machine

Method

1   Prepare a solution of IgG in TBS containing 1% w/v BSA and adjust to 0·3 mg ml^{-1}. (*Aliquot and store at* $-20°$ *for use*)

2   Prepare standard IgG solutions in the range 2 ng–2 μg ml^{-1} in TBS containing 0·1% w/v BSA.

3   Add 50 μl aliquots of standard IgG to 50 μl of an appropriate dilution (determined above) of anti-IgG serum (in triplicate).

4   Mix samples and incubate for 16 h at room temperature.

5   Add 50 μl of ^{125}I-Fab (diluted in 20% chicken serum to half dilution used above) and incubate for 4 h at room temperature.

6   Precipitate complex by the addition of 200 μl of PEG solution (23% w/v in TBS). Incubate and harvest precipitates as in steps 4–7 above.

7   Plot the inhibition of binding of ^{125}I-labelled Fab on a linear scale (i.e. c.p.m in precipitate) against the concentration of un-labelled IgG added on a log scale.

Use this standard curve to determine the concentration of IgG in unknown solutions

9.4   ENZYME LINKED IMMUNOSORBENT ASSAYS

When assaying antibodies or antigens it is often convenient to have either the antigen or antibody immobilized by attachment to a solid surface. Polystyrene beads, red cells, agarose beads etc. can be used as the support but it is more convenient to use a plastic test tube or microtitre plate as the carrier for the antigen or antibody. Frequently antigen is first bound to the solid phase followed by addition of the antibody under test. After washing, antibody bound to antigen is revealed by adding a labelled antibody directed against the first immunoglobulin. This label may be a radioisotope, such as ^{125}I, or an enzyme, such as horse radish peroxidase. Enzyme labels are replacing radiolabels for many applications due to restrictions on the use of radioisotopes in routine laboratories. In contrast to the short half lives of the common radio labels enzyme-labelled antibodies are stable and may be stored for periods in excess of 1 year.

9.4.1   CONJUGATION OF HORSE RADISH PEROXIDASE TO IMMUNOGLOBULIN

Materials

Horse radish peroxidase (Appendix II)
Anti-immunoglobulin serum, IgG fraction (Appendix II or Section 7.6)
0·1 M Sodium periodate
0·001 M Sodium acetate buffer, pH 4·4 (Appendix 1)
0·1 M Sodium carbonate buffer, pH 9·5 (Appendix I)
Sodium borohydride (4 mg ml^{-1}) in distilled water
0·1 M Borate buffer, pH 7·4 (Appendix I)
Glycerol

Method
1   Dissolve 4 mg horse radish peroxidase in 1 ml distilled water.
2   Add 200 μl freshly prepared sodium periodate solution and stir

237

gently for 20 min at room temperature. *The mixture should turn a greenish brown colour.*

3   Dialyse against sodium acetate buffer, overnight at 4°.

4   Add 20 μl of sodium carbonate buffer *to raise the pH to approximately 9–9·5* and immediately add 1 ml of the IgG fraction to be conjugated.

5   Add 100 μl of freshly prepared sodium borohydride solution (4 mg ml^{-1} in distilled water) and leave at 4° for 2 h. *This reduces any free enzyme.*

6   Dialyse against borate buffer.

7   Add an equal volume of 60% glycerol in borate buffer and store at 4°.

This conjugate should be stable for at least 1 year. Although it is not usually necessary to separate conjugated Ig from unconjugated Ig or enzyme, this may be done by gel filtration on G200 Sephadex (Section 7.2.4).

9.4.2   IMMUNOSORBENT ASSAY

Materials and equipment

Antigen, e.g. human serum albumin (Appendix II)

0·05 M carbonate-bicarbonate buffer, pH 9·6 (Appendix I)

Phosphate buffered saline PBS (Appendix I) containing 0·05% v/v Tween 20 (PBS-Tween)

Hydrogen peroxide (20 vol)

0·1 M, citrate phosphate buffer pH 5·0 (Appendix I)

Sulphuric acid, 12·5%

O-phenylene diamine (Appendix II)

Horse radish peroxidase-anti-immunoglobulin conjugate, e.g. anti-mouse Ig conjugate (Section 9.4.1).

Test sera, e.g. sera from mice immunized with human serum albumin

Micro-ELISA plates (Appendix II) or other polystyrene microtitre trays

Spectrophotometer (Appendix II)

Method

1   Dilute the antigen in carbonate-bicarbonate buffer. *The optimum concentration should be determined for each antigen but a concentration of 5–10 μg ml^{-1} works well for most antigens.*

2   Add 200 μl to each well of a micro-ELISA plate and incubate at 4° for 3 h in a humid chamber.

3   Wash out the antigen and fill the wells completely with PBS-Tween.

4   Incubate at room temperature for 3 min and then empty by inverting and shaking.

238

5 Repeat the washing step twice.

6 Dilute the test serum in PBS-Tween. *The optimum dilution must be determined, it will be about 1 : 1000.*

7 Add 200 μl diluted test serum and incubate for 2 h at room temperature in a humid chamber.

8 Repeat washing procedure as in steps 3 and 4.

9 Add 200 μl conjugate diluted in PBS-Tween. *The exact dilution must be determined by experiment but when using conjugates made with DAKO immunoglobulins a dilution of about 1 : 1000 to 1 : 10 000 is usually suitable.*

10 Incubate overnight at 4° in a humid chamber.

11 Repeat washing procedure as in steps 3 and 4.

12 While the plate is incubating during washing prepare the substrate by adding 34 mg O-phenylene diamine and 50 μl hydrogen peroxide (20 vol) to 100 ml of citrate phosphate buffer pH 5·0. *This substrate should be made up freshly each time and used immediately. Keep in a dark bottle while it is being pipetted.*

13 Add 200 μl substrate to each well and leave in the dark at room temperature for 30 min to develop colour.

14 Stop the reaction by adding 50 μl of sulphuric acid (12·5% initial concentration).

15 Read the absorbance at 492 nm in a spectrophotometer.

Technical notes

1 Strictly, each assay should include dilutions of a standard reference serum for the calibration of unknown samples. In practice, however, the test is quite reproducible and some workers record their results directly in absorbance units.

2 The same assay may be performed using isotopically labelled antibody. In this case each well would be cut out and counted in a γ-ray spectrometer after step 10, instead of processing for enzyme activity.

3 2,2-azinodi- (3-ethyl benzthiazoline sulphonic acid) (ABTS) may be used as an alternative to O-phenylenediamine. Dissolve 50 mg ABTS in 100 ml of 0·1 M citrate phosphate buffer, pH 5·0, and add 50 μl hydrogen peroxide. Use this in step 12 above. Stop the reaction with 50 μl per well of sodium fluoride solution (80 mg in 25 ml distilled water). Read the absorbance at 650 nm.

9.5 **RADIO LABELLING TECHNIQUES**

Isotopically labelled antigen or antibody molecules can be detected with great sensitivity and quantitated with relative ease. The techniques described below allow the introduction of a radioactive tracer without a significant alteration in the immunological properties of the labelled molecules.

Many labelling techniques are available, we have selected those with the widest application.

9.5.1 IODINATION OF PROTEINS: CHLORAMINE T METHOD

Applications: iodination of antigens or antibodies, either in solution or bound to a solid phase immunoadsorbent.

Materials and equipment

All reagents must be prepared just before labelling.
Protein for iodination, 500 μg ml^{-1} in 0·1 M Tris-HCl, pH 7·4 (Appendix I)
Chloramine T, 1 mg ml^{-1} in Tris-HCl buffer
Sodium metabisulphite, 2 mg ml^{-1} in Tris-HCl buffer
5×10^{-5} M potassium iodide in Tris-HCl buffer
Sodium ^{125}iodide, carrier free (Appendix II)
Phosphate buffer (PBS) (Appendix I) containing 0·25% w/v gelatin (Appendix II)
Sephadex G-50
Gamma counter

Method

1   Mix 100 μl of protein (500 μg ml^{-1} initial concentration) with 0·5 mCi^{125}I and 10 μl of chloramine T (1 mg ml^{-1}, initial concentration).
2   Incubate for 2–4 min at room temperature.
3   Add 10 μl of sodium metabisulphite solution (2 mg ml^{-1} initial concentration) and mix thoroughly.
4   After 2 min, add 10 μl of potassium iodide solution.
5   Separate the labelled protein from the free iodine using a column of Sephadex G-50 equilibrated with PBS containing 0·25% gelatin (Section 1.2.3).
6   Elute the column with PBS containing gelatin and collect 0·5 ml fractions.
7   Determine the cpm of each fraction using a gamma counter. Identify the first peak of radioactivity, this is the labelled protein.
8   Store at 4° for use.

Technical note

This technique may be used to iodinate antibodies attached to an antigen immunoadsorbent. (This protects the active site). The free

240

iodide is removed by washing with buffer, and the labelled antibody recovered by acid elution (Sections 8.1.2 and 8.1.4).

9.5.2   IODINATION OF PROTEINS:
         IODOGEN METHOD

Applications: iodination of antigen or antibodies in solution. Iodination of cell membranes.

Preparation in advance

Materials and equipment

Iodogen (1, 3, 4, 6-tetrachloro-3a, 6a diphenylglycoluril) (Appendix II)
Methylene chloride
Test tube, 10×75 mm, plastic (compatible with solvent)
Water bath at 37°.

Method

1   Prepare a solution of Iodogen ($20~\mu g~ml^{-1}$) in methylene chloride.
2   Add 20 μl of the above solution ($0.4~\mu g$ Iodogen) to a test tube.
3   Evaporate the methylene chloride, by rotating the tube slowly in a water bath at 37°, to leave a thin film of Iodogen in the bottom of the tube.
4   Store in the dark at room temperature.
Tubes coated as above may be used for several weeks.

Iodination technique

Materials and equipment

Protein for iodination ($2~mg~ml^{-1}$) in borate-saline buffer, (pH 8.3, ionic strength 0.1 (Appendix I)
Potassium iodide ($11~\mu g~ml^{-1}$) in borate saline buffer
Sodium ^{125}iodide, carrier free (Appendix II)
Iodogen coated tubes, prepared as above

Method

1   Place the Iodogen coated tube on ice and add 50 μl of protein solution ($2~mg~ml^{-1}$ initial concentration).
2   Initiate the reaction by the addition of 10 μl of potassium iodide solution ($11~\mu g~ml^{-1}$ initial concentration) and 14 μCi $^{125}I^{-}$, and adjust final volume to 100 μl by the addition of borate-saline buffer.

241

3 Incubate for 5 min with gentle stirring.
4 Terminate the reaction by decanting the protein solution.
5 Separate the labelled protein from the free iodine by gel chromatography (Section 1.2.3).

Technical notes

1 This reaction has been found to be more efficient than the chloramine T method for the iodination of rabbit IgG.
2 A similar method may be used for the iodination of cells. Typically, use 4×10^6 cells, 6·6 μg of potassium iodide and 100 μCi $^{125}I^-$ in a total volume of 400 μl of phosphate buffered saline (Appendix I). Add mixture to a tube coated with 50 μg of Iodogen. Incubate for 15 min on ice with gentle stirring. Terminate the reaction by decanting the cells and wash three times in phosphate buffered saline by centrifugation (150 g for 10 min at 4°).
This technique does not alter cell viability, as assessed by the uptake of trypan blue.
3 In the iodination of sheep erythrocytes: typical incorporation of ^{125}I into membranes was 0·34%, uptake by cytosol protein was 0·04%.

9.5.3   BIOSYNTHETIC LABELLING OF HYBRIDOMA-DERIVED ANTIBODY

Applications: labelling of secreted proteins in actively synthesizing cells, especially hybridoma cells.

Materials and equipment

Hybridoma cells (Chapter 11) from tissue culture
Horse or fetal bovine serum, dialysed against phosphate buffered saline (Appendix I)
Radioactive labelling medium—
   either ^{3}H-leucine (20 μCi ml^{-1}) (Appendix II)
   or ^{14}C-leucine (5 μCi ml^{-1}) (Appendix II)
   in leucine-free tissue culture medium containing 5% dialysed serum
Plastic test tubes, conical, sterile

Method

1 Count the cell suspension (Section 2.4).
2 Add 2×10^5 cells to a sterile, conical test tube and centrifuge at 150 g for 10 min at room temperature.

242

3 Remove the supernatant and add 0·2 ml of labelling medium.

4 Incubate overnight at 37° in a humid incubator gassed with 5% CO_2 in air.

5 After incubation, centrifuge (150 g for 10 min at room temperature) and remove the supernatant.

6 Store at $-20°$ for use.

Technical notes

1 This technique does not require large amounts of antibody.

2 ^{14}C-leucine gives a higher energy emission than ^{3}H-leucine and so is counted more efficiently in a scintillation counter. It is, however, more expensive.

3 Because of their different rates of radioactive decay, ^{14}C and ^{3}H labelled antibodies have a much longer lifetime for use than ^{125}I labelled antibodies.

9.5.4   CELL SURFACE IODINATION:
         LACTOPEROXIDASE TECHNIQUE
         (see also Section 9.5.2 technical notes)

Application: iodination of cell surface proteins.

Materials and equipment

Phosphate buffered saline (PBS—Appendix I)
Cells, for iodination (10^8 cells ml^{-1}) in PBS
Lactoperoxidase (0·2 mg ml^{-1}) in PBS
Glucose oxidase (2·0 IU ml^{-1}) in PBS
50 mM glucose in PBS
Sodium ^{125}iodide, carrier free (Appendix II)

Method

1 Wash cells three times in PBS by centrifugation (150 g for 10 min at room temperature) to remove exogenous material, count and adjust to 10^8 cells ml^{-1}.

2 To 100 μl of cell suspension (10^8 cells ml^{-1}, initial concentration) add 10 μl lactoperoxidase (0·2 mg ml^{-1} initial concentration) in PBS, 10 μl glucose oxidase (2 IU ml^{-1} in PBS, initial concentration) and 500 μCi ^{125}I$^-$.

3 Initiate the reaction by the addition of 10 μl of 50 mM glucose in PBS and incubate for 10 min at room temperature.

4 Add 10 ml of PBS.

5 Wash three times in PBS by centrifugation (150 g for 10 min at 4°).

243

Technical notes

1 Because the lactoperoxidase enzyme cannot cross the plasma membrane of viable cells, only surface proteins are iodinated. Internal and external proteins are labelled if the cells are dead.

2 Total uptake of radioiodine may be enhanced by the addition of 5 μl of 5×10^{-6} M potassium iodide solution. However, this is said to increase cytoplasmic uptake of $^{125}I^-$.

3 Lactoperoxidase may be 'poisoned' by the addition of 10 mM sodium azide and the reaction terminated precisely.

FURTHER READING

FELBER J.P. (1978) Radioimmunoassay in the clinical chemistry laboratory. *Advances in Clinical Chemistry* **20**.

HAY F.C., NINEHAM L.J. & ROITT I.M. (1976) Routine assay for the detection of immune complexes of known immunoglobulin class using solid phase C1q. *Clin. exp. Immunol.* **24**, 396.

PEETERS H. (1978) Protides of the biological fluids 26th Colloquium. (Complete volume on immune complexes).

THORELL J.I. & LARSON S.M. (1978) *Radioimmunoassay and related techniques*. C.V. Mosby, St. Louis.

SEDLACEK H.H. & SEILER F.R. (eds.) (1979) *Immune complexes*. Behring Institute Mitteilungen, No, 64.

WORLD HEALTH ORGANISATION (1977) *The Role of Immune Complexes in Disease*. WHO Technical Report Series No. 607. Geneva.

10 Techniques in cellular immunology

Many of the values given in this chapter, especially for cell numbers and expected responses, can only be taken as a guide. Cells do not behave in an exactly similar manner between laboratories and so each system must be standardized for research purposes.

10.1 T-B COOPERATION WITH HAPTEN-CARRIER CONJUGATES

The basic principles involved in this section have already been dealt with in Section 3.1.2. However, the use of chemically defined antigens provides a much more powerful research tool with which to investigate the specific requirements of T-B cooperation.

Mitchison showed very convincingly that the antibody response to a hapten, for example dinitrophenyl, DNP, depends on it being CHEMICALLY COUPLED to a carrier molecule, for example, fowl gamma-globulin (FγG) or Keyhole Limpet Haemocyanin (KLH). It is obvious that B cells recognize and respond to the hapten; in this experiment we will investigate the nature of the cells recognizing the carrier.

Initial preparations

Throughout this chapter you will use mice primed to DNP–FγG or DNP–KLH. Prepare the hapten-carrier conjugates as described in Section 1.3, and adsorb them onto alum as in Section 1.4.4.

Inject groups of 15–20 inbred mice intraperitoneally according to the protocol below (cf. also Section 1.8 for choice of mouse strain).

Use the mice 2–3 months after priming. If required, the mice may be boosted a second time according to the same schedule.

Protocol

Group	Antigen on alum	Amount (μg)	Adjuvant
I	DNP–FγG	400	4×10^9 B. pertussis
II	DNP–KLH	400	4×10^9 B. pertussis
III	FγG	400	4×10^9 B. pertussis

245

ASSAY FOR DNP PLAQUE-FORMING CELLS

This assay was modified by Cunningham from the haemolytic plaque assay (Section 3.1.2) and can be used to enumerate antibody forming cells against soluble antigens conjugated to the surface of indicator erythrocytes, in this case dinitrophenyl (DNP) or trinitrophenyl (TNP).

PREPARATION OF DNP OR TNP CONJUGATED ERYTHROCYTES

Three methods are available to sensitize the indicator erythrocytes (e.g. sheep or horse RBC):

1 **Chemical**—The trinitrophenyl group (TNP) may be coupled directly to the erythrocytes. This is a much more gentle reaction than dinitrophenylation; TNP crossreacts strongly with DNP.

2 **Dinitrophenylated, non-complement fixing antibodies.** Chicken antibodies do not fix mammalian complement and so DNP chicken anti-erythrocyte antibodies may be used to sensitize indicator cells at sub-agglutinating doses. However, in using this assay method for DNP plaques, one cannot then use $F\gamma G$ as a carrier molecule.

3 **Dinitrophenylated fragments of mammalian anti-erythrocyte antibodies.** Rabbit IgG anti-SRBC, for example, will fix guinea-pig complement and so the dinitrophenylated Fab fragment must be used to sensitize erythrocytes. DNP-Fab will still bind to the erythrocytes but cannot induce agglutination or fix complement.

We will describe methods 1 and 3 in detail. In the past, the third method has been more widely applied, but for class purposes method 1 is probably preferable.

10.1.2   TRINITROPHENYLATION OF ERYTHROCYTES

Materials

Erythrocytes, horse or sheep (Appendix II)
2,4,6-Trinitrobenzene sulphonic acid (Appendix II)
Glycyl-glycine
0·28 M Cacodylate buffer, pH 6·9 (Appendix I)
Phosphate buffered saline, PBS (Appendix I)

Method

1 Wash erythrocytes three times with PBS by centrifugation (300 g for 10 min).

2   Resuspend 4 ml of packed cells in 16 ml cacodylate buffer, and react with trinitrobenzene sulphonic acid according to the protocol.

3   Mix TNP solution with cells for 30 min on a magnetic stirrer at room temperature.

4   Add 50 ml of a solution of glycyl-glycine (initial concentration 2 mg ml^{-1}) in cacodylate buffer to each aliquot to react the free TNP sulphonate.

5   Wash three times in PBS by centrifugation (300 g for 10 min) and store at 4°.

Determine the optimum conditions for sensitization according to Section 10.1.4.

Protocol

Tube number:	1	2	3	4
mg TNP in 2 ml buffer	25	30	35	40
sheep erythrocytes, 20% suspension	5 ml ————————————→			

10.1.3   DNP Fab' ANTI-SHEEP ERYTHROCYTE (SRBC) SENSITIZATION

PREPARATION OF Fab' ANTI-SRBC

The antiserum prepared in Section 5.4.1b is suitable for this purpose. The method described has been found to be convenient but it is not the only method that may be used to prepare Fab or Fab'.

Materials and equipment

Rabbit anti-SRBC hyperimmune serum (Section 5.4.1b)
Other materials and equipment as in Sections indicated

Method

1   Isolate the IgG fraction of the antiserum by DEAE-cellulose ion exchange chromatography (Section 7.3.1).

2   After concentration, dialyse the IgG anti-SRBC against 0·1 M sodium acetate and digest with pepsin (Section 7.7.2) to obtain the F(ab')$_2$ fragment.

3   Apply the digest to a G-100 or G-150 Sephadex column equilibrated with PBS, recover the F(ab')$_2$ peak (Section 7.7.2), concentrate and dialyse against PBS.

Store a small sample at −20° for testing later.

4   Reduce F(ab')$_2$ with 0·02 M dithiothreitol for 30 min at 37°.

5   Alkylate with 0·05 M iodoacetamide for 10 min at room temperature.

247

6   Dialyse Fab' mixture overnight against PBS.

Reduction and alkylation of the $F(ab')_2$ is usually sufficient to prevent haemagglutination and so it is not necessary to fractionate the mixture any further.

7   Dinitrophenylate the Fab' anti-SRBC as described in Section 1.3.1a, and determine the average number of DNP groups per Fab' molecule.

Test each preparation by haemagglutination (Section 5.4.1) and haemolysis (Section 6.3) according to the protocol.

Protocol

Prepara- tion number	Description	Haemag- glutinin titre	Haemo- lysin titre
1	Rabbit anti-SRBC whole serum		
2	IgG anti-SRBC		
3	$F(ab')_2$ anti-SRBC		
4	Fab' anti-SRBC		
5	Fab' anti-SRBC + goat or sheep anti-rabbit immunoglobulin		
6	DNP–Fab' anti-SRBC		
7	DNP–Fab' anti-SRBC + goat or sheep anti-rabbit immunoglobulin		

Ideally the haemagglutination and haemolysis test should be carried out after each stage of the procedure, and the procedure continued if the results of the tests are satisfactory.

A typical haemagglutination result is shown in Fig. 10.1.

10.1.3a   SENSITIZATION OF INDICATOR CELLS

Materials

Sheep erythrocytes (Appendix II)
DNP–Fab' anti-SRBC
Phosphate buffered saline, PBS (Appendix I)

Method

1   Wash SRBC three times in PBS by centrifugation (300 g for 10 min) and adjust to a final concentration of 40% v/v.
2   Sensitize aliquots of SRBC according to the protocol (p. 249).
3   Incubate at 37° for 30 min, mixing occasionally.
4   Wash five times with PBS by centrifugation to remove unbound protein.
5   Adjust cell concentration to 20% v/v and store at 4°.

Determine the optimum conditions for sensitization as described in Section 10.1.4.

248

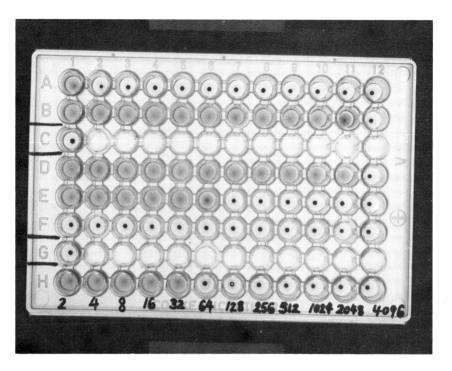

Fig. 10.1. Haemagglutination test with rabbit anti-sheep erythrocyte serum
Antigen–sheep erythrocytes (SRBC)

Doubling dilutions of antiserum along the tray starting at 1 : 2.

Column A: Pre-immunization bleed showing low-titre 'natural' or heterophile antibodies.

Column B: Antiserum after two injections of 5×10^8 SRBC in Freund's
   complete adjuvant and 5 intravenous boosts with 10^8 SRBC. Antiserum
   collected 12 weeks after first challenge.

Column C: SRBC alone, control for spontaneous agglutination.

Column D: IgG fraction of antiserum isolated by DEAE-cellulose ion exchange chromatography.

Column E: $F(ab')_2$ fraction.

Column F: Fab' fraction.

Column G: SRBC alone.

Column H: Fab' fraction plus one drop of 1 : 40 dilution goat anti-rabbit
   IgG.

Protocol

Aliquot number	1	2	3	4	5	6
µl of DNP-Fab' anti-SRBC (initial concn. 1 mg ml^{-1}) added	1	5	10	20	100	200
sheep erythrocytes 40% v/v suspension (ml)	1	$\longrightarrow$				

Technical notes

1 Use 2–3-week-old SRBC but fresh HRBC.
2 The sensitized erythrocytes are stable for 1 week at 4°. It is, however, advisable to wash the cells each time before use.

10.1.3b PREPARATION OF ASSAY CHAMBERS

Materials and equipment

Glass microscope slides
Adhesive tape, double sided (Appendix II)
Photographic roller

Method

1 Wash slides overnight in a strong detergent solution and rinse thoroughly in distilled water. Soak overnight in absolute ethanol. Air dry the slides.
2 Place 20 slides in a line with their long edges adjacent and stick double-sided tape along each edge and along the centre of the row.
3 Remove the backing from the tape and add a second row of slides to complete the sandwich.
4 Roll the slides firmly with a photographic roller to seal the chambers.
5 Separate adjacent slides.

10.1.4 ANTI-DNP ASSAY

Materials and equipment

DNP–FγG or DNP–KLH primed mice (Section 10.1)
DNP or TNP sensitized SRBC (Section 10.1.2 or 10.1.3)
Tissue-culture medium (Appendix I)
Fetal bovine serum
Guinea-pig serum, as complement source (Fresh or preserved serum Appendix II)
Assay chambers (Section 10.1.3b)
50 : 50 mixture, paraffin wax and petroleum jelly on hot plate
Microtitre tray, U-shaped (Appendix II)
Dropping pipettes (18 g needle with end cut square attached to 1 ml syringe barrel or Appendix II)

Method

1 Remove the spleens from 2–3 mice and prepare a single-cell suspension as described in Sections 1.7.3 and 2.4.
2 Adjust to 10^7 lymphocytes ml^{-1}.

3   Place one drop of medium into each hole of the microtitre tray to be used.

4   Add one drop of 20% sensitized erythrocyte suspension.

5   Add 0·1 ml of spleen cell suspension.

6   Add one drop of neat guinea-pig serum absorbed with sheep erythrocytes (see Section 10.9.1. Technical note 2).

7   Mix the suspension in each hole of the tray and load into an assay chamber with a Pasteur pipette.

8   When both chambers are full, seal edges by dipping into paraffin wax: petroleum jelly mixture.

9   Incubate at 37° and examine at 30, 45, 60 and 90 min.

10   Remove all the assay chambers as soon as plaques are clearly visible to the naked eye.

11   Count the number of plaques per chamber using a low-power binocular microscope.

12   Calculate the number of plaques per total spleen for each group, and plot a graph of p.f.c. against volume or concentration of sensitizing agent, as shown in Fig. 10.2.

Use this optimum volume or concentration of sensitizing agent in all future assays.

Technical notes

1   It is advisable to remove clumps from the spleen suspensions by settling them through 1 ml of fetal bovine serum instead of filtering through nylon wool.

2   It is not necessary to perform replicates of each assay point.

3   Use 37° incubator without forced air circulation, any vibration will prevent uniform settling of the RBC.

4   Use a low angle of incidence for the light when counting the plaques under the microscope. The plaques will appear as dark holes in the birefringent layer of erythrocytes.

In the assay described above, direct (mainly IgM) plaques were detected; indirect (mainly IgG) plaques may be detected by the addition of a developing serum, e.g. anti-mouse immunoglobulin, as described below.

Indirect plaques

Materials and equipment

Optimally sensitized erythrocytes (Section above and Fig. 10.2)
Rabbit anti-mouse immunoglobulin (Section 1.4.2 or Appendix II)
Other materials and equipment as given for previous section

Method

1   Dilute the anti-immunoglobulin serum with PBS as shown in the protocol (p. 252).

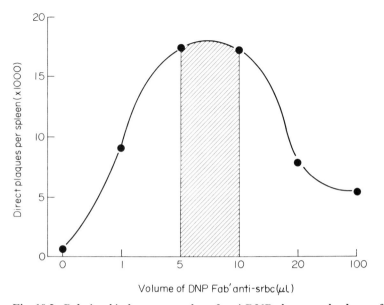

Fig. 10.2. Relationship between number of anti-DNP plaques and volume of DNP. Fab′ anti-SRBC used to sensitize indicator cells
The optimal volume for sensitization, within the shaded area, should be used in all future assays.

Protocol

Tube number	1	2	3	4	5
ml PBS	0·8⎱ mix	mix			
ml antiserum	0·2⎰				
dilution	1 : 10	1 : 20	1 : 40	1 : 80	1 : 60

0·5 ⟶

0·5

2   Add one drop of each dilution to one hole of the microtitre tray.
3   Repeat the assay as in previous section, but OMIT the 1 drop of medium from each hole of the tray, this has been replaced by the anti-immunoglobulin serum.
4   Determine the dilution of developing serum giving the maximum number of plaques.

Technical note

The IgG plaques are taken to be the difference between the total number of developed plaques and the number of direct plaques.

Some anti-Ig sera inhibit IgM plaques while developing IgG plaques. If this is found to be the case in your system, then no correction of the number of developed plaques is required.

Test for the inhibition of direct plaque formation as follows:
Determine IgM (direct) plaques with and without anti-Ig using either: (a) spleen cells from an animal 4 days after antigen priming, or (b) spleen cells from an animal primed with a highly substituted carrier (see Section 1.3.1 for explanation).

Having spent a great deal of time standardizing reagents, the experimental assay is extremely rapid.

10.2 HAPTEN-CARRIER COOPERATION WITH A HETEROLOGOUS CARRIER

Preparation required: Inbred mice must be primed to DNP–KLH or FγG respectively 2–3 months before this experiment (see Sections 1.5 and 10.1).

Materials and equipment

Mice primed as above
Inbred mice for X-irradiation (cf. Section 1.8.3)
DNP–HSA, DNP–KLH, DNP–FγG and FγG soluble antigens (Section 1.3)
Materials for plaque assay (Section 10.1.4)

Method

1   Prepare spleen-cell suspensions from donor mice primed with (a) DNP–KLH or (b) FγG.
2   Treat 10^8 FγG-primed spleen cells with anti-Thy.1 and complement or normal AKR serum and complement at 37° for 30 min (see Sections 10.8.5 and 10.9).
3   X-irradiate the recipient mice with 800–850 R and reconstitute them according to the protocol (p. 254).
4   Assay the mice for direct and indirect DNP plaques on the 7th day after cell transfer.
5   Calculate the total number of plaques per spleen for each recipient and the geometric mean for each group (see Section 4.1.2c).

You should now be aware that B cells primed to a hapten on carrier 1 can respond to the same hapten on carrier 2 by cooperating with a second population of cells primed to carrier 2. Identify the experimental groups which support this statement.

(a) What is the nature of the cooperating cell in this second population?

(b) What is the chemical requirement for hapten-carrier cooperation? (Cf. groups 2 and 4)

(c) What is the rationale for including groups 3 and 6 in this experiment?

253

Group	X-irradiated recipients per group*	Number of cells given i.v. in 0·2 ml	Intraperitoneal challenge (soluble antigen)
1	3–5	2×10^7 DNP–KLH spleen	10 μg DNP–KLH
2	3–5	2×10^7 DNP–KLH spleen $+ 2 \times 10^7$ FγG spleen	10 μg DNP–FγG
3	3–5	2×10^7 FγG spleen	10 μg DNP–FγG
4	3–5	2×10^7 DNP–KLH spleen $+ 2 \times 10^7$ FγG spleen	10 μg DNP–HSA + 10 μg FγG
5	3–5	2×10^7 DNP–KLH spleen $+ 2 \times 10^7$ anti-Thy. 1 + complement-treated FγG spleen	10 μg DNP–FγG
6	3–5	2×10^7 DNP–KLH spleen $+ 2 \times 10^7$ normal AKR serum + complement-treated FγG spleen	10 μg DNP–FγG
7	3–5	none	10 μg DNP–FγG or 10 μg DNP–KLH

* Never less than 4 mice group^{-1} for research purposes.
Group 7 is the control for the efficacy of X-irradiation and may be omitted after the initial experiment.

10.3 LYMPHOCYTE CIRCULATION

Lymphocytes do not circulate in a random manner. It is known, for example, that there is a functional division of lymphocytes into the so-called recirculating and non-recirculating pools. Hence a full knowledge of the factors affecting the passage of cells from one pool to the other during the immune response is essential. In addition, cells show set migration patterns during ontogeny, moving, for example, from the central to the peripheral lymphoid organs.

The traffic pattern of lymphocytes may be followed using isotopically labelled cells as detailed below.

10.3.1 ONTOGENIC MIGRATION PATTERNS

Dividing cells in the bursa or thymus may be labelled by an intra-organ infusion of ^{3}H-thymidine or ^{131}iododeoxyuridine. In this procedure it is essential to minimize the effect of 'spill over' of the labelled material into the peripheral tissues, and so the animal is 'flooded' by an intravenous injection of non-radioactive DNA analogue.

Isotopically labelled cells in the peripheral lymphoid organs may then be identified by autoradiography of tissue sections as described in Section 10.10.

LYMPHOCYTE 'HOMING'

If lymphocytes are removed from an animal, isotopically labelled *in vitro* and returned to a syngeneic recipient they show definite migration patterns, localizing within different organs at different times.

Basic technique

Materials and equipment

Inbred mice (Section 1.8.2 and Appendix II)
Sodium ^{51}chromate (Appendix II)
Gamma counter

Method

1 Prepare a lymph node suspension from 2–4 donor mice.
2 Count and adjust the suspension to 10^8 viable lymphocytes ml^{-1}.
3 Incubate 1 ml of cells with 30 μCi Na^{51}Cr for 30 min at 37° in tissue culture medium buffered with HEPES (20 mM) and containing 5% fetal bovine serum.
4 Wash the cells 5 times by centrifugation and resuspend in 2 ml of medium.
5 Inject 5×10^6 cells intravenously into each of 12 recipients, and retain an aliquot of 5×10^6 cells for γ-counting.
6 Kill 3 recipient mice at 4, 24, 48 and 72 h post injection.
7 Remove the thymus, spleen, mesenteric lymph nodes and liver from each recipient and count the amount of isotope in each organ. (^{51}Cr *is a high energy γ-emitter and so whole-organ counting is possible.*)
   Count also the aliquot of 5×10^6 original cells.
8 Calculate the amount of radioactivity in each organ as a percentage of the original counts injected.
9 Plot a graph of % radioactivity against time for each organ.

Interpretation of results

The % radioactivity per organ is an estimate of the proportion of lymphocytes localizing in that organ. The ratio of counts localizing in the spleen relative to the liver is a good estimate of the viability of the original lymphocyte suspension. If the suspension has a high viability the index is high, and vice versa. As will be seen later (Section 10.8.3), however, this spleen/liver localization also changes if cells are coated but not necessarily killed, with anti-membrane antibodies (due to *in vivo* immune adherence and possibly opsonization).

Lymphocyte suspensions with high viability pass from the blood and localize predominantly in the spleen. Eventually cells leave the spleen and enter the lymph nodes, as shown by the change in radioactivity of each organ with time. As expected no re-injected cells were detected in the thymus. Compare your data with that shown in Fig. 10.3.

Time after intravenous injection (h)	Number of recipients	Mean % radioactivity			
		Liver	Spleen	Thymus	Lymph node
4	3	6	35	0	9
24	3	7	18	0	17
48	3	7	15	0	13
72	3	8	13	0	12

Fig. 10.3. Organ distribution of ^{51}Cr-labelled lymphocytes injected into syngeneic recipients (data from J. Sprent)
These data were obtained with thoracic duct lymphocytes which have almost 100% viability. It is necessary to combine dead-cell removal (Section 10.9) with the method outlined in the text to obtain comparable results.

Suggested experimental procedure

Compare the localization and migration patterns of the following cells:
1   Normal lymph node cells.
2   B lymph node cells derived from nu/nu mice (Section 1.8.2) or thymectomized, bone marrow reconstituted mice (Section 10.6).
3   T lymph node cells prepared by anti-immunoglobulin column affinity chromatography (Section 8.2.1).

10.3.3   INTRA-ORGAN DISTRIBUTION OF CELLS

A similar technique can also be used to examine the distribution of labelled cells within each organ. It is necessary, however, to use a different isotope as high-energy γ-emissions cannot be captured by a photographic emulsion.

Materials and equipment

Inbred mice (Section 1.8.2 and Appendix II)
Tritiated uridine (Appendix II)
Materials for autoradiography (see Section 10.10)

Method

1   Prepare a lymph node suspension from 2–3 donor mice.

2   Count cells and adjust to 5×10^7 cells ml^{-1} in tissue-culture medium buffered with HEPES (20 mM) and containing 5% fetal bovine serum.

3   Add ^{3}H-uridine to a final concentration of 25 μCi ml^{-1} and incubate at 37° for 30 min.

4   Wash the cells three times by centrifugation and inject 1×10^7 cells intravenously into each of 4 recipients.

5   Kill recipients at 0·5, 4, 8 and 24 h after injection.

6   Remove the spleen and mesenteric lymph nodes from each recipient and fix for histological sectioning.

7   Prepare sections of each organ and dip in photographic emulsion for autoradiography (Section 10.10).

8   After development of the autoradiographs, stain the tissue sections in haematoxylin and eosin.

Labelled cells may be identified by the presence of black grains of silver over their nucleus and cytoplasm. Examine the slides at low power and determine the change in distribution of labelled cells within the spleen and lymph node with time. Use this technique to compare the differing localization characteristics of T and B cells as suggested in Section 10.3.2.

10.4   MANIPULATION OF THE IMMUNE SYSTEM

Much of the modern immunological knowledge has been gained by removing some part of the lymphoid system and observing the result. Initially studies were limited to the intact animal deprived of some major lymphoid organ, for example, the thymus or bursa. More recently techniques have been developed for the reconstitution of immunologically deprived mice; the mouse is immunosuppressed by X-irradiation and then used as a life support system for the cells under test.

10.4.1   SUPPRESSION OF THE IMMUNE RESPONSE BY X-IRRADIATION

The dose of X-rays required to kill most types of non-dividing cells is much greater than that required to kill actively dividing cells. One of its major effects is to induce chromosomal breaks and so the cells are not able to complete mitosis. Lymphocytes, however, are unique among mammalian cells in being susceptible to X-ray induced death during interphase. They have a D_{37} of only 100 R.

The dose-dependent immunosuppressive effect of X-irradiation can be demonstrated in a primary immune response against sheep erythrocytes. This experiment is also designed to determine the lethal and immunosuppressive X-ray doses of recipient animals for other experiments (see Technical notes).

Materials and equipment

Mice (preferably inbred, Section 1.8.2)
Sheep erythrocytes (SRBC) (Appendix II)
X-ray machine or γ-source
Materials for haemolytic plaque assay (Section 3.1.2)

Method

Irradiate and prime the mice according to the protocol.

Protocol

	Group (3–5 animals per group)							
	1	2	3	4	5	6	7	8
Irradiation dose (R)	0	0	200	400	600	800	850	900
Immunizing antigen– SRBC intravenously	0	2×10^7						→

1   Challenge the animals with antigen immediately before or after X-irradiation.
2   Assay the anti-SRBC haemolytic plaque response 5 days after antigen challenge (Section 3.1.2).
3   Calculate the total number of plaques per spleen for each animal and the geometric mean for each group.
4   Plot a graph of the X-ray dose against the log mean plaque response.

Technical note

For most inbred strains of mice there should be very few deaths during the period of assay due to X-irradiation over the range indicated. For long-term survival, however, it is necessary to reconstitute the mice with bone marrow as X-irradiation not only suppresses lymphoproliferation, but also proliferation of the haemopoietic system. Bone-marrow reconstitution is dealt with in Section 10.6.

10.4.2   RADIORESISTANCE

Experiments suggest that T and B cells shows a differential radio-resistance in the whole animal. Thus, if an animal is primed with sheep erythrocytes and X-irradiated 4 days later, functional T cells remain, whereas B-cell activity is suppressed.

Materials and equipment

Inbred mice (Section 1.8.2)
Sheep erythrocytes (SRBC) (Appendix II)
Materials for haemolytic plaque assay (Section 3.1.2)

Protocol

Group	Recipients per group	Previous treatment	Cells transferred	SRBC challenge
1	3–5	2×10^7 SRBC + 800R*	none	2×10^7
2	3–5	2×10^7 SRBC + 800R*	thymocytes	2×10^7
3	3–5	2×10^7 SRBC + 800R*	spleen treated with anti-Thy.1 + complement	2×10^7
4	3–5	2×10^7 SRBC + 800R*	spleen treated with normal mouse serum + complement	2×10^7

* 800R 4 days after SRBC challenge

Method

1   Prime recipient mice with 2×10^7 sheep erythrocytes intravenously. X-irradiate (800–850R) 4 days after priming.
2   Prepare spleen and thymocyte suspensions from normal donor mice.
3   Treat aliquots of the spleen suspension with anti-Thy.1 and complement or normal mouse serum and complement (Sections 10.8.5 and 10.9).
4   Reconstitute the X-irradiated mice according to the protocol.
5   Assay all mice for anti-SRBC haemolytic plaques 8 days after cell transfer (Section 3.1.2).
6   Calculate the total plaque-forming cells per spleen for each individual and the geometric mean for each group.

With reference to the experiments in Section 10.2 and the known specificity of the anti-Thy.1 serum, you should be able to identify the radiosensitive and radioresistant lymphocyte population.

This is an extremely useful method by which to prepare helper cells (cf. Section 4.2).

Technical notes

1   We have assayed at only one time point, both T and B cells have phases of relative radioresistance after antigen stimulation.
2   Differential radioresistance is not shown by T and B cells *in vitro*.

259

SURGICAL AND CHEMICAL MANIPULATION OF THE LYMPHOID SYSTEM

Removal of a central lymphoid organ during embryonic or early post-natal life results in a severe depression or complete absence of the dependent peripheral lymphoid population. Historically, the chicken was a very important model for this type of investigation as its sites of T and B differentiation are anatomically distinct.

The central lymphoid organs are active during embryonic life and so at birth there is a well-established peripheral lymphoid population. Accordingly, any techniques concerned with the ablation of the central lymphoid organs must be carried out as early as possible in ontogeny. If ablation is delayed until the peri- or post-natal period, it must be accompanied by generalized immunosuppression, usually X-irradiation. The remaining central lymphoid organ is then allowed to repopulate the peripheral lymphoid tissue, with or without bone-marrow therapy to overcome the X-irradiation. There are, however, at least two exceptions to this rule of generalized immunosuppression:

(a) **Hormonal bursectomy.** If 7-day-old chick embryos are treated with 2 mg of testosterone propionate the bursa fails to develop and so cannot process stem cells to B lymphocytes. Unfortunately, hormonal bursectomy induces a malformation of the dorsal cloacal musculature and the birds, being unable to void their faeces adequately, tend to die.

(b) **Cyclophosphamide bursectomy.** Newly hatched chicks are given an intravenous injection of 2 mg of cyclophosphamide on each of the 4 days following hatching. Injection can be performed via the knee veins. This procedure is usually accompanied by a 25–50% mortality at 8 weeks. The degree of B-cell suppression is not increased by surgical removal of the bursal rudiment or by earlier administration of the drug.

10.5.1   SURGICAL BURSECTOMY

This technique can only be used on birds, the equivalent site of B-cell differentiation has yet to be identified in mammals.

Materials and equipment

Chicks, on day of hatching
Surgical instruments
X-ray machine or γ-source

Method

1   Anaesthetize the chick with ether and squeeze abdomen between finger and thumb to void faeces.

2   Remove feathers between tail and cloaca, and swab area with 70% alcohol.

3   With chick on its abdomen, hold the tail with forceps and make a small incision with fine-pointed scissors in the centre line, midway between tail and cloaca.

4   Insert the closed scissors firmly into the incision, keeping the points up.

5   Open the scissors *in situ* (horizontally). This will enlarge the original incision and free the bursa from its dorsal attachment.

6   Pull the bursa through the incision using blunt forceps and dissect away the surrounding tissue with fine forceps until the bursa is attached to the rectum alone. (*Take care to identify and avoid the ureters which run close to the bursa.*)

7   Cut the bursa free; close to the rectum. Cautery is not necessary.

8   Close the incision with 3 single sutures.

9   X-irradiate the chicks 1 day after surgery. An X-ray dose of 700–800R through 1 mm Al and 1 mm Cu is usually sublethal for chicks and is successful in suppressing peripheral lymphocytes.

Technical notes

1   There should be no post-operative death. Mortality results only from X-irradiation. It may be necessary to vary the X-ray dose used depending on strain, health and housing conditions of birds.

2   If the bursa breaks during reflection it is inadvisable to complete the operation as organ remnants are able to reform a dwarf, but fully functional, bursa.

3   Bursectomized birds are usually used at 8 weeks of age, when the T-cell system has regenerated.

4   Although bursectomized birds are usually immunosuppressed for a primary response they often give a normal secondary response, presumably due to the expansion of a residual population of peripheral B cells.

Hypo- or agammaglobulinaemic birds may be selected on the following basis:

1   Serum immunoglobulin levels as determined by Mancini single radial diffusion in agar (Section 5.3.3a) using rabbit anti-chicken immunoglubulin (Section 1.4.5).

2   Anti-sheep erythrocyte haemagglutination titre (Section 5.4.1). Often bursectomized birds have high levels of serum immunoglobulins, but are unable to produce an antibody response to antigenic challenge. The significance of this observation is obscure at the present time.

3   Percentage of immunoglobulin-bearing lymphocytes in blood, as detected by immunofluorescence (Section 2.5.1).

The above tests may be used to screen live birds for further experiments. At eventual sacrifice, however, a macroscopic examination must be made for bursal rudiments.

Note

A similar technique has been developed for the surgical bursectomy of 17–18-day-old embryos, but it requires considerable skill.

10.5.2   SURGICAL THYMECTOMY

Surgical removal of the thymus is the only technique available for thymectomy in both birds and mammals.

10.5.2a   **Neonatal thymectomy of the mouse**

The operation must be performed within the first 24 h of neonatal life for the maximum depression of T cells.

Materials and equipment

Neonatal mice, and mothers
Surgical instruments

Method

1   Cool the mouse in a refrigerator until it stops moving. (An anaesthetic is not used as the difference between the anaesthetic and lethal dose is marginal in neonatal mice.)
2   Support the animal in a harness as shown in Fig. 10.4.
3   Open in skin by a longitudinal incision in the midline overlying the sternum.
4   Make a triangular cut in the rib cage at the anterior end of the sternum. Remove the underlying fibrous tissue to expose the thymus.
5   Suck out both thymus lobes using a fine-glass tube attached to a vacuum line. (*Do not suck too hard or enter too deeply to avoid the heart following the thymus into the suction tube.*)
6   Close the wound with 2 or 3 fine-silk sutures.
7   Warm the mouse gently under a lamp.

With practice post-operative mortality is low. Cannabalism may be reduced by fostering the operated mice onto docile mothers.

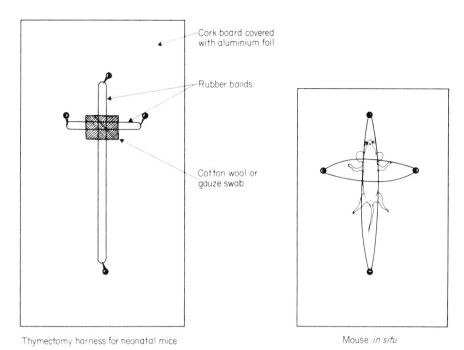

Thymectomy harness for neonatal mice

Mouse *in situ*

Fig. 10.4. Harness for the thymectomy of neonatal mice

10.5.2b   Neonatal thymectomy of chickens

The anatomical distribution of the avian thymus is quite unlike that of the mammal. It consists of a series of 6–8 paired lobes running beside the carotid arteries in the neck. In addition there is often a thymic infiltrate of the thyroid gland.

Materials and equipment

Chickens, on day of hatch
Surgical instruments
X-ray machine or γ-source

Method

1   Anaesthetize the chick using 0·1 ml of a 12 mg ml^{-1} solution of sodium pentobarbital given intraperitoneally.
2   Remove the feathers from either the dorsal or ventral surface of the neck and swab the area with 70% alcohol.
3   Open the neck via either a dorsal or ventral incision. (*If a ventral incision is made, it is necessary to reflect the crop and oesophagus.*)
4   Expose the carotid arteries and identify the thymus lobes to their anterior and posterior extent.

263

5 Using a glass tube connected to a vacuum line, break the fascia covering the thymus lobes and suck out each lobe.

It is advisable to remove all subcutaneous fat to ensure that no thymic tissue remains.

6 Close the wound with a series of single sutures.

7 Allow the chicks to recover in an incubator.

8 X-irradiate the next day, as in Section 10.5.1.

Technical note

Because of their high body temperature, chicks are sensitive to hypothermia while under anaesthesia. It is therefore advisable to perform the operation under a lamp.

The effectiveness of thymectomy may be assessed in the following ways, in addition to a macroscopic examination at eventual sacrifice.

1 Ability of immunized birds to give a positive wattle test to ppd.

2 High percentage of immunoglobulin-bearing lymphocytes in the blood (Section 2.5.1).

3 Poor or absent skin graft rejection (Section 3.2.2a). In the chicken it is convenient to graft onto the scaley part of the leg to avoid the problem of feathers.

10.5.2c **Adult bursectomy and thymectomy**

Adult bursectomy and thymectomy is without immediate general effect in both mammals and birds. After 1–2 years some of the B- or T-cell functions decline. The effectiveness of adult thymectomy in the mouse has been increased by treating the operated animal with 2 injections of anti-lymphocyte serum (Section 10.8.1) or by combining lethal X-irradiation with bone-marrow reconstitution (Section 10.6).

ADULT THYMECTOMY (MOUSE)

Materials and equipment

Mice
Surgical instruments
Ethanol, 70% v/v in water

Method

1 Anaesthetize the mouse with a safe inhalation anaesthetic.

2 Stretch the animal out on an operating board (as in Fig. 10.4, but adjust harness to fit an adult animal). Attach a pinned wire loop to the upper incisors to hold the head back.

3 Swab the ventral surface of the upper thorax and neck with ethanol.

4   Make a midline longitudinal incision (about 2 cm long) through the skin just above the anterior end of the sternum.

5   Open the skin, separate and deflect the salivary glands (*handle gently to avoid bleeding*).

6   Make an anterior-posterior cut through the right clavicle just adjacent to the sternum.

7   Repeat for the left clavicle, deflect and cut off the triangular piece of anterior sternum.

8   Remove the fascia overlying the thymus.

9   Place a thumb under the mouse's diaphragm and press so that the contents of the thorax force the thymus into a more convenient position for manipulation.

10   Remove the left and right lobe of the thymus using a wide-mouthed pipette attached to a vacuum trap.

11   Release the arms and pinch the skin together with the finger and thumb, thus exerting a slight lateral pressure on each side of the thorax.

12   Close the incision with a Michel clip.

Technical notes

1   Once the triangular piece of anterior sternum has been removed it is necessary to work rapidly. If too much air enters the thoracic cavity lung collapse will occur.

2   Post-operative mortality should be less than 10%.

10.6   **RECONSTITUTED MICE**

Historically the 'B-mouse' (thymus deprived, X-irradiated and bone-marrow reconstituted) was of great importance but has now been replaced by inbred nu/nu mice (Section 1.8.2) which are virtually devoid of mature T cells.

Materials and equipment

6-week-old CBA male mice
CBA donors for bone-marrow cells
X-ray machine or γ-source

Method

1   Thymectomize the recipient mice (as above).

2   3–6 weeks after thymectomy irradiate the mice; use highest possible X-ray dose. *This can be up to 1100R under 'clean' conditions.*

3   Prepare a suspension of bone-marrow cells from the femurs of the donor mice. Remove each femur, cut off the ends and blow out

265

the marrow with tissue-culture medium from a syringe and needle. Disperse the cells with a Pasteur pipette.

4   Count the cells and treat with anti-Thy.1 and complement to remove any mature T lymphocytes (Sections 10.8.5 and 10.9).

5   Inject 5×10^6 syngeneic bone-marrow cells into the tail vein of each thymectomized, irradiated mouse.

6   The mice may be used 8–10 weeks later.

Assay the effectiveness of B-cell reconstitution and T depletion using anti-immunoglobulin membrane immunoflourescence (Section 2.5.1) and complement-mediated anti-Thy.1 killing (Sections 10.8.5 and 10.9.1).

10.7   THORACIC DUCT CANNULATION OF MICE

There is a continuous circulation of small lymphocytes from the blood into other peripheral organs and thence into the tissues in general. From here the cells finally return to the blood via the lymphatic vessels, the most important of which is the thoracic duct. Cells in the thoracic duct are part of the so-called recirculating pool of lymphocytes and represent non-dividing, G_0 cells that are either virgin or memory cells. There is doubt at present as to whether the virgin cells are permitted to enter the recirculating pool for any prolonged period of time or whether it is purely the abode of memory cells. It is known, however, that cells selectively leave the recirculating pool if the animal is challenged with antigen and congregate at the site of greatest antigen concentration.

Much of the information on cell 'trafficking' patterns has been gained by thoracic duct cannulation as a means of obtaining recirculating lymphocytes, principally in the mouse, rat and sheep.

Strictly speaking the cysterna chyla, rather than the thoracic duct is cannulated in mice. This is a relatively wide, flaccid vessel lying behind the kidney between the inferior vena cava and the lumbar muscles.

Technique

Initial preparations

1   Give each mouse 0·2 ml of cream by injection into the oesophagus 20 min before the operation. The lipid soon appears as a translucent milkiness in the lymph and enables the cysterna chyla to be easily visualized.

2   Prepare anaesthetic as follows:

Dissolve 10 g tribromomethanol in 10 ml of amyl alcohol and store in a light-tight bottle at 4°. Dilute this solution 1 : 50 and use 0·01 ml g^{-1} total body weight to induce anaesthesia.

Materials and equipment

Mice, 6–8-week-old
Boak cannulas (Appendix II)
Cotton buds or Q tips (Appendix II)
Surgical instruments and Michel clips
Tissue adhesive (Appendix II)
Tissue-culture medium and balanced salt solution (BSS) (Appendix I)

Method

1 Shave the left flank of the anaesthetized mouse.

2 Place the mouse on a cork board (under an adjustable light) with the shaved side uppermost and with the head to the left.

3 Swab the flank with alcohol, lift the skin with forceps and excise a strip of skin from the thigh region to the costal margin of the rib cage. *It is important to make the excision both extensive and in the mid-lateral region.*

4 Open the peritoneal cavity with a 2–3 cm incision in the abdominal musculature parallel to the inferior border of the spleen.

5 Place four retractors (*made from the wire holding Michel clips, and attached to the heads of dissecting pins*) in the incision and pin out so that the abdominal cavity is exposed through a square hole measuring about 2 cm × 2 cm.

6 Free the kidney from the fatty tissue holding it onto the lumbar muscle by blunt dissection using two cotton buds. Draw the kidney ventrally to expose the cysterna chyla. *It lies in a furrow between the inferior vena cava and the lumbar muscles.*

7 Prepare the cannula by cutting the tip with a scalpel blade at a point just after the short arm becomes parallel with the long arm. *Optimum lymph flow is obtained if the tip is cut to produce an 'arrow shape'.*

8 From the right, place an 18-gauge needle through the posteriorly retracted abdominal muscles and insert, from the left, the uncut (long) arm of the cannula. Withdraw the needle so that the cannula can be drawn into position with the cut (short) arm overlying the duct and the long arm over and parallel with the mouse's tail.

9 Fill the cannula with BSS from a syringe and 25-gauge needle, be sure to avoid air bubbles. Remove the syringe and keep the cannula horizontal with the hooked end under the upper-left retractor.

10 Make a small hole in the cysterna chyla using a pair of sharp-tipped jeweller's forceps; with the forceps closed place the tips just through the wall of the vessel and open the tips slightly, at the same time pulling the mesentery ventrally with a cotton bud. The hole produced should be about 1 mm in diameter and will be clearly

seen if air can be drawn into the hole by firm ventral traction with the cotton bud.

11 Hold the curved end of the cannula with the jeweller's forceps and place the tip into the hole made in the vessel.

12 Hold the cannula in position with a cotton bud and test whether lymph can enter the cannula freely by lowering the long arm below the horizontal. *The siphoning effect of the saline in the cannula should draw the lymph into the cannula.* Return the cannula to a horizontal position and apply one drop of tissue adhesive over the general region where the cannula enters the duct. Exercise great care in applying the adhesive which will 'set' in about 20–30 sec, do not let it enter the lymph vessel.

13 Remove the retractors and close the wound with 3–4 Michel clips through the skin. For overnight collection, it is not necessary to close the abdominal musculature separately.

14 Place adhesive tape around the mouse's abdomen, but not around the cannula, so that the mouse can be suspended from above and allowed to run on the outside of a vertical wheel (see Technical note at end of section).

15 Infuse the mouse via the tail vein with a balanced salt solution at 0.5–1.0 ml h^{-1} to promote lymph flow.

16 Collect the thoracic duct lymph into 2 ml of tissue-culture medium containing 10% fetal calf serum and two drops of preservative free heparin. Use 15 ml plastic tubes standing on ice in a thermos flask.

17 Check cannulas constantly within the first 3 h of the operation to see that the lymph is flowing—remove fibrin clots with a horse hair or a fine nylon thread. *A simple test that the lymph is flowing is to raise the cannula—this should cause the lymph to run backwards freely.*

During a 16 h collection it should be possible to obtain between 2.0–10.0×10^7 lymphocytes per mouse, depending on the age, health, etc, of the mouse.

Technical note

If the mice are allowed to run on the outside of a tread mill during drainage this promotes lymph flow and increases cell yield. It is also essential that mice are kept warm and given water and food *ad libitum*.

10.8   CELL-SPECIFIC ANTIGENS AND ANTISERA

Cells in general carry a whole array of surface antigens that can be recognized by appropriate antisera or antibodies (Chapter 11). Although these antigens may be conveniently considered under the following headings, it must be stressed that we are not attempting a classification, any particular antigen may occur under one or more heading.

1 **Species antigens.** By definition these antigens are carried by all cells within a single species. They may be recognized by antibodies raised by cross-species immunization. It is probable that closely related species, for example, mouse and rat, share many of these antigens.

2 **Constitutive and tissue antigens.** These antigens are in some way associated with the rôle of the cell. Accordingly, human, rat and amphibian nuclei share many antigens as do human and rat gastric and hepatic cells. These antigens are often of importance in immunopathological disorders where they 'elicit' autoantibodies (Section 4.4).

3 **Histocompatibility antigens.** These antigens were originally recognized as being important in graft rejection (Section 3.2.2). Although some of these antigens can be recognized by antisera (serological determinants) some cannot; these latter antigens (lymphocyte determinants) have been identified by the mixed lymphocyte reaction (Section 10.11.4). Histocompatibility antigens are coded for by the 'major histocompatibility complex' (MHC) of gene loci: H-2 in mouse and HL-A in man.

It has now been recognized that many other cell-surface antigens can bring about graft rejection, for example, skin specific tissue antigens.

4 **Stage-specific differentiation antigens.** These antigens are qualitatively or quantitatively modulated during cell differentiation. T and B cells, for example, differ qualitatively in these antigens: Thy.1 in the mouse (Section 10.8.5) and T and B heteroantigens in the chicken. Moreover, T lymphocytes themselves show a differential expression of the Thy.1 antigen during ontogeny; thymocytes express a greater surface density of Thy.1 than mature T-lymphocytes. Thymocytes are also known to have a lower surface density of H-2 than peripheral lymphocytes.

10.8.1 ANTI-LYMPHOCYTE SERUM

Anti-lymphocyte sera (ALS) have been used to suppress the cells mediating the immune response in both human and animal situations. ALS are potentially more specific immunosuppressive agents than, for example, X-irradiation which also suppresses haemopoietic function.

For *in vivo* use the heteroantiserum is fractionated to obtain γ-globulin or IgG to reduce the amount of foreign protein injected into the recipient. Additionally, the antiserum is ultracentrifuged to remove soluble aggregates and so reduce its immunogenicity to an extent where it might become tolerogenic (Section 4.3).

269

Materials

Mice, preferably inbred, 4–6 weeks of age
Rabbits

Method

1   Remove thymi from mice and prepare single-cell suspension.
2   Inject 10^9 viable lymphocytes into the marginal ear vein of the rabbit.
3   Two weeks later repeat the injection, however, the rabbit must first receive an anti-anaphylactic agent, e.g. 25 mg promethazine hydrochloride given intravenously.
4   Two weeks later exsanguinate the rabbit by cardiac puncture.
5   Separate the serum, inactivate the complement components at 56° for 45 min and store at $-20°$.

10.8.2   MODE OF ACTION OF ALS *IN VIVO*

ALS are able to kill both T and B cells in *in vitro* assays (Section 10.9); surprisingly, however, there is a marked T-cell specificity when used *in vivo*. Hence in mice, the system most extensively studied, T-dependent areas of the spleen and lymph nodes are markedly depleted, and only T-dependent, but not T-independent, humoral responses are suppressed after ALS treatment. Accordingly, adult thymectomy accompanied by ALS treatment is as effective at suppressing the T-cell pool as neonatal thymectomy.

It is known that ALS do not penetrate lymphoid tissues appreciably and so only cells in the recirculating pool, mainly T cells, are susceptible to ALS killing. Although ALS can kill lymphoid cells with the aid of complement, it is likely that immune adherence and opsonization (Section 6.5.1) followed by phagocytosis by the reticuloendothelial system is the main mechanism by which immunosuppression is effected (Section 10.8.3).

10.8.3   *IN VIVO* IMMUNE ADHERENCE

As will be seen in Section 10.9 it is possible to lyse T and B lymphocytes directly using ALS with complement. It is unlikely, however, that this is the main mechanism by which ALS suppression is achieved *in vivo* because, especially for clinical use, much lower concentrations of ALS (γ-globulin or IgG fraction) are used than are required to fix enough complement for cell lysis. At the lower antibody concentrations enough complement is probably bound to bring about immune adherence to macrophages (and erythrocytes in primates) via C3. The ALS coated cells could then be removed by the reticulo-endothelial system (RES).

270

Materials and equipment

Anti-lymphocyte and normal control serum (Section 10.8.1)
Other materials as in Section 10.3.2

Method

1 Prepare a lymphocyte suspension and label with ^{51}Cr as in
Section 10.3.2.
2 Treat labelled lymphocytes with ALS or NRS according to the
protocol. Total final volume 0·5 ml.
3 Wash the cells twice by centrifugation and resuspend in 1·0 ml
of medium.
4 Inject 5×10^6 cells intravenously, and retain an aliquot of
5×10^6 cells from tube 1 for γ-counting.
5 Kill the mice 4 h post-injection and count the γ-emissions from
spleen and liver. Count also the 5×10^6 cells from tube 1.
6 Calculate the amount of radioactivity in each organ as a percentage of the original counts injected. Calculate also the spleen/liver
ratio.
    Interpret the results with reference to Section 10.3.2.

Protocol

Tube number:	1	2	3	4	5	6
ALS or NRS final dilution	0	1 : 50	1 : 100	1 : 200	1 : 400	1 : 800
Lymphocytes-^{51}Cr 10^8 ml^{-1}	0·5 ml					$\longrightarrow$

10.8.4 ANTIBODIES TO MEMBRANE ANTIGENS

Antisera against polymorphic cell surface antigens may be
produced reproducibly by immunization between congenic strains
of animals (almost invariably mice, Section 10.8.5). Because the two
strains of animals are identical except for the locus carrying the two
allelic genes, only the antigens of interest (alloantigens) will be
recognized as foreign and elicit an antibody response.

However, in species where no polymorphic antigens have been
recognized (almost every species, except mice), the production of
antibodies to specific cell surface antigens relies on an across species
immunization (heteroimmunization, producing a heteroantiserum).
Under these conditions, antibodies against the antigen of interest
are likely to be a minor contaminant in a complex antiserum reacting with many cell surface determinants.

271

In the 'bad old days' (before 1975) it was necessary to perform extensive cross-absorption to remove all the unwanted antibody activity. (All too often the cross-absorption was so extensive that the antiserum finally contained no antibody to anything.)

It is now possible to use cell fusion to produce lines of hybridoma cells secreting monoclonal antibody (see Chapter 11). Although the positive selection of antibody producing cells is almost as time consuming as the negative selection of 'monospecific' antibodies, once the cell line has been established one has it for ever (potentially).

Hybridoma produced antibodies are now commercially available to several alloantigens (Appendix II).

10.8.5 ANTISERA TO LYMPHOCYTE MEMBRANE ALLOANTIGENS

Several useful alloantigens have been recognized on mouse lymphocytes and plasma cells. These antigens are strain-specific differentiation antigens and occur on subpopulations of cells, for example, the Thy.1 antigen which occurs only on thymocytes and T lymphocytes. Thy.1 occurs as two alleles:

gene Thy.1^a, gene product Thy 1.1 on T cells of AKR, RF and several substrains
gene Thy.1^b, gene product Thy 1.2 on T cells of most other inbred and outbred strains.

Antisera may be raised to these antigens by cross-immunizing H-2 compatible mice with thymocytes.

Materials

AKR and C3H or CBA mice
Alternatively use AKR/J and AKR/Cum mice. These are congenic strains differing only at the Thy.1 locus.

Method

1   Prepare a thymocyte suspension from AKR donors and wash twice by centrifugation.
2   Inject 3×10^7 thymocytes intraperitoneally into each C3H or CBA recipient weekly for 10 weeks.
3   Take a sample bleed from the tail of immunized mice on week 11, pool serum and test by cytotoxicity (Section 10.9).

A specimen titration curve is given in Fig. 10.5. Exsanguinate the mice when a high-titre antiserum has been obtained.

Notes

As the mice (AKR, C3H and CBA) are histocompatible at the major histocompatibility complex (MHC) no anti-H-2 antibodies are

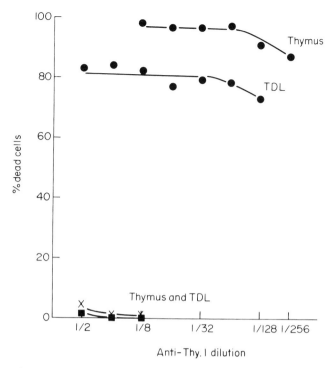

Fig. 10.5. Complement-mediated cytotoxicity with anti-Thy.1 serum
●——● anti-Thy.1 plus complement.
×——× normal AKR serum plus complement.
■——■ anti-Thy.1 serum alone.
Percentage immunoglobulin positive lymphocytes by immunofluorescence: thymus 0·3% thoracic duct lymphocytes 18·9%.

produced by this immunization procedure. Several other contaminating antibodies have been identified, however, such as anti-thymocyte autoantibody and anti-immunoglobulin allotype anti-body. In the assay systems described in the book these contaminating antibodies are not detected and so the anti-Thy.1 serum may be used specifically to detect, kill or inhibit T cells and their functions.

Reif and Allen who first discovered the Thy.1 antigen in 1963 also detected its presence in nervous tissue. Recently T cell specific heteroantisera have been raised by immunizing rabbits with mouse-brain homogenates. Monoclonal antibodies, produced by hybridomas, are now available against the Thy.1 antigens (Appendix II).

10.8.6 INDIRECT IMMUNOFLUORESCENCE WITH ALLOANTISERA

It is not possible to take advantage of the increased sensitivity of indirect immunofluorescent staining using alloantisera. The fluorescently conjugated second antiserum, for example, rabbit anti-

273

mouse immunoglubulin, would detect both the bound alloantibody and the immunoglobulin receptors carried on B lymphocytes (see Section 2.5). This problem has recently been circumvented using DNP-coupled alloantisera which can be detected by an anti-DNP serum conjugated with one of the fluorochromes. The method is also applicable to antibodies produced by cell hybridomas (Chapter 11).

Materials and equipment

As in the sections indicated below, but in addition,
Anti-Thy.1 serum, C3H anti-AKR or vice versa, or anti-H2 serum (Section 10.8.5)
Normal mouse serum
Goat or rabbit anti-DNP (Details below)
Rabbit anti-mouse immunoglobulin (Section 1.4.2)

Method

1   Prepare goat or rabbit anti-DNP using $DNP_{30\ 35}\ F\gamma G$ (Dinitrophenylate the $F\gamma G$ as described in Section 1.3.1a). Give two injections of the hapten-carrier conjugate in Freund's complete adjuvant as described in Section 1.4 and boost with alum precipitated antigen (Section 1.4.4) until a strong precipitation line is seen in Ouchterlony immunodiffusion (Section 5.3.3b) against either DNP–HSA or DNP–BSA.
2   Prepare either an anti-Thy.1 or an anti-H-2 serum as described in Section 10.8.5.
3   Prepare a 50% saturated ammonium sulphate precipitate of the alloantiserum, and a $33\frac{1}{3}\%$ saturated ammonium sulphate precipi-

Protocol: For anti-Thy.1 staining of thymus and spleen

Tube number	Alloantiserum	Dilution	Fluorescent conjugate (1 : 10 dilution)
1	DNP anti-Thy.1	1 : 4	anti-DNP
2	DNP anti-Thy.1	1 : 8	anti-DNP
3	DNP anti-Thy.1	1 : 16	anti-DNP
4	DNP anti-Thy.1	1 : 32	anti-DNP
5	DNP normal mouse serum	1 : 4	anti-DNP
6	DNP normal mouse serum	1 : 8	anti-DNP
7	anti-Thy.1	1 : 4	anti-mouse Ig
8	anti-Thy.1	1 : 8	anti-mouse Ig
9	anti-Thy.1	1 : 16	anti-mouse Ig
10	anti-Thy.1	1 : 32	anti-mouse Ig
11	normal mouse serum	1 : 4	anti-mouse Ig
12	normal mouse serum	1 : 8	anti-mouse Ig

tate of the anti-DNP serum (Section 1.2.2) and dialyse each against PBS (Section 1.2.3).

4   Conjugate the alloantibody with DNP as described in Section 1.3.1b, BUT use 100 mg of dinitrobenzenesulphonate per 100 mg of protein.

5   Conjugate the anti-DNP precipitate with a fluorochrome as described in Section 1.6.

6   Repeat the ammonium sulphate precipitation and DNP conjugation using normal mouse serum.

The antisera may be standardized as shown in the protocol (p. 274); staining mouse lymph node and thymus cells by the indirect immunofluorescence technique described in Section 2.5.1.

Data from a representative experiment is shown in Fig. 10.6.

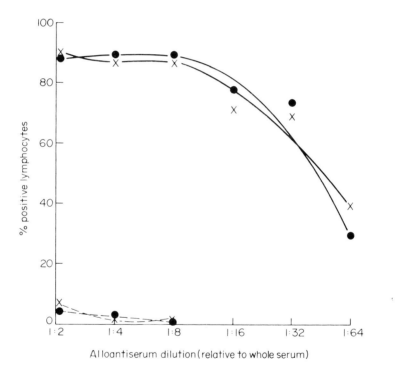

Alloantiserum dilution (relative to whole serum)

Fig. 10.6. Staining of mouse thymus cells by DNP anti-Thy.1.
× — × DNP C3H anti-Thy.1 AKR detected by fluorescein-labelled goat anti-DNP-ovalbumin.
× --- × Normal C3H serum followed by anti-DNP conjugate.
● — ● Anti-Thy.1 detected by fluorescein-labelled rabbit anti-mouse immunoglobulin.
●--- ● Normal C3H serum followed by anti-mouse immunoglobulin conjugate. As can be seen from the graph, the two curves of staining can be superimposed, and so the two staining techniques are probably defining the same populations with equal sensitivity. Similar results have been found for lymph-node staining. (Data by courtesy of Anthony Finch.)

1 Under the conditions described, each molecule of mouse gamma-globulin should bind 15–20 DNP groups.

2 Tubes number 7–10 in the protocol are included as a positive control to detect any loss of antibody activity induced by DNP conjugation of the alloantisera.

3 Store the DNP conjugates in the dark at 4°, do not freeze.

4 It is possible to undertake double-labelling studies using two alloantibodies each conjugated with different haptens and detected with the relevant anti-hapten antibody labelled with different fluorochromes. Conjugates of penicilloyl-antibody have also been used, detected by rhodamine labelled rabbit anti-penicilloyl-ovalbumin.

10.9 COMPLEMENT-MEDIATED CYTOLYSIS

This technique is probably one of the *in vitro* equivalents of cytotoxic hypersensitivity (Section 4.5.2); antisera directed against cell-surface antigens are used to kill cells carrying these antigens with the aid of complement.

We will describe two techniques that differ in the means by which cell death is assayed.

10.9.1 DYE EXCLUSION TEST

This test is an extension of the method used to estimate cell viability described in Section 2.4.1.

Materials

Anti-lymphocyte serum, ALS (Section 10.8.1)
Rabbit anti-mouse immunoglobulin (Section 1.4.2)
Guinea-pig serum (Complement) (Appendix II)
Nigrosin dye (Appendix II)
Inbred mice, 4–6 weeks old

Method

1 Absorb the complement with mouse spleen and erythrocytes; approximately 0·1 ml packed cells ml^{-1} of serum, for 30 min at 4°.

2 Centrifuge the absorbed complement. Use immediately or store at $-20°$.

3 Prepare thymus and lymph node suspensions from mouse donors. Estimate viability and adjust to 5×10^7 viable lymphocytes ml^{-1}. (*See Technical note for removal of dead cells.*)

4   Prepare cell and serum mixtures according to the following protocol, and incubate at 37° for 30 min.

Protocol

Tube number	1	2	3	4	5	6
ALS dilution*	1 : 20	1 : 40	1 : 80	1 : 160	1 : 320	1 : 640
or						
NRS dilution*	1 : 20	1 : 40				
Lymph node cells $(5 \times 10^7 \text{ ml}^{-1})$	0·1 ml ⟶					
Absorbed guinea-pig serum (1 : 5 initial dilution)	0·1 ml ⟶					

Repeat this protocol using thymus cells with the same dilutions of ALS and NRS.* Final dilution.

Assay 1 (see protocol above)

Cells: lymph node

Antisera; ALS and pre-immunization serum (NRS)

Assay 2 (see protocol below)

Cells: lymph node

Antisera: anti-immunoglobulin (if asays 1 and 2 are performed simultaneously a second NRS control is not required).

5   After incubation stand the tubes in ice to prevent further complement fixation and cell lysis.

6   Count the number of viable cells in each suspension as described in Section 2.4.1.

7   Calculate the number of viable cells ml^{-1} and from this the percentage lysis for each tube according to the following equation:

$$\% \text{ lysis} = \frac{Cn - Ca}{Co} \times 100$$

where Cn = No. live cells in NRS

Ca = No. live cells in ALS or anti-Ig

Co = Original no. live cells.

Protocol

Tube number	1	2	3	4	5
Anti-immunoglobulin dilution*	1 : 10	1 : 20	1 : 40	1 : 80	1 : 160
Lymph node cells $(5 \times 10^7 \text{ ml}^{-1})$	0·1 ml ⟶				
Absorbed guinea-pig serum (1 : 5 initial dilution)	0·1 ml ⟶				

Repeat this protocol using thymus cells with the same dilutions of anti-immunoglobulin. * Final dilution.

8   Plot a graph of % lysis against antiserum dilution for each tissue and antiserum.

Interpretation of results

1   You should find that ALS (anti-thymocyte serum) kills all nucleated cells in the thymus and lymph node suspension to a high dilution of antiserum. This lack of T-cell specificity is, of course, to be expected as lymphocytes share many surface antigens.
2   The percentage of cells killed by the anti-immunoglobulin serum should coincide with the expected % of B cells in the tissue used. (See Fig. 2.1.)
3   If the killing of thymocytes by anti-immunoglobulin or NRS exceeds 5%, then there are probably anti-species antibodies present, not related to the original immunizing procedure. In this case it is necessary to absorb ALL sera with liver membranes (see Section 1.6.6).

Technical notes

1   The sensitivity of this assay depends upon a high initial cell viability. Frequently 20–30% dead cells are encountered in lymph node suspensions. Dead cells may be removed by the following procedure.

Materials and equipment—

Phosphate buffered saline, PBS (Appendix I)
0·308 M glucose in water
Siliconized Pasteur pipettes
10 ml conical centrifuge tubes

ALL STEPS MUST BE CARRIED OUT AT 4°

(a) Mix 1 volume of PBS with 19 volumes of the glucose solution (low-ionic strength buffer).
(b) Spin down the lymphocytes and resuspend to 2–4×10^7 ml^{-1} in low-ionic strength buffer.
(c) Cut the end from a siliconized Pasteur pipette just below the drawn-out shoulder and loosely pack with cotton wool (about 5 mm in length).
(d) Add 4 ml of cell suspension to each pipette (allow it to flow through under 1 g). Collect the effluent in a siliconized tube.
(e) Layer 1 ml of fetal bovine serum below the cell suspension and centrifuge at 220 g for 15 min at 4°.
(f) Resuspend the cells in normal medium and perform a viability count.

2   The guinea-pig serum complement source must be absorbed

with spleen and red cells before use as it is frequently itself cytotoxic. It was discovered that an agarose absorption may also be used to remove anti-mouse antibodies. Use 100 mg of agarose ml^{-1} of serum, absorb for 60 min at 4°.

3   Low dilutions of serum, for example, in anti-Thy.1 killing, are frequently anti-complementary. Anti-complementarity may also be a problem with antibodies purified by acid elution from immuno-adsorbents (Section 8.1) due to aggregated protein. This may be avoided by washing the cells twice by centrifugation after antibody treatment; the diluted complement is then added.

4   In this assay it is advisable to count the number of viable cells after lysis rather than the number of dead cells, especially if centrifugation steps are included after killing. Dead cells are often broken up and lost during centrifugation.

10.9.2 ^{51}Cr-LABELLED CELL LYSIS

Estimating cell death by dye inclusion, although simple, is rather time consuming and so not many assays can be performed simultaneously. If the cells are labelled with ^{51}Cr it is possible to estimate cell death by the amount of isotope released. In this case it is an advantage to centrifuge the cells after killing to enhance cell dissolution and isotope release.

Materials and equipment

Sodium ^{51}chromate (Appendix II)
Inbred mice, 4–6 weeks old
Gamma counter

Method

1   Prepare thymus and lymph node suspensions in tissue-culture medium containing HEPES (20 mM) and 5% fetal bovine serum.

2   Adjust to 5×10^7 lymphocytes ml^{-1} and add 100 μCi of sodium ^{51}chromate to 1 ml of each cell suspension. Incubate at 37° for 40 min.

3   Wash cells twice with medium and allow to stand on ice for 30 min.

4   Wash cells three times with medium and resuspend to 5×10^6 lymphocytes ml^{-1}.

5   Mix 0·1 ml of each cell suspension with antibody and complement (see protocols, Section 10.9.1) and incubate at 37° for 30 min.

6   After incubation adjust final volume to 0·5 ml, mix well and centrifuge (150 g for 10 min at 4°).

7   Remove 0·1 ml of supernatant and count amount of released isotope in gamma counter.

279

Many investigators determine the maximum (100%) ^{51}Cr release by lysing an aliquot of cells, either by freezing and thawing or with 10% Saponin. Under the labelling conditions described this is usually 1000–1400 cpm (for 5×10^6 cells).

For some applications, however, this is not a realistic value. This technique may be used, for example, for quantitative absorption experiments by which the relative amount of cell-surface antigen on different cell types may be compared. A fixed number of cells is used to absorb a fixed concentration of antiserum and the original and absorbed antisera are then assayed on ^{51}Cr-labelled cells. In this case it is advisable to determine the dilutions of original antiserum giving a plateau release value, and to use this as the 100% ^{51}Cr release. Alternatively one may work more sensitively with the dilution of antiserum required to give 50% of this maximum release (cf. Section 6.1).

The technical notes given in Section 10.9.1 also apply to this technique.

10.10 AUTORADIOGRAPHIC LABELLING OF LYMPHOCYTES

In Section 2.5.1 a series of experiments were performed to investigate the surface components of lymphocytes using fluorochrome-labelled antibodies. The sensitivity of this approach can be greatly increased by substituting a radioactive isotope for the fluorochrome. In addition, autoradiography is semi-quantitative, the relative number of grains per cell is dependent upon the number of labelled antibody molecules bound and in turn on the number of surface determinants detected. It is therefore possible to estimate the relative distribution of the determinants throughout the cell population, and within the same experiment, the relative concentration and distribution of determinants between two cell populations.

In this way it has been shown that B cells vary widely in the number of available immunoglobulin molecules on their surface (see Fig. 10.7) and that T and B cells differ quantitatively in their membrane content of immunoglobulin.

The basic autoradiographic method as described below may be used under any situation where a radioactive isotope is introduced into or onto a cell or tissue.

Example: labelling of chicken lymphocytes

Materials and equipment

Chickens, 1 day old
Anti-immunoglobulin antibody—either purified by acid elution (Section 8.1) or an IgG fraction (Section 7.3)

Control—either an irrelevant purified antibody (e.g. anti-KLH) or
   normal rabbit IgG (NRIgG)
Chloramine T
Sodium metabisulphite
Sodium ^{125}iodide (Appendix II)
Sephadex G-25 (Appendix II)
Glass tubing, internal diameter 6·0 mm
Ilford K5 nuclear emulsion (Appendix II)

Although strictly one should titrate the concentration of antibody
used until a plateau value of labelled cells is attained, it has been
found in practice that 50 μg of pure anti-immunoglobulin antibody
or 100 μg of IgG anti-immunoglobulin per 10^7 lymphocytes is a
vast excess.

Specimen experimental protocol

Anti-immunoglobulin labelling of bursa cells from 6 1-day-old
chicks:
   Antiserum: rabbit anti-chicken light chain (anti-LC) purified by
acid elution from immunoadsorbent of chicken IgG (Section 8.1).
Control serum: rabbit anti-Keyhole limpet haemocyanin (anti-
KLH) antibody prepared in a similar manner.

CALCULATION OF INITIAL CONCENTRATION OF REAGENTS
FOR PROTEIN IODINATION

Oxidation conditions: Use 1 mCi of ^{125}I per 200 μg of protein in
100 μg ml^{-1} chloramine T (final concentration). The protein concentration must be at or above 5 mg ml^{-1} to avoid excessive
denaturation.

Specimen calculation

Rabbit anti-chicken LC and anti-KLH at 20 mg ml^{-1} initial
   concentration
Wish to label 6 aliquots of bursa cells at 50 μg of antibody
   aliquot^{-1} = 300 μg protein, ∴ use 1·5 mCi ^{125}I.
^{125}I (I.M.S. 30) supplied at 100 mCi ml^{-1} ∴ use 15 μl
To maintain 5 mg ml^{-1} protein concentration must calculate permissible volume of chloramine T as follows:

   Protein used = 15 μl at 20 mg ml^{-1}; maximum permissible oxidation volume: 60 μl at 5 mg ml^{-1}.

Final oxidation mixture

15 μl protein + 15 μl ^{125}I + 20 μl chloramine T (Total volume
   50 μl; protein concentration 6 mg ml^{-1})

281

Chloramine T used at 100 μg ml^{-1} final concentration $\therefore$ initial concentration must be 250 μg ml^{-1}, i.e. prepare an initial solution of 25 mg chloramine T in 100 ml PBS.

Reaction stopped by a twofold excess, by weight, of sodium metabisulphite.

Final mixture

15 μl protein + 15 μl ^{125}I + 20 μl chloramine T + 50 μl sodium meta-bisulphite. Total volume = 100 μl

Final concentration of metabisulphite = 200 μg ml^{-1}; initial concentration must be 400 μg ml^{-1}, i.e. prepare an initial solution of 40 mg sodium metabisulphite in 100 ml PBS.

Method

1 Partially seal the end of 2 pieces of glass tubing, length 30 cm, internal diameter 0·6 cm, and plug with cotton wool.
2 Pour two columns of Sephadex G-25, height 10 cm.
3 Determine void volume and expanded sample volume of each column using 0·3 ml blue dextran (initial sample volume). Equilibrate columns with PBS (Section 1.2.3).
4 Pipette out protein for iodination into pointed glass tubes.
5 Add calculated volume of sodium ^{125}iodide (CARE).
6 Add chloramine T and oxidize for 3 min at room temperature.
7 Terminate reaction by addition of sodium metabisulphite.
8 Adjust final volume to 0·3 ml with PBS.
9 Pass the iodination mixture through the Sephadex G-25 column.
10 Monitor the column effluent for the first appearance of radioactivity. (*This should be just after the void volume has left the column.*)
11 Collect the labelled protein in the expanded sample volume.

The radioactively labelled protein may be stored overnight at 4° before use.

Cell labelling

1 Add 50 μg of iodinated protein (either anti-LC or anti-KLH) to aliquots of 10^7 bursal lymphocytes.
2 Incubate at 4° for 30 min.
3 Centrifuge each aliquot of cells through a 2 ml discontinuous gradient of 50% and 100% fetal bovine serum in tissue culture medium (225 g for 15 min at 4°).
4 Suck off the supernatant and resuspend the cells in 1 ml of tissue-culture medium.
5 Layer the cells onto a second gradient and centrifuge.

6   Finally resuspend the cell pellet in a few drops of fetal bovine serum and prepare smears as described in Section 2.3.1.

7   Check that the smears are adequate using a phase-contrast microscope, and adjust the cell concentration with fetal bovine serum if required.

8   Prepare at least 6 smears per cell aliquot, and label the slides for identification.

9   Fix the slides (Section 2.3.1), wash in running tap water for 30 min and finally air dry.

10   Dip the slides in a 1 : 5 solution (v/v) of Ilford K5 nuclear emulsion and dry slides in front of a fan or over silica gel overnight (IN A PHOTOGRAPHIC DARKROOM).

11   Leave slides to expose in light-tight containers at 4°. (*Do not store near radioactive materials.*)

Exposure time

1   Under the conditions described, one sample slide should be removed from each group after 4–5 days.

2   Develop, fix and wash the sample autoradiographs and then stain in May–Grünwald–Giemsa (Section 2.3.2).

3   Examine the slides under oil immersion. If the autoradiographs in the control groups show more than 8–10 grains per cell develop all the slides. If, however, the control staining is low, examine the anti-LC treated cells. If the grain counts are clearly above the control values, develop all the slides.

4   Sample the autoradiographs at least every 4 days until satisfactory positive labelling is achieved with a low number of grains on control cells.

5   At the end of the exposure period (usually 10–14 days under the conditions described), select at least two slides per group for grain counting. Use the following criteria:

(a) the cells must be sufficiently spread so that the grains between two adjacent cells do not overlap.

(b) the cell density must be similar on anti-LC and control slides within each group.

(c) the emulsion over the cells must be free from 'fogging' of any source (see Rogers 1969, in references at end of chapter).

6   Count the number of grains over at least 200 cells per group. Record and rank the grain counts as shown in Fig. 10.7.

7   Calculate the frequency of cells within each ranked group.

CALCULATION OF PERCENTAGE OF POSITIVE CELLS

The number of cells showing positive labelling, i.e. grains above those expected by the non-specific binding of labelled protein and other non-specific sources, may be calculated by the following equation:

For each grain count category:

$$C_p = (C_a - C_c) \times \frac{1}{1 - C_c} 100$$

where: C_p = % positively labelled cells
C_a = proportion cells labelled with antiserum
C_c = proportion cells labelled with control serum.

Calculate the % positive cells in each category for each group. Plot a graph of cell frequency against grain counts.

A specimen result and calculation is shown in Fig. 10.7.

Fig. 10.7. Anti-light-chain labelling of chicken bursa cells
Cells: 1-day-old white leghorn bursa
Antiserum: ^{125}I-anti-LC antibodies
Control: ^{125}I-anti-KLH antibodies

	Proportion of labelled cells:										
Number of grains:	0 5	6 11	12 17	18 23	24 29	30 35	36 41	42 47	48 53	54 59	> 60
Anti-LC	0·08	0·15	0·17	0·17	0·10	0·10	0·08	0·06	0·02	0·03	0·40
Anti-KLH	0·95	0·05									
% positive cells	0	11	17	17	10	10	8	6	2	3	4

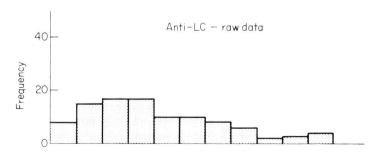

Fig. 10.7 continued

284

Fig. 10.7 continued

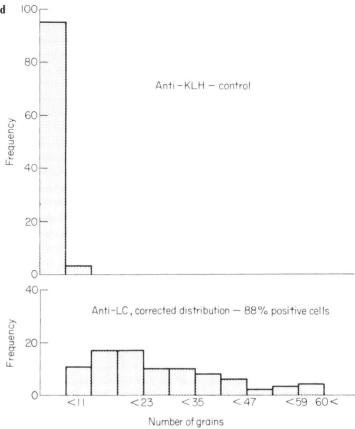

10.11 T LYMPHOCYTES *IN VITRO*

Unlike the *in vitro* assays for B cells described in section 3.1, the *in vitro* T-cell assays we will describe require considerable time and expertise. They usually involve working with cells in culture, often up to 5 or more days, and so it is essential to use sterile techniques throughout.

10.11.1 MITOGENIC RESPONSE

Like B cells, when T cells meet their specific antigen they are stimulated to undergo division. This mitogenic response is usually accompanied by a morphological change to a blast cell.

The degree of lymphocyte stimulation may therefore be assayed either by determining the percentage of blast cells in the culture or by measuring the amount of radioactive DNA analogue incorporated into newly synthesized DNA. It is important to note, however, that blast transformation, DNA synthesis and cell proliferation are not synonymous. Several instances have been reported where incorporation of DNA analogue has occurred without cell division. The *in vitro* mitotic response has been shown to have an approximate correlation with the *in vivo* situation, for example, a normal individual would have a lower mitotic response to ppd (purified protein derivative of tubercle bacilli) than a Mantoux-positive individual. In addition, an immunodeficient individual with poor Mantoux reactivity would have a low *in vitro* mitotic response to ppd.

Many plant substances, known collectively as lectins or phytomitogens have the ability to induce blast cell transformation and mitosis in a manner similar to antigen. The mitogen binds to a specific cell-surface receptor, as does antigen, and the signal thus generated causes the nucleus to be de-repressed and the lymphocyte enters the cell cycle. Unlike antigens, however, mitogens stimulate a large proportion of lymphocytes. Again, as for antigen stimulation of lymphocytes *in vitro*, it has been possible to show an approximate correlation between the *in vitro* response to mitogens and the immune status of the individual.

Phytohaemagglutinin (PHA) has been the most extensively studied of the phytomitogens. Available evidence suggests that soluble PHA stimulates only T cells. There are, however, mitogens available that stimulate both T and B cells (Pokeweed mitogen) or B cells alone (lipopolysaccharides, such as *E. coli* endotoxin). The ability of mitogens to stimulate T and/or B cells selectively varies not only with species but also with the cell source, suggesting that only a subpopulation of T and/or B cells are capable of responding to mitogen stimulation.

We will describe an *in vitro* technique to assay the response of human peripheral blood to PHA.

Materials and equipment

Human peripheral blood
Phytohaemagglutinin, PHA (Appendix II)
Triosil 75 (Appendix II)
Ficoll (Appendix II)
Tissue culture medium containing antibiotics (Appendix I)
Fetal bovine serum (Appendix II)
^{3}H-thymidine (Appendix II)
5 ml plastic tubes, Falcon (Appendix II)
37° incubator
Cylinder of 5% CO_2 in air

ALL PROCEDURES MUST BE CARRIED OUT UNDER STERILE CONDITIONS

Method

1 Defibrinate blood (Section 1.7.2)
2 Prepare a density gradient by mixing 9·9% Triosil 75 with 8·0%

286

Ficoll (cf. Section 1.7.1, alternatively use 'Lymphoprep', Appendix II).

3 Layer an equal volume of defibrinated blood onto the gradient and centrifuge at 300 g for 15 min at 4°.

4 Most of the leucocytes will be found at the serum-density gradient interface. Remove the cells with a Pasteur pipette and wash three times by centrifugation.

5 Count lymphocytes and adjust to 2×10^6 ml^{-1}.

6 Set up lymphocyte cultures with PHA according to the protocol.

7 Incubate the tubes in a 37° CO_2 incubator.

If gassed incubator is not available, place the tubes in a glass dessicator and flush with 5% CO_2 in air. The high CO_2 tension is required for the bicarbonate-CO_2 buffering system. The maximum uptake of ^3H-thymidine occurs about 72 hours after PHA stimulation. If you intend to conduct a complete experiment it is essential that you investigate both the full dose response curve and the kinetics of the response in your own culture system.

8 4 hours before harvesting add 1·0 μCi of ^3H-thymidine to each culture.

Protocol

| | Tube number (3–5 replicates of each tube) | | | | |
	1	2	3	4	5
1 ml PHA diluted to:	0	1 : 10	1 : 20	1 : 40	1 : 80
Volume of lymphocytes (2×10^6 ml^{-1} initial concentration)	1 ml				→
Final PHA concentration	0	1 : 20	1 : 40	1 : 80	1 : 160

Harvesting and counting cultures

Filter papers, Whatman 3MM, 2·1 cm (Appendix II)
Phosphate buffered saline (Appendix I)
Chloroform
Trichloracetic acid, 10% aqueous solution
Scintillation fluid (Appendix I)
Scintillation vials
β-counter

Method

1 Wash cells 2–3 times in PBS by centrifugation.

2 Resuspend cell pellet in 0·4 ml PBS.

3 Support filter discs (1 for each culture tube—and numbered in pencil) on a pin in a cork board.

4 Place 0·2 ml of cell suspension onto the corresponding disc.

5 Air dry discs with a fan.

6 Wash all discs in 10% cold TCA to precipitate the protein. (At this stage all the discs may be combined.)

7 Wash discs in PBS and then absolute alcohol.

8 Rinse in the chloroform and allow to dry.

9 Place each disc in a scintillation vial containing scintillation fluid and count β emissions in a scintillation counter.

Assessment of results

Calculate the geometric mean cpm for each group of replicates (Section 4.1.2c).

There are basically two ways of recording data:

(a) By simply giving the mean cpm for stimulated and unstimulated cultures.

(b) As an index of stimulation, this is calculated by the following equation:

$$\text{Index of stimulation} = \frac{\text{cpm PHA cultures}}{\text{cpm unstimulated cultures}}$$

In the experiment described here either method of data presentation is acceptable as we simply wish to compare the mitogenic response to different concentrations of PHA. If, however, we wished to compare different types of cells, each having their own unstimulated control, the situation is more complex. Often the serum supplement used for culture is itself mitogenic and so backgrounds may be abnormally high in some cultures but not others. Spleen cultures, for example, show a much higher background incorporation than blood lymphocyte cultures. In this case an index of stimulation would not be a useful way in which to present the data as the background variation would be hidden.

Technical notes

1 It may be necessary to test several batches of FBS as they vary in their ability to 'support' in vitro cultures.

2 ^{131}Iodo-deoxyuridine may be used instead of ^{3}H- or ^{14}C-thymidine. This DNA analogue has the advantage that it is not re-utilized in a culture and so is a measure of incorporation alone, without the complication of turnover. In addition, as it is a gamma emitter, it does not require scintillation fluid for counting.

3 In the experiment above, we used only a 4-h pulse with ^{3}H-thymidine instead of the more usual 16–20-h pulse. We do this not only to shorten the time in culture after isotope addition, thus reducing any effect of bacterial infection, but also to avoid re-utilization of isotope released from cells. This latter consideration is, however, minimal under these conditions as there is a vast excess of free thymidine.

4 Occasionally a high 'background' incorporation may be encountered when culturing cells from penicillin-sensitive individuals due to the antibiotic in the culture medium.

10.11.2 MICROCULTURE TECHNIQUE

Although similar in principle to the macrotechnique described above (Section 10.11.1), this technique uses only 10^5 responding cells per culture. The reduced cell number allows a greater number of variables to be tested per experiment. In addition, the introduction of semiautomated procedures has greatly reduced the time required for harvesting.

Materials and equipment

Blood, containing heparin (10 IU ml^{-1}). *The heparin must be preservative free.*
Tissue culture medium (Appendix I) containing heparin 10 IU ml^{-1}. (Use throughout)
'Lymphoprep' (Appendix II)
^{3}H-Thymidine (Appendix II) use at 10 μCi ml^{-1} in tissue culture medium
Scintillation fluid
Microculture trays, 96-wells, flat bottoms (Appendix II)
Hamilton precision automatic syringe (Appendix II)
Cell harvesting machine (Appendix II)
Beta counter

1 Centrifuge heparinized blood (10 IU ml^{-1}) at 400 g for 10 min at room temperature. Remove and KEEP the plasma. Add an equal plasma volume of tissue culture medium to the cell pellet and mix thoroughly.
2 Carefully layer 10 ml of reconstituted blood onto 10 ml 'Lymphoprep'.
3 Centrifuge at 400 g (interface force) for 30 min at room temperature. *A misty layer of lymphocytes will be visible at the interface.*
4 Remove lymphocytes using a pasteur pipette and mix with an equal volume of tissue culture medium.
5 Centrifuge at 400 g for 15 min at room temperature and pour off the supernatant.
6 Wash twice in tissue culture medium by centrifugation (400 g for 10 min at room temperature).
7 Remove an aliquot of cells and determine the number of viable lymphocytes ml^{-1} (Section 2.4). Adjust to 2×10^6 lymphocytes ml^{-1}.
8 Prepare cultures in microwells according to the following protocol:

Control wells	Stimulated wells
100 μl tissue culture medium	50 μl tissue culture medium
	* 50 μl stimulant
50 μl lymphocyte suspension	50 μl lymphocyte suspension
50 μl autologous plasma	50 μl autologous plasma
200 μl total volume	200 μl total volume

* Mitogen, antigen or allogeneic cells, at optimum concentration.

9   Set up triplicate cultures of each treatment using a 'Hamilton' precision automatic syringe.

10   Seal plates and place in a humidified incubator gassed with 5% CO_2 in air.

11   The magnitude of the mitotic response is determined by the addition of 50 μl of ^{3}H-TdR to each well before harvesting.

As an approximate guide:

For PHA cultures: add ^{3}H-TdR 40–48 h after the initiation of culture, incubate for 4 h at 37° before harvesting.

For mixed lymphocyte: (cf. Section 10.11.7) or antigen stimulated (for example, Candida or ppd) cultures: add ^{3}H-TdR 5 days after the initiation of culture, incubate for 18 h at 37° before harvesting.

12   Harvest the cultures using a semiautomatic cell harvesting procedure (for example, see cell harvesting machines Appendix II).

13   Dry filter strips from harvesting machine at 37° for at least 3 hours.

14   Remove discs from the filter strips and place each disc in a counting vial containing scintillation fluid.

15   Count β emissions in a scintillation counter, assess results as in Section 10.11.1.

10.11.3   MIXED LYMPHOCYTE REACTION

A mitotic response is also obtained when cells taken from two inbred strains or from two outbread individuals of any species are mixed in *in vitro* culture. This so-called mixed lymphocyte reaction (MLR) is often used clinically to select donor-recipient combinations for tissue transplantation.

Like the g.v.h. reaction (Section 3.2.3) the majority of the RESPONSIVE (as opposed to responding) cells are T-lymphocytes. Again, like the g.v.h. reaction, it has not been possible to demonstrate unequivocally an effect of previous immunization on the magnitude of the response between strains with a 'strong' H2 difference. It is, however, possible to increase the magnitude of the response by previous sensitization across 'weak' H2 differences.

It is important, in the context of the MLR, to distinguish between responsive and responding cells because of the phenomenon known as BACK STIMULATION. It was found that F_1 cells gave a mitotic response when mixed with X-irradiated or mitomycin-treated parental cells. In MLR genetics the F_1 cannot recognize the parent cells as being foreign. The mechanism proposed to explain this back stimulation was that the blocked parental cells recognize the F_1 cells as foreign and produce 'mitogenic factors' which non-specifically induce proliferation in the immunologically unresponsive F_1 cells.

MLR cultures may be performed using culture conditions similar to those described for PHA (Section 10.11.1) but mix 10^6 cells from each of two donors to yield the total of 2×10^6 per culture. In this case a two-way MLR will result, i.e. donor A will recognize B and vice versa. In many situations it is an advantage to have a uni-directional response and so parent and F_1 mixtures can be used (cf. Section 3.2.3), or, more simply, the proliferation of either cell type may be blocked with X-irradiation or mitomycin C.

A suggested experimental protocol is given in Section 10.11.5, these cultures are then used as a source of cytotoxic effector cells.

10.11.4 CELL-MEDIATED CYTOTOXICITY

T lymphocytes will respond to foreign cell-surface antigens by blast-ogenesis. Later in this response, effector cells are generated that will specifically lyse relevant target cells *in vitro*. This *in vitro* killing is generally regarded as being analogous to one type of cell-initiated tissue damage *in vivo*.

Classically the phenomenon of T-cell-mediated cytotoxicity was elucidated using lymphocytes sensitized to DBA/2 alloantigens and assayed on ^{51}Cr-labelled P815Y (DBA/2) mastocytoma cells. A similar system can be used to investigate T-cell killing against any system of alloantigens using PHA transformed blast cells labelled with ^{51}Cr.

Effector cells may be generated by either (a) immunizing C3H mice, for example, with DBA/2 spleen cells or (b) initiating a g.v.h. reaction (Section 3.2.3) in, for example, irradiated (DBA × C3H)F_1 using C3H cells and (c) in the course of a MLR (Section 10.11.5).

10.11.5 MLR AND CELL-MEDIATED CYTOLYSIS (CMC)

Materials and equipment

CBA or C3H and DBA/2 mice (Section 1.8.2 and Appendix II)
P815Y mastocytoma cells
Sodium ^{51}chromate (Appendix II)
X-ray machine or γ-source
Gamma counter

Mixed lymphocyte reaction

1   Prepare spleen-cell suspensions from C3H and DBA/2 mice.
2   Irradiate DBA/2 cells (3000 R); these will be used as MLR stimulator cells. Irradiate immediately before putting into culture. *The stimulatory capacity of irradiated cells falls within a few hours if they are allowed to stand at 4°.*
3   Prepare MLR cultures using irradiated DBA/2 and C3H cells (Section 10.11.1). Mix 10^6 of each cell type, culture in 3 ml of medium in 5 ml Falcon plastic tubes as in protocol A.

Prepare sufficient replicates of each tube to provide cells for the CMC assay on the 4th day of MLR culture (see Protocol B) (*viability of MLR cultures varies—this must be standardized for each laboratory*) and in addition prepare 3 replicates of tubes 1–3 for the assay of DNA synthesis in the MLR culture.

4   On the 4th day of the MLR culture collect cells for the CMC assay (Protocol B).
5   On the 5th day of the MLR culture add ^{3}H-thymidine to 3 replicates of tubes 1–3 to assay for DNA-synthesis (Section 10.11.1).

A. MLR protocol

	Tube number		
	1	2	3*
X-irradiated cells	2×10^6 DBA/2	10^6 DBA/2	10^6 C3H or CBA
C3H or CBA responder cells	0	10^6	10^6

* This is a better control than unirradiated cells alone as irradiated cells might exert a slight inhibitory activity upon the generation of possible CMC cells.

B. CMC protocol

	Tube number (3 replicates)					
	1	2	3	4	5	6
^{51}Cr labelled mastocytoma cells	10^5	⟶				
MLR lymphocytes from tube number						
1	50×10^5	—	—	—	—	—
2	—	50×10^5	20×10^5	10×10^5	—	—
3	—	—	—	—	50×10^5	—

(We have given absolute number of MLR cells rather than the usual lymphocyte target ratio. In fact the efficiency of target-cell killing is not ratio-dependent over a wide range.)

Cell-mediated cytolysis

1 Label mastocytoma cells with ^{51}Cr (Section 10.9.2).
2 Count number of viable lymphocytes recovered from MLR (protocol A).
3 Prepare cell mixtures in 2 ml of medium as shown in Protocol B.
4 Culture for 6 h at 37° in a CO_2 incubator.
5 Resuspend the cells after culture and centrifuge (150 *g* for 10 min at 4°).
6 Remove 1 ml of the supernatant from each tube for gamma counting.

CALCULATION OF ISOTOPE RELEASE
(= target-cell destruction)

1 Lyse an aliquot of 10^5 original ^{51}Cr-labelled mastocytoma cells either by freezing and thawing (three times at 37° and $-20°$) or with 10% Saponin.
2 Spin-down insoluble material from the lysate and count radio-activity in the supernatant. *Use this value as the maximum (100%) isotope release.*
3 Calculate spontaneous release from the labelled mastocytoma (Tube 6, in triplicate) as a percentage of the total counts released by Saponin. *The mean of these 3 determinations will be used to correct the release observed in lymphocyte-target mixtures (Tubes 1–5).*
4 Calculate experimental release for each lymphocyte-target mixture as a percentage of the total counts released by Saponin (Tubes 1–5, in triplicate).
5 Calculate specific release as follows:

$$\% \text{ specific release} = \frac{100[R_E - R_S]}{100 - R_S}$$

where R_E = mean % experimental release
R_S = mean % spontaneous release.

6 Plot a graph of % specific release for each group against the number of MLR-derived cells used to lyse the mastocytoma cells. Calculate also the standard deviation of each group (Section 4.1.2b).

Technical Note

In experimental determinations of CMC it is advisable to assay at 4, 6 and 8 h rather than at the single time-point as suggested here.

10.11.6   CMC WITH PHA BLASTS

As mentioned earlier (Section 10.11.4) the applicability of CMC may be extended to any system of alloantigens using ^{51}Cr-labelled PHA blasts as target cells.

PHA blasts may be produced 'en masse' as follows:

Materials and equipment

Inbred mice

Tissue-culture media containing fetal bovine serum and antibiotics (Appendix I)

100 ml glass bottles, 'medical flats' or Falcon plastic bottles (Appendix II)

See also Section 10.11.1

Method

1 Prepare cell suspensions from mouse lymph node.

2 Count cells and adjust to $3-5 \times 10^6$ ml^{-1}.

3 Add optimal concentration of PHA (determined in Section 10.11.1).

4 Add 20 ml of cell suspension to each bottle and gas for 60 sec with 5% CO_2 in air.

5 Place bottles on their sides in a 37° incubator.

The kinetics of the response are essentially similar to that seen in Section 10.11.1.

6 After 72 h, pool cells, wash three times in tissue-culture medium and label with ^{51}Cr (Section 10.9.2).

7 Use for CMC as in Section 10.11.5.

Note

It is now known that in certain mouse-strain combinations a MLR may be observed without the generation of detectable cytotoxic effector cells, for example, between C3H and CBA/J or CBA/H and CBA/J mice which differ only at the M-locus. Intriguingly, the MLR in this situation is unidirectional and the stimulus is only provided by B cells.

10.12 **SOLUBLE FACTORS PRODUCED BY LYMPHOCYTES**

When lymphocytes are activated, either by mitogens or antigen, they produce a range of soluble mediators, in addition to antibody. These mediators are known collectively as LYMPHOKINES irrespective of the mode of generation or their subsequent action. The various lymphokines are classified according to their mode of action, usually *in vitro*, for example:

Lymphototoxin—kills nucleated cells.

Macrophage activating factor—enhances macrophage mobility and phagocytosis.

Mitogenic factor—stimulates mitosis in lymphocyte populations.

Migration-inhibition factor (MIF)—inhibits macrophage migration.

By inspection of the brief list given above, it is obviously important to be able to distinguish these mediators from (a)|'meat'—e.g. some substance which simply induces more physiological conditions in the system under test, thereby enhancing but not initiating, some pre-existing phenomenon, and (b) poison—self-explanatory. This is not, however, always simple.

The inhibition of macrophage migration by lymphokines from activated lymphocytes has been studied in detail and shows an approximate correlation with *in vivo* immune status.

10.12.1 MACROPHAGE MIGRATION INHIBITION

Materials and equipment

Guinea-pigs, normal and immunized with BCG (*Mycobacterium tuberculosis*)
Purified protein derivative of *M. tuberculosis*, ppd (Appendix II)
Tissue-culture medium with 10% fetal bovine serum (Appendix I)
Siliconized 0·75 mm capillary tubes
Mackaness-type chambers (Section 6.5.1)
Paraffin wax or 'seal-ease' (latter, Appendix II)
Silicone grease

Method

1   Obtain a suspension of peritoneal exudate cells from normal and immune guinea-pigs (Section 1.7.5).
2   Count cells and adjust to 5×10^7 nucleated cells ml^{-1}.
3   Fill capillaries with cell suspension and seal one end either with softened paraffin wax or 'seal-ease' dental plasticine.
4   Pack capillaries into flat-bottomed plastic tubes and centrifuge at 150 g for 5 min at 4°.
5   Meanwhile prepare chambers by placing a small amount of silicone grease against side, and smear rim with silicone grease.
6   Half fill chambers with medium containing the appropriate antigen dilution (see protocol over page).
7   Cut capillary just to the cell side of the cell-medium interface.
8   Place sealed end of capillary into silicone grease in migration chamber. *Check that the whole tube is on the bottom of the chamber.*
9   Fill the chamber with medium and antigen, and seal with a cover-slip. Exclude all air bubbles.
10   Incubate the chamber at 37° overnight.
11   Place migration chambers in a photographic enlarger and trace area of migration onto a sheet of paper.
12   Cut out the pencilled area and weigh.

The degree of migration inhibition is calculated as follows:

$$\% \text{ migration} = \frac{\text{Weight of migration area immune cells}}{\text{Weight of migration area normal cells}} \times 100$$

A value of less than 80% is considered as a significant inhibition.

295

Technical notes

1 There is a wide scatter of data within replicates with this technique. At least 5 replicates must be used for each antigen dilution.

2 Because of the danger of bias in tracing the area of migration, it is essential that the whole experiment should be coded and read blind.

3 Many antigens are stimulatory or inhibitory depending on dose. It is therefore essential to perform a full-dose response curve at each test. Because of this it is inadvisable to use immune cells without antigen as a control.

Protocol

	Chamber number (5 replicates)				
	1	2	3	4	5
ppd concentration (μg ml^{-1}) (a) immune or (b) normal cells	0	50	100	250	500

10.12.2 INTERFERONS

The attention of immunologists has increasingly been drawn towards the mode of action and potential therapeutic effects of the interferons.

Interferon was first identified by its ability to inhibit virus replication (type I or viral interferon). Later, a second molecular species (type II or immune interferon) was discovered. Although immune interferon has antiviral effects, of greater potential importance is its ability to modulate (inhibit or stimulate) cell growth and function, especially of lymphoid or tumour cells. Lymphocytes and macrophages produce interferon after antigen or mitogen stimulation.

Both type I and type II interferon are standardized in terms of their antiviral activity, using assays similar, in principle, to the one described below. Methods for the production of interferon are beyond the present scope of the book, see reference at end of chapter for further details.

Antiviral assay: this bioassay takes 3 days.

Materials and equipment

L-929 cells (adherent cultures)
Interferon

Tissue culture medium (Appendix I)
Fetal bovine serum (FBS)
Phosphate buffered saline, PBS (Appendix I)
Encephalomyocarditis (EMC) virus
Ethanol-citrate buffer, see Technical notes.
Neutral red 0·01% w/v in PBS, see Technical notes.

Method

1   Place 1 ml aliquots of L-929 cells (2×10^5 cells ml^{-1}) into each well of the culture plate and incubate at 37° in a humid incubator gassed with 5% CO_2 in air. *If required, adjust the cell plating concentration to ensure that the cells are confluent after overnight incubation.*

2   Dilute out the samples to be tested for interferon activity, start at 1 : 10 and make doubling dilutions in tissue culture medium containing 2% FBS.

Assay for interferon activity using the following protocol for each culture plate:

Protocol

Treatment	L-929 cells	Interferon	EMC virus
1	+	0	−
2	+	1 : 10	−
3	+	1 : 10	+
4	+	1 : 20	+
5	+	1 : 40	+
↓		etc	
n	+	0	+

Use 2–3 replicates of each treatment

3   Remove the supernatants from the confluent L-929 cell cultures and replace with 1 ml of interferon dilution or tissue culture medium, according to the protocol above.

4   Incubate overnight at 37°.

5   Remove the supernatants from all cultures and wash twice with PBS.

6   Add 1 ml of EMC virus suspension (1500 virus plaque forming units ml^{-1} in tissue culture medium containing 2% FBS) or tissue culture medium according to the protocol.

7   Incubate overnight at 37°.
    After overnight incubation, the cytopathic effect of the virus should be discernable in the control wells (treatment 'n' in protocol) using an inverted microscope.

8   Remove the supernatant from all wells and add 1 ml neutral red dye to each. *This is a vital stain and is taken up only by living cells.*

297

9 Incubate in the dark for 2 h.

10 Remove the excess dye and wash three times with PBS. Finally invert the plate to empty completely.

11 Add 1 ml of ethanol-citrate buffer to each well to extract the dye.

12 Mix each sample well using a Pasteur pipette and read absorbance at 550 nm using a spectrophotometer.

EMC virus kills the cells and so reduces the uptake of neutral red. Pretreatment of the cells with interferon prevents viral replication and inhibits cell death, this is reflected by an increase in dye uptake. Thus, the interferon activity of each sample may be quantitated from the dye uptake of cells treated with interferon before infection relative to cells infected with virus alone.

$$\% \text{ antiviral activity} = \frac{Ai - Av}{Ac - Av} \times 100$$

where Ai = absorbance due to neutral red extracted from cells treated with interferon

Av = absorbance due to neutral red extracted from untreated cells infected with virus (treatment 'n' in protocol)

Ac = absorbance due to neutral red extracted from uninfected cells (treatment 1 in protocol).

Technical notes

1 Treatments 1 and 2 must not give significantly different results. Treatment 2 is a control for direct effects of interferon on cell viability.

2 The cells must reach confluence and cease growing before assay for antiviral effects, thus avoiding any direct action of interferon in inhibiting cell division.

3 Standardized preparations of mouse and human interferon are now widely available. These may be used for the construction of a standard curve for the calibration of samples of interferon with unknown activity.

4 Neutral red solution, dissolve powder in a minimal volume of 0·1 M sodium hydroxide and dilute to a 1% w/v stock solution using PBS. For use: dilute to a 0·01% w/v solution with PBS.

5 Ethanol-citrate buffer, dissolve 11·348 g of citric acid and 13·5 g of tri-sodium citrate in 1 l of water (final pH 4·2). For use: mix 1 volume of ethanol with 1 volume of citrate.

10.13 **ANTIBODY-DEPENDENT CELL-MEDIATED CYTOTOXICITY**

Antibody-dependent cell-mediated cytotoxicity (ADCMC) is a phenomenon in which target cells, coated with very small amounts of antibody, are killed by non-immune effector cells. The effector

298

cells (K cells) have receptors for the Fc regions of the antibody and appear to recognize immune complexes specifically. The exact killing mechanism is unknown, but it involves cell to cell contact and is possibly the result of the release of lysosomal enzymes.

The full nature of the effector cells remains to be elucidated, but it is known that different types of cell mediate the killing depending on the character of the target. With red cell targets the effector cells tend to be of the granulocyte/macrophage lines; but with tumour target cells, cells of the lymphocyte line seem to predominate as effectors.

CYTOTOXIC ASSAY

Materials

Mouse (Appendix II)
Chicken (Appendix II)
Rabbit anti-chicken erythrocyte serum (diluted 1 : 6000 in tissue culture medium plus 10% FBS, Appendix I)
Tissue culture medium
Fetal bovine serum (Appendix II)
Sodium ^{51}chromate (Appendix II)
Sheep erythrocytes (SRBC) (Appendix II)

Method

(A) TARGET CELLS

1   Take 0·2 ml of blood from the chicken into a heparinized syringe. *The main wing vein is a convenient site for venipuncture to obtain small volumes of blood.*
2   Dilute 0·1 ml of blood with 1·9 ml of Eagle's MEM containing 10% FBS.
3   Use 0·1 ml of diluted blood and add 0·1 ml of sodium ^{51}chromate (specific activity see Appendix II).
4   Gas with 5% CO_2 in air.
5   Incubate at 37° for 1 hour.
6   Wash 4 times with medium containing 5% FBS. Centrifuge at 90 *g* for 7 minutes at 4°.
7   Wash SRBC in tissue culture medium 4 times by centrifugation (450 *g* for 10 min).
8   Adjust SRBC concentration to 10^7 ml^{-1}.
9   Add 10^5 labelled chicken red cells to each ml of sheep red cells.

(B) EFFECTOR CELLS

1   Remove the spleen from the mouse and prepare a single cell suspension (Section 1.7.3).
2   Adjust to 2·5 × 10^6 leukocytes ml^{-1}.

(c) CYTOTOXIC ASSAY

1   Set up culture tubes according to protocol below.

Protocol

Tube (in triplicate)	Spleen cells (μl)	Antibody (μl)	^{51}Cr-labelled chicken red cells (μl)
A	100	100	100
B	100	0	100
C	0	100	100
D	0	0	100
E	100 μl distilled water	100 μl distilled water	100

2   Cap the tubes and incubate them, leaning at an angle of 30–45°, in a gassed CO_2 incubator or a desiccator (5% in air) for 18 hours.
3   Add 1 ml medium to each tube and then spin (90 g) for 10 minutes.
4   Remove 0·8 ml supernatant from each tube and assess this for ^{51}Cr release in a gamma counter.

Note

Tube A shows the ^{51}Cr release due to spleen cells plus anti-target antibody. The other cultures are controls. Tube B gives the amount of release due to spleen cells alone, while C measures the release due to antibody. Spontaneous death of the erythrocytes is monitored by tube D.

Calculations

The calculation of the amount of cytotoxicity is complicated as there is some difficulty in choosing the correct control value against which to calculate the experimental ^{51}Cr release. This is because spleen cells, in the absence of antibody, exert a protective effect over the chicken erythrocytes. It will be seen that the ^{51}Cr release in tube B is usually less than the spontaneous release in tube D. Therefore, for the control culture, one may choose either effectors plus target cells (B) or target cells plus antibody (C).

The calculation of percentage cytotoxicity may then be as follows:

$$\text{percentage } ^{51}\text{Cr release} = \frac{A - C}{E - C} \times 100$$

or

$$= \frac{A - B}{E - B} \times 100$$

Letters in formulae correspond to culture tubes in the protocol.

10.14   ENUMERATION OF HUMAN T AND B LYMPHOCYTES

Although techniques for the assessment of the humoral immune system are well established in the clinical laboratory, the assessment of cellular immune function is still a developing area. There are many 'semi-experimental' techniques awaiting or undergoing clinical evaluation.

10.14.1   B LYMPHOCYTES

Peripheral blood B lymphocytes are usually estimated by anti-immunoglobulin immunofluorescence (as in Section 2.5.1) using lymphocytes prepared by density gradient centrifugation (Section 10.11.1).

10.14.2   LYMPHOCYTES

T lymphocyte specific antibodies are not yet generally available. T lymphocytes are usually detected by their ability to form spontaneous (no immunological specificity—cf. Section 2.6) rosettes with sheep erythrocytes.

Materials and equipment

Human blood containing heparin (10 IU ml^{-1})
'Lymphoprep' (Appendix II)
Phosphate buffered saline (PBS—Appendix I)
Sheep erythrocytes
Nigrosin dye in PBS (0·1% w/v)
Fetal bovine serum (FBS)

Method

1   Obtain venous blood in heparin (10 IU ml^{-1}) and perform a total and differential leucocyte count (Section 2.4).
2   Isolate lymphocyte fraction as described in Section 10.11.2. Count viable lymphocytes (Section 2.4.1), calculate and record total

301

yield. (*If total yield is low, < 60% the ratio of T : B lymphocytes will be significantly altered.*) Adjust to 5×10^6 lymphocytes ml^{-1}.

3 Wash sheep erythrocytes by centrifugation (400 g for 10 min at room temperature) and adjust to a 2·5% v/v suspension in PBS.

4 Mix 0·1 ml of the lymphocyte suspension with 0·1 ml of sheep erythrocytes and centrifuge at 225 g for 5 min at room temperature.

5 Incubate for 2 h at 4°.

6 Add 50 μl of FBS and 50 μl of nigrosin solution.

7 Resuspend cell mixture by gently tapping the tube and pipette a sample into a haemocytomer.

8 Count 200 lymphocytes and determine the percentage of cells with 3 or more erythrocytes attached. (*These are T lymphocytes.*)

9 Calculate the absolute number of *T* lymphocytes ml^{-1} of original blood.

Technical notes

1 Use plastic tubes and siliconized glass pipettes.

2 Heat the FBS at 56° for 30 min to inactivate complement and absorb with washed sheep erythrocytes (0·5 volume of packed erythrocytes) for 2 h at 4°. Centrifuge at 400 g for 15 min, to recover serum and store in small aliquots at $-20°$.

FURTHER READING

BARON S. & DIANZANI F. (eds.) (1977) The Interferon System: A current review to 1978. *Tex. Reports Biol. Med.* vol. 35.

COHEN S., PICK E. & OPPENHEIM J.J. (1979) *The Biology of the Lymphokines.* Academic Press, New York.

ROGERS A.W. (1969) *Techniques of Autoradiography.* Elsevier, Amsterdam.

ROSE N.R. & BIGAZZI P.E. 1973. *Methods in Immunodiagnosis.* J. Wiley, New York.

SPRENT J. (1975) Recirculating Lymphocytes. In *The Lymphocyte: Structure and Function.* Marcel Dekker, New York.

11   Hybridoma cells and monoclonal antibody

With hindsight, it is impressive that immunological research has advanced so rapidly using a tool so ill-defined as an antiserum, where the active ingredient, antibody, is a minor component in a complex mixture of serum proteins. In addition, unless one uses antigens that stimulate a very limited number of lymphocyte clones, the antibody itself is a heterogeneous mixture of molecules with a wide range of binding affinities. It is not surprising, therefore, that an antiserum lacks the degree of definition required for many of the current immunochemical techniques, where an increase in assay sensitivity is often counteracted by a decrease in serological specificity.

The non-specific or cross-reactive binding reactions shown by antibody or other components in an antiserum can be a serious problem when antisera are used to identify or quantitate antigens either in research, for example, the study of differentiation or tumour antigens, or in the clinical laboratory, for immunodiagnosis. Although it is possible to ensure that an antiserum is 'monospecific' by careful controls or cross-absorption, such standardisation is usually limited to one test system and indeed, often only to one laboratory.

The need for homogenous antibodies as reproducible reagents was fulfilled by the rescue and propagation of hybrid cell tumours representing clones of single plasma cells. Köhler and Milstein fused plasmacytoma cells with normal plasma cells to produce hybrid cells (later called hybridomas) that secreted *both* myeloma and antibody immunoglobulin. By antigen-specific screening of culture supernatants and cloning of secreting cells, these investigators were able to produce potentially immortal cell lines synthesizing homogenous antibody of exquisite specificity.

The technology of hybridoma production has undergone a rapid expansion and diversification since these original experiments. We will describe our version of the techniques currently in vogue.

11.1   OUTLINE OF TECHNIQUE

Spleen cells, prepared from immunised mice or rats, are induced to fuse with murine plasmacytoma cells using polyethylene glycol. Many cells show cytoplasmic fusion, a lower proportion complete

303

the nuclear fusion required to produce tetraploid (or greater, depending on the number of fusing cells) hybrids. Although this procedure results in a heterogenous mixture of fused and unfused cells, there is a preferential association of ontogenetically similar cells: plasmacytoma cells tend to 'rescue' large, recently activated B lymphocytes.

After aliquoting into culture wells, the cell mixture is cultured in a selective medium that positively selects for fusion hybrids. The culture supernatants are tested for antibody activity after 1–3 weeks and positive cultures cloned by conventional cell cloning techniques.

Basis of fusion and selection

To understand the choice of cells and manipulation of the system it is necessary to consider the contribution of each component of the hybrid cell:

1   The plasmablast parent is terminally differentiated, dies in culture but provides the genetic information for the required antibody.
2   The plasmacytoma parent confers potential immortality on the hybrid cell, but will itself grow in culture.

Thus, once plasma cells from an appropriately immunized animal have been fused with tumour cells *in vitro* it is necessary to eliminate unfused tumour cells (or tumour–tumour hybrids) and then select those hybrid cells secreting antibody of the required specificity.

Elimination of plasmacytoma cells

This problem was overcome by the use of a plasmacytoma cell line deficient in the enzyme responsible for the incorporation of hypoxanthine into DNA.

By way of explanation, cells can synthesize DNA in two ways, either by 'de novo' synthesis or via the so-called 'salvage' pathway using exogenous or endogenous sources of preformed bases:

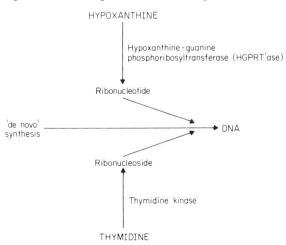

If plasmacytoma cells are grown in the presence of a purine analogue, for example, 8 azaguanine or 6 thioguanine, the HGPRT'ase enzyme catalyses the incorporation of the purine analogue into DNA where it interferes with normal protein synthesis and so the cells die.

The gene coding for the HGPRT'ase enzyme is on the X chromosome and so only a single copy per cell is expressed. Eventually cells will arise that are deficient in the HGPRT'ase gene and therefore do not incorporate the purine analogue. These HGPRT'ase deficient cells are unable to utilise hypoxanthine and so synthesise ribonucleotides only by 'de novo' synthesis.

In 1967 Littlefield introduced a selective medium containing aminopterin (or amethopterin, methotrexate), hypoxanthine and thymidine (HAT medium). Aminopterin is an analogue of folic acid and binds very tenaciously to folic acid reductase, thus blocking the co-enzymes required for 'de novo' synthesis of DNA. To grow in this medium a cell must make DNA via the 'salvage' pathway.

Thus, if plasmacytoma cells, deficient in HGPRT'ase, are fused with normal lymphoid cells and then placed in HAT medium, only the hybrids between plasmacytoma and normal cells will grow; the plasmacytoma cell provides immortality and the plasma cell provides the HGPRT'ase enzyme.

Origin of plasmacytoma lines for fusion

The vast majority of fusion experiments have been performed using sublines of P3/X63-Ag8, which is itself an 8-azaguanine resistant subline of the plasmacytoma MOPC 21 (induced in a BALB/C mouse by the injection of mineral oil). This cell line is special in that it tends to fuse spontaneously (with itself) and can grow at very low cell densities, thus facilitating the recovery of fusion hybrids. However, this line has the disadvantage that it synthesises and secretes the MOPC 21 myeloma protein (a fully sequenced IgG1, K) and so hybrid cells will secrete myeloma and antibody molecules, as well as inactive hybrid molecules.

Spontaneous variants of P3/X63-Ag8 have been selected that neither synthesize nor secrete immunoglobulin molecules, but still retain the ability to rescue normal antibody producing cells. These are listed below, all are resistant to 8-azaguanine:

NS1-Ag4-1. Synthesizes, but does not secrete, K light chain. Hybrids can still secrete a mixed molecule of antibody heavy chains with myeloma light chains.

P3/X63-Ag8-6.5.3. Does not synthesize or secrete immunoglobulin chains.

SP2/0-Ag14. Non-secreting variant of a hybrid cell formed by the fusion of a lymphoid cell (secreting anti-sheep erythrocyte antibody) with P3/X63-Ag8.

For obvious reasons, we recommend one of the non-synthesizing, non-secreting variants for any fusion work. Although there are some commercial suppliers (Appendix II), it is usual to beg the 'parent' cell lines from one of the many laboratories doing routine fusions.

11.2   MAINTENANCE OF PLASMACYTOMA CELLS FOR FUSION

The efficiency of fusion and recovery of hybrids is greatest when the plasmacytoma 'parent' cells are uniformly viable and growing exponentially. The times and cell densities given below should only be used as a guide, it is necessary to determine the growth characteristics of each plasmacytoma line upon receipt.

Materials and equipment

Plasmacytoma line (if necessary, recover from frozen state, Appendix I)
Tissue culture medium with serum supplement (Appendix I)
Plastic culture flasks (Appendix II), 10 ml culture volume
Incubator, humidified and gassed with 5% CO_2 in air

Method

1   Add 10^5 plasmacytoma cells to 10 ml of tissue culture medium and place in a humid incubator gassed with 5% CO_2 in air.
2   Each day, resuspend the cells and determine the number ml^{-1} using a haemocytometer.
3   Plot a growth curve of cell number v time.
4   As soon as the growth rate starts to decline, dilute the cells, by transferring $0.2-1.0$ ml aliquots of the resuspended culture to flasks containing 10 ml of fresh medium.
5   When the cells have again reached their exponential growth phase, select viable cultures for storage under liquid nitrogen (Appendix I).

Technical notes

1   These cell lines will reach a maximum density of approximately 10^6 cells ml^{-1}. Exponential growth should be maintained by diluting the culture 1 : 10 with fresh medium every 3–5 days. Under these conditions the cells will have a doubling time of 16–20 h.
2   The plasmacytoma cells grow either in suspension or lightly adherent. Release the adherent cells by tapping the culture flask or by gentle pipetting.
3   Check by phase contrast microscopy that the cells are 'healthy'.

They should be phase bright and of regular shape with clear outlines. Although most lines are cloned, considerable size variation is common. Cell viability (Section 2.4) should be between 90 and 95%.

4 As with all cell lines in long-term culture, care must be taken to avoid cross-contamination between cultures.

5 The rate of reversion to HAT resistance varies with cell lines and is a relatively rare event. Eliminate revertants by culturing the cells in medium containing 8-azaguanine or 6-thioguanine (2×10^{-5} M) every 3–6 months.

6 As with all long term maintenance of cell lines *in vitro* it is advisable to check periodically for *Mycoplasma* infection. Commercial kits are available (Appendix II) for the demonstration of *Mycoplasma* DNA using a fluorescent dye.

11.3   **TARGET CELLS FOR FUSION**

Most of the plasmacytoma cells used for fusion have a BALB/c haplotype, but will fuse efficiently with mouse or rat cells without regard to histocompatibility barriers. It is important to note, however, that if it is intended to propagate the hybridoma cells *in vivo*, it is technically simpler to use immunised BALB/c mice as spleen cell donors. In addition, although the murine plasmacytoma lines can fuse to almost any species, for example, human or frog, stable hybrid lines are only rarely obtained in other than rodent fusions (see Technical notes below).

It is difficult to suggest specific immunization protocols, most have been determined empirically and vary not only with the type of antigen used but also with the 'folklore' of the laboratory. Plasmacytoma cells seem to fuse preferentially with recently activated B lymphoblasts, and so one might expect that the immunization scheme giving highest serum antibody titres might not necessarily give the highest rate of positive hybrids.

Few problems have been encountered with cell or particulate antigens, almost any immunization scheme will give a 10–20% recovery of positive hybrids (percentage calculated as a function of total hybrid cells growing in culture). There is, however, some evidence to suggest that mice given only 1 or 2 injections of cell-associated antigen might produce more positive hybrids than hyperimmunized mice. Most investigators tend to fuse 2–4 days after a final intravenous injection of antigen on the rationale that this should localize recently activated B lymphocytes in the spleen.

The initial problem encountered in the production of hybrids secreting antibody against soluble antigens has recently been overcome by Stähli *et al* 1980 using human chorionic gonadotrophin in a very aggressive immunization protocol. The protocol was designed to keep the memory B lymphocytes in an activated, dividing state and to limit the number of terminally differentiated plasma cells.

307

The production of specific hybrids was increased from an initial rate of less than 1% to an impressive 18–40%. 6-week-old mice were immunized as below:

Time before fusion	Antigen concentration (μg)	Adjuvant	Route of administration
—48 weeks	50	complete Freund's adjuvant + 10^9 B pertussis	i.p.
—32	50	incomplete Freund's adjuvant	i.p.
—27	10	incomplete Freund's adjuvant	i.p.
— 4 days	400	saline alone	i.p.
— 3	400	saline alone	*i.p. and i.v.
— 2	400	saline alone	*i.p. and i.v.
— 1	400	saline alone	i.p.
0	Fusion		

* 200 μg by each route.

Note: Although serum antibody titres do not necessarily correlate with the ultimate fusion efficiency, it is always worthwhile to monitor serum levels to ensure that the mouse strain can respond to the antigen.

Recent experience indicates that hybridomas against soluble proteins might not be as great a problem as previously thought. For example, we have found that a short immunization of mice using human IgG is effective for the isolation of hybridomas secreting specific anti-human IgG antibody. The immunization protocol used was:

i.p.—100 μg human IgG in complete Freund's adjuvant 7 days before fusion, followed by:

i.v.—boost with 100 μg soluble IgG 4 days before fusion.

Again, this stresses the importance of an empirical approach for the determination of the best immunization conditions.

11.4 FUSION PROTOCOL

Initial preparations

1 Immunize mice against required antigen.
2 Prepare plasmacytoma cell cultures for fusion (*set up a sufficient culture volume to yield 10^7 cells for each spleen to be fused*).

For efficient fusion, the plasmacytoma cells should be uniformly viable and in the exponential phase of growth. To ensure that this is so, we routinely replace the culture medium, at the same cell density, the day before the cells are used for fusion.

Materials and equipment—

Plasmacytoma cells in culture
Tissue culture medium (Appendix I)
Serum (Appendix I)
Tissue culture flasks (Appendix II)

Prepare cultures of plasmacytoma cells and, 24 h before use, harvest the cells by centrifugation (150 g for 10 min at room temperature) and reculture in an equal volume of tissue culture medium plus serum supplement.

3   Polyethylene glycol solution.

Materials

Polyethylene glycol, molecular weight 1500
Phosphate buffered saline (PBS) (Appendix I)

Method

1   Add 50 g PEG to warm PBS (in a 37° water bath) and adjust to 100 ml.

2   Dispense 5 ml aliquots into 10 ml glass bottles and autoclave at 120° for 15 min.

3   Store at 4° for use.

Techniques

Materials and equipment

Mice (immunized as above)
Plasmacytoma cells in culture (as above)
Tissue culture medium and serum (Appendix I)
L-glutamine (200 mM initial concentration)
Polyethylene glycol (PEG 1500), 50% w/v in phosphate buffered saline (as above)
Ethanol, 70% v/v in distilled water
Water bath at 37°
Culture plate, 96 microwells (Appendix II)
Conical test tubes, 50 ml, sterile
Conical test tubes, 15 ml, sterile
Petri dishes, 5 cm, sterile
Pasteur pipettes, sterile
Scissors, 2 pairs, sterile
Forceps, fine, sterile
Forceps, blunt, 2 pairs, sterile
Time clock

Method

1   Prepare tissue culture medium as follows:
(a) 100 ml medium, add 10 ml serum and 1·0 ml L-glutamine.
(b) 200 ml medium, add 2·0 ml L-glutamine.
2   Kill mouse by cervical dislocation and swab its left side with ethanol.
3   Open skin to expose peritoneum, discard scissors and forceps.
4   Use fresh forceps and scissors to open the peritoneum and remove the spleen, transfer to a petri dish containing serum-free tissue culture medium.
5   Prepare a suspension of spleen cells free of clumps (Section 3.1.2).
6   Wash spleen cells three times by centrifugation (250 g for 10 min at 4°) and resuspend in 5 ml of serum-free tissue culture medium.
7   Determine the number of viable lymphoid cells ml^{-1} (Section 2.4).

B. PREPARATION OF PLASMACYTOMA CELLS

1   Resuspend the cells and pool the suspensions into a 50 ml conical tube.
2   Wash the cells three times by centrifugation (250 g for 15 min at room temperature) in serum-free tissue culture medium.
3   Resuspend the final pellet in serum-free tissue culture medium, count the number of viable cells (Section 2.4) and adjust to 1×10^6 cells ml^{-1}.

C. FUSION

1   Mix 10^8 spleen cells with 10^7 plasmacytoma cells in a 50 ml conical tube and centrifuge at 500 g for 7 min at room temperature.
2   Decant the supernatant carefully, finally inverting the tube to drain completely.
3   Mix cell pellet by gently tapping the tube and allow to equilibrate to 37° in a water bath. Similarly allow PEG solution and tissue culture medium with 10% serum to equilibrate to 37°.
4   Add 0·8 ml of PEG to resuspended cells, mix gently and incubate at 37° for 1 min.
5   Add 1·0 ml of serum-free medium over 1 min with gentle shaking.
6   Add 20 ml of serum-free medium over 5 min. *Dilution must be done very slowly as the cells are very sensitive to mechanical damage when in the PEG solution.*
7   Centrifuge at 200 g for 10 min at room temperature.
8   Remove supernatant and resuspend the cell pellet in 10 ml of tissue culture medium containing 10% serum.

9 Aliquot 50 μl of cell suspension into each well of a 96-well culture plate.

10 Dilute the remaining cell suspension with 2 volumes of medium containing 10% serum and aliquot 50 μl into each well of a second 96-well culture plate.

11 Dilute the remaining cell suspension with 2 volumes of medium containing 10% serum and aliquot 50 μl into each well of a third 96-well culture plate.

12 Place all the plates in a humid 37° incubator gassed with 5% CO_2 in air.

The plates are now incubated for 24 h before the addition of the HAT selective medium.

Technical notes

1 Although murine plasmacytoma cells have been fused with avian, amphibian and human lymphocytes in a similar manner, they rarely produce stable, antibody secreting hybrids because of a rapid loss of chromosomes. Indeed, in mouse-human hybrids, the elimination of human, but not mouse, chromosomes occurs so frequently that this technique has been extensively used for gene mapping (see further reading).

2 The method of plating out the fusion mixture may be varied depending on the frequency of hybrid formation, the frequency of hybrids secreting the desired type of antibody and the method of detecting antibodies. If the frequency of hybrids is low, as with soluble proteins, for example, them 2 ml cultures can be dispensed into 24 well culture wells. We have found that the dilution technique described above limits the number of independent clones that grow out and so reduces the chance of a positive clone (secreting the desired antibody) being lost by 'overgrowth' of non-secreting hybrids.

11.4.1 PREPARATION OF STOCK SOLUTION OF HAT MEDIUM

Materials

Hypoxanthine (6-hydroxypurine) (molecular weight 136·1) 10×10^{-2} M

Thymidine (molecular weight 242·2) $1·6 \times 10^{-3}$ M

Aminopterin (4-amino-folic acid; 4-aminopteroyl glutamic acid) (molecular weight 440·4) $4·0 \times 10^{-5}$ M

Note: Aminopterin is highly toxic and a potent carcinogen.

Method

A 100-fold concentrated stock solution of hypoxanthine and thymidine.

1 Dissolve 136·1 mg hypoxanthine and 38·8 mg thymidine in 100 ml twice distilled water at 50°.
2 Sterilize by membrane filtration and store in 2–5 ml aliquots at −20°.

The hypoxanthine might precipitate out of solution during storage. Redissolve by heating in a boiling water bath.

B   100-fold concentrated solution of aminopterin.
1 Add 1·76 mg aminopterin to 90 ml of twice distilled water.
2 Add 1 M sodium hydroxide dropwise until the aminopterin dissolves and then titrate to pH 7·5 with 1 M hydrochloric acid.
3 Adjust final volume to 100 ml with twice distilled water.
4 Sterilize by membrane filtration, dispense into 2–5 ml aliquots and store at −20°.

Technical notes

1 Aminopterin must be protected from light.
2 This stock can be frozen and thawed several times for use, provided sterility is maintained.
3 Aminopterin may be purchased as a sterile 10^{-4} M solution from Flow Laboratories (Appendix II).

11.4.2   USE OF HAT MEDIUM

Materials

Stock solution of hypoxanthine and thymidine (HT), as above.
Stock solution of aminopterin (A), as above.
Tissue culture medium containing L-glutamine (Section 11.4) and
    10% serum (Appendix I)
Plates containing fused cells (Section 11.4)

Method

1 Add 2 ml of HT and 2 ml of A stock solutions to 100 ml of tissue culture medium containing 10% serum.
2 Add 50 μl of HAT medium to each well containing fused cells.
3 Return plates to 37° incubator.

Technical notes

1 The HAT medium used above is **double strength** so that the final concentration in the cultures is as follows:
    hypoxanthine $1·0 \times 10^{-4}$ M
    thymidine $1·6 \times 10^{-5}$ M
    aminopterin $4·0 \times 10^{-7}$ M
This medium will appear to kill all the cells in the plate but do not despair, hybrids usually grow without any problem.

2   You will need to feed each well with 25 μl of **single strengtn** medium only once per week. Prepare single strength medium by adding 1 ml of each of the HT and A stock solutions to 100 ml of tissue culture medium containing 10% serum.

Vigorously growing hybrids are usually visible in the high cell density plates, i.e. those prepared from the undiluted suspension of fused wells at 1–2 weeks after fusion (indicated by a change in the pH indicator dye). Examine all the plates under an inverted microscope and select the plate containing the cell dilution that allows one clone to grow in each 2–3 wells. Discard the plates that received the more concentrated cell suspensions, they will probably have several clones per well.

Depending on the source of plasmacytoma cells and frequency of fusion, hybrids may not show optimal growth when cultured alone. This problem may be overcome by plating cells onto feeder layers of macrophages.

11.4.3   PREPARATION OF MACROPHAGE FEEDER LAYERS

Materials and equipment

Mice
Tissue culture medium containing 10% serum (Appendix I)
Microculture plates, flat bottomed, 96 wells (Appendix II)
Incubator, humidified and gassed with 5% CO_2 in air.

Method

1   Prepare a suspension of peritoneal exudate cells from untreated mice (Section 1.7.5).
2   Wash the cells once in tissue culture medium by centrifugation (150 g for 10 min at room temperature).
3   *If the cells are histoincompatible with the fusion hybrids, irradiate the peritoneal exudate cells with 2000 rad.*
4   Count (Section 2.4) and adjust the cells to 2×10^5 ml^{-1}.
5   Dispense 100 μl aliquots into each well of a microculture plate.
6   Incubate in a humid 37° incubator gassed with 5% CO_2 air.

The feeder layers may be used for plating out of fusion mixtures after 24 h or up to 7 days.

Technical note

Each mouse should yield about 5×10^6 peritoneal exudate cells, of which about 50% will be lymphocytes.

313

SCREENING OF FUSION WELLS FOR
ANTIBODY ACTIVITY

The initial screen for antibody activity should be carried out as soon as growth of hybrid cells is seen under the microscope or when the pH indicator dye has become yellow.

Although we have diluted the cells to limit the number of independent hybrid cells per well, it is important to realise that several hybrids may grow, perhaps at different rates, each producing their own clone of cells. This might affect the screening assay in two ways:

1   A positive clone (secreting the desired antibody) may be detected soon after fusion, but then might be lost by overgrowth of a negative or other positive clones.

2   No activity may be detected during the first assay due to the cells of a positive clone being in a minority. It is, therefore, essential to test negative supernatants on two or three occasions.

Once antibody activity has been detected in any particular well, it is essential to clone and re-test the cells as soon as possible.

The type of assay to be used is determined by the nature of the antigen and the type of antibody desired. During initial screening, for the selection of positive hybrids for cloning, speed, convenience and reproducibility are essential. Positive wells must be detected rapidly and then cloned out rapidly to avoid overgrowth. Convenience is required so that a large number of supernatants can be screened to identify the wells containing the antibody with the required properties.

It is absolutely essential that the assay be established and standardized *before* any hybridization is undertaken.

Binding assays have the advantage that they will, by definition, detect all antibody activity against a particular antigen. Thus, unless one wishes to select for a particular effector function, for example, agglutination or complement fixation, solid-phase radio- or enzyme-linked immunoassays are preferable. We will describe a radioimmunoassay developed in our laboratories for the detection of antibodies to surface components of *Trypanosoma cruzi* (the causative agent of South American Sleeping Sickness). A similar assay has been described by Stocker and Heusser 1979 (see further reading) for the detection of antibodies to mouse alloantigens. Modifications of this assay for soluble antigens are given in the technical notes section.

11.5.1   SOLID-PHASE RADIOIMMUNOASSAY FOR CELL-SURFACE ANTIGENS

A. Preparation of cell-coated assay plates

Materials and equipment

Cells carrying antigen of interest

Glutaraldehyde

Phosphate buffered saline (PBS—Appendix I)

PBS containing bovine haemoglobin, 5% w/v and sodium azide, 0·2% w/v.

Microtitre plate with U-shaped wells, flexible polyvinyl chloride (Appendix II)

Method

1 Harvest the cells and wash three times in PBS by centrifugation (150 g for 10 min at 4°).

2 Count (Section 2.4) and adjust the cell numbers to 2×10^7 ml^{-1}.

3 Dispense 50 μl aliquots of fresh 0·25% glutaraldehyde in PBS into each well of the microtitre plate.

4 Add 50 μl of cell suspension to each of 95 wells of the plate and centrifuge at 100 g for 5–10 min at 4°. *The 96th well is used as a control for non-specific binding in the final assay.*

5 Remove the glutaraldehyde solution by tapping the inverted plate over a sink.

6 Flood the plate with PBS and roll a glass rod over the surface to remove air bubbles. Empty the plate, as in 5, and repeat the washing procedure twice. *Washing may also be performed by immersing the plate in a beaker of PBS.*

7 Flood the plate with PBS containing bovine haemoglobin (5% w/v) and sodium azide (0·2% w/v). Again, roll a glass rod over the surface to remove air bubbles.

8 Incubate the plate for 1 h at room temperature. *This will saturate the protein binding sites on the plastic.*

9 The plates may be used immediately or stored up to 10 weeks without removing the haemoglobin buffer.

Technical notes

1 Soluble proteins will adsorb directly to these polyvinyl plates. Add 50 μl of protein solution (at 50–200 μg ml^{-1}) in PBS to each well and incubate for at least one hour at room temperature. Remove the supernatant (and keep for re-use) and wash three times with PBS containing bovine haemoglobin (5% w/v) and sodium azide (0·2% w/v). The protein solution must be free of detergent as this will inhibit binding.

2 Stocker and Heusser (1979) have also linked antibody to the plate and used this to adsorb viable cells which are then fixed in glutaraldehyde.

3 The relatively low concentration of glutaraldehyde used to fix the cells does not seem to alter surface antigens.

B. Radio-iodinated anti-mouse immunoglobulin antibody

Prepare antibody to mouse immunoglobulin by affinity chromatography (Section 8.1.2) and label with ^{125}I using 'Iodogen' (Section 9.5.2).

Alternatively label anti-mouse immunoglobulin antibody while it is still attached to the affinity column (Section 8.1.2) using the chloramine T technique (Section 9.5.1). Elute the ^{125}I-labelled antibodies with 0·2 M glycine-HCl buffer (Appendix I) containing carrier protein.

11.5.2 BINDING ASSAY

Materials and equipment

Cultures of fused cells
Assay plates coated with cells
Phosphate buffered saline (PBS—Appendix I)
PBS containing bovine haemoglobin (5% w/v) and sodium azide (0·2% w/v).
^{125}I labelled anti-mouse immunoglobulin antibody (Section 9).
Plate sealers (Appendix II)
Vacuum trap for radioactive washings
Nichrome wire, electrically heated, for cutting up plates.
Gamma counter

Method

1   Remove the haemoglobin buffer by tapping the inverted test plate.
2   Remove 50 μl of supernatant from each hybrid well to be tested and transfer to the assay plate according to the following protocol:

Well number	Test antigen	Antibody	^{125}I-anti-mouse immunoglobulin
1	+	hybrid supernatant	+
↓		↓	
93	+	hybrid supernatant	+
94	+	*positive control	+
95	+	*negative control	+
96	−	*positive control	+

* See Technical notes, item 3

3   Incubate for 1 h at room temperature.
4   Wash the plate three times by immersing it in PBS and emptying it into a sink.
5   Add 25 μl of haemoglobin buffer containing 5×10^4 cpm ^{125}I

labelled anti-mouse immunoglobulin antibody to each well and incubate for 1 h at room temperature.

6   Remove the unbound radioactive antibody using a Pasteur pipette attached to a suction trap.

7   Wash five times by adding three drops of PBS to each well and then suck the solution into a vacuum trap.

8   Leave plates to dry in a fume cupboard.

9   Cut up the tray with an electrically heated Nichrome wire to release the wells. *For convenience, a plate sealer can be stuck to the bottom of the tray during cutting.*

10   Load the wells directly into a gamma counter with forceps.

Technical notes

1   The baseline counts in wells 95 and 96 should be less than 200 cpm.

2   Provided the baseline counts are reproducible, a count of more than 500 cpm usually indicates antibody activity in the test supernatant.

3   Because hybridoma supernatants have low total protein concentrations they give much 'cleaner' results in these assays compared with conventional antisera. Accordingly, the best controls are positive and negative supernatants from already established hybrids. Although, in initial experiments, it is often possible to beg hybrid supernatants with unrelated antibody activity to serve as negative controls, it is usually necessary to use diluted conventional antisera as positive controls.

4   When working with parasites we have often found that antigens are not expressed uniformly by all members of a population. Under these conditions it is necessary to use a binding assay that gives information on the population distribution of binding, for example, indirect immunofluorescence using either a UV microscope (Section 2.5.1) or a fluorescence-activated cell sorter (Section 8.4).

5   *As soon as positive cultures have been identified the cells should be cloned and, if possible, some of each uncloned positive well should be expanded by culture and stored in liquid nitrogen as an insurance against a failure during cloning.*

6   This is intended as a screening assay. Quantitation may be achieved as explained in Section 9.3.

Note: Do not transfer the hybrids directly from HAT to normal tissue culture medium, sufficient aminopterin may be carried over to prevent a resumption of 'de novo' synthesis of DNA. Instead, grow the cells in HT and tissue culture medium for 3–5 days before transferring to medium alone.

11.6   CLONING OF HYBRIDS

Antibody-secreting hybrid cells from positive culture wells must be cloned to ensure that the antibody is homogenous and monospecific. In practical terms, cloning is necessary to ensure that non-producers, arising either in the original fusion wells or as spontaneous variants, do not outgrow the antibody secreting hybrids.

Cloning, the initiation of a cell line from a single progenitor, may be achieved (a) in soft agar, (b) by limiting dilution, or (c) if the hardware is available, by using the fluorescence-activated cell sorter (Parks *et al* 1979).

11.6.1   CLONING IN SOFT AGAR

Initial preparations

Soft agar stock solution

Materials

Agarose (Appendix II)
Water, twice distilled

Method

1   Prepare a 2% w/v solution of agarose in twice distilled water and aliquot into glass bottles.
2   Autoclave at $120°$ for 15 min and store at $4°$ for use.

Technique

Materials and equipment

Hybrid cells
Agarose solution 2% w/v, as above
Tissue culture medium, double strength, with 20% serum (Appendix I)
Culture plates, 24 well (Appendix II)
Water bath at $44°$

Method

1   Melt the agarose in boiling water and allow it to equilibrate in a $44°$ water bath. Similarly equilibrate the tissue culture medium to $44°$.
2   Mix equal volumes of agarose and tissue culture medium, and return the mixture to the water bath. *The agarose will solidify if this is not done rapidly.*
3   Dispense 1 ml of the agarose tissue culture medium into each well of the tissue culture plate and allow it to solidify. *Allow two cloning wells for each positive hybrid culture.*

318

4   Count the hybrid cells (Section 2.5) and prepare suspensions at 2×10^3 cells ml^{-1} and 1×10^3 cells ml^{-1}.
5   For each cell suspension: mix 0·5 ml of cells with 1·0 ml of the agarose tissue culture medium mixture.
6   Add 0·6 ml of the cell-agarose mixture to a subbed well.
7   Repeat for all cells to be cloned.
8   Allow the agarose to solidify and incubate the plate in a humid incubator gassed with 5% CO_2 in air.

Cell colonies will grow within 1–2 weeks and will be visible as white spots in the agarose, each spot representing an individual clone.

9   Pick off ten discrete colonies per well using sterile Pasteur pipettes and transfer to liquid culture (Section 11.7).

Technical notes

1   The underlay agarose is used to ensure that the cell clones grow away from the well bottom. This aids manipulation of clones during isolation.
2   Only discrete cell colonies must be isolated.
3   The cloning efficiency of this technique is usually between 20–70% (percentage of original cells that grow as colonies). If optimal growth is not achieved then a feeder layer of macrophages may be used, under the agarose (Section 11.4.3).
4   Not all of the colonies isolated will grow to produce lines of antibody secreting cells. It is necessary, therefore, to screen and select for antibody activity (Section 11.5). If an assay can be designed which allows the detection of antibody secreting colonies in soft agar (for example, see Sharon *et al* 1979) then it is possible to select antibody secreting clones directly.

11.6.2   CLONING BY LIMITING DILUTION

Initial preparations

Prepare macrophage feeder layers in 96 well, flat bottom microculture plates (Section 11.4.3). Allow one plate for each positive hybrid well to be cloned.

Materials and equipment

Hybrid cells for cloning
Microculture plates with macrophage feeder layers (Section 11.4.3)
Incubator, 37°, humid and gassed with 5% CO_2 in air

Method

For each positive hybrid well:
1   Harvest and count the cells.
2   Prepare cell suspensions at 10 and 5 cells ml^{-1}.

319

3 Add 100 μl aliquots of the 10 cells ml^{-1} suspension to each of 48 wells. Repeat into remaining wells for the suspension at 5 cells ml^{-1}.
4 Incubate the plates in a humid 37° incubator gassed with 5% CO_2 in air. *Colonies should be visible after 1–2 weeks.*
5 Test supernatants for antibody activity (Section 11.5) and select positive wells for culture.

Technical notes

1 The initial distribution of cells per well follows Poisson statistics, thus although about 60% of the wells will receive only one cell (and therefore initiate a true clone), a significant proportion will receive 2 or more cells. Cloning must be repeated to ensure the homogeneity of any interesting hybrid line.
2 It is advisable to reclone both the plasmacytoma and hybridoma lines at regular intervals. This will eliminate any variant cells, especially spontaneous non-secreting variants before they overgrow the culture.

11.7 INITIATION AND MAINTENANCE OF CELL LINES

Freshly isolated hybrid cell cultures often grow slowly and are less tolerant of low cell densities than their plasmacytoma parent. The volume of the cell culture must be expanded slowly, at a rate that can only be determined empirically because hybrid lines show different growth rates. In general, colonies or cloning wells should be transferred to a maximum of 0.5 ml of medium (again with a feeder layer if necessary) and diluted with an equal volume of fresh medium as the pH indicator dye just begins to turn an orange-yellow.

If hybridoma lines are allowed to grow up to stationary phase in static flasks or spinner culture vessels they can produce up to 1 μg ml^{-1} of antibody protein. Although the antibody is pure, the spent medium contains many other serum proteins.

Large amounts of hybridoma derived antibody may be prepared by injecting these tumorogenic lines into histocompatible (or immunoincompetent) mice.

Materials

Mice, histocompatible (or nude, athymic Section 1.8.2)
Hybridoma line from *in vitro* culture
Pristan (2, 6, 10, 14-tetramethylpentadecane) (Appendix II)

Method

1 Inject 0.5 ml pristan into the peritoneal cavity of each mouse.
2 After 7 days, inject 10^7 hybridoma cells i.p. into each mouse.

Most hybridoma lines will produce solid tumours or ascities within 2–3 weeks.

3   Use a syringe and 19 g needle to drain off the ascitic fluid. Clarify the ascitic fluid by centrifugation (500 g for 15 min at 4°).

4   Assay the ascitic fluid from individual mice by electrophoresis (Section 5.3.4a), store those samples showing a prominent peak of paraprotein in the gammaglobulin region.

5   Repeat 3 and 4 for the lifetime of the mouse.

Technical notes

1   Ascitic fluid often contains up to 1 mg ml^{-1} of specific antibody protein. There are, of course, other proteins, including immunoglobulins of unknown specificity.

2   The serum of these tumour bearing mice also contains large quantities of hybridoma derived antibody.

3   It is inadvisable to maintain a hybridoma by serial passage in mice because of the risk of accumulating non-secreting cells. Instead, inject large batches of mice with recently cloned hybridoma cells from *in vitro* culture.

11.8   ANTIBODY PURIFICATION

Although culture or ascitic fluid containing a high titre of monoclonal antibody is sufficiently pure for many applications, it still contains many irrelevant proteins, some of which may be immunoglobulin molecules of unknown specificity.

If the appropriate antigen is available and suitable, the simplest way to isolate antibody, of the highest purity, is to use affinity chromatography. Alternatively immunoglobulin may be isolated by the techniques described either in Chapter 7 or below.

11.8.1   ANTIGEN IMMUNOADSORBENTS

Protein antigens (not necessarily in a pure form) may be linked to a support matrix, such as cyanogen bromide-activated Sepharose (Section 8.1) and packed into a column. Ascitic fluid or culture supernatant is then simply allowed to filter through the column, which is then washed to remove unbound proteins and the antibody eluted under the most gentle conditions compatible with antibody release (see Section 8.1.5 for choice and advantages of elution buffers).

11.8.2   CELL SURFACE IMMUNOADSORBENTS

The purification of antibody against cell surface components is technically more difficult. If the appropriate cells can be immob-

321

ilized on a support matrix and cross-linked by glutaraldehyde, it is possible to use cell-column chromatography for the isolation of specific antibody.

Preparation of cellular immunoadsorbent

Materials and equipment

Cells carrying appropriate antigen
Concanavalin A (Con A) (Appendix II)
Glutaraldehyde
Phosphate buffered saline (PBS) (Appendix I)
Sephadex G50 (Appendix II), coarse, swollen in PBS (Section 7.2.2).

Method

1   Add 50 mg of Con A in PBS to Sephadex and stir at room temperature.
2   After 30 min allow the Sephadex to settle and remove the excess Con A by decantation.
3   Add packed cells and mix slowly for 15 min at room temperature. *The exact proportions of cells and matrix will vary according to the availability of the cells and the concentration of antigen at the cell surface. Typically, use 4 ml of packed cells to 50 ml of swollen Sephadex.*
4   Add 100 ml of glutaraldehyde solution (3% in PBS) and stir gently for 1 h at room temperature.
5   Wash Sephadex-cell mixture with PBS by three cycles of mixing and decantation.
6   Pour mixture into a column and wash overnight with PBS for use.

Isolation of antibody

1   Add ascitic fluid or culture supernatant to the top of the affinity column and allow it to filter through slowly (5–10 ml h^{-1}).
2   Wash with PBS until the absorbancy of the effluent is less than 0.01 at 280 nm.
3   Elute antibody with 0.05 M glycine-HCl, 0.5 M NaCl, pH 3.0, and adjust pH and concentration of eluate (as in Section 8.1.2).
4   Re-equilibrate the column with PBS containing sodium azide (0.2% w/v).
5   Test eluted antibody for activity (Section 11.5.1) and store at −20°.

Technical notes

1   The cell columns may be stored at 4° in PBS containing sodium azide (0.2% w/v) and re-used over several weeks. Before use, pre-elute the column with acid buffer and re-equilibrate with PBS.

322

2   Antibodies prepared by acid elution from immunoadsorbent invariably contain soluble complexes formed by denaturation under acid conditions. If required, these may be removed by gel chromatography (Section 7.2).

11.8.3   ISOLATION OF IMMUNOGLOBULIN

If antibody cannot be isolated directly, it is possible to prepare an immunoglobulin fraction of the ascitic fluid or culture supernatant using either affinity or ion exchange chromatography.

Anti-immunoglobulin columns

The IgG (Section 7.3) or antibody (Section 8.1) fraction of goat or rabbit anti-mouse immunoglobulin may be linked to Sepharose (Section 8.1.1) and the affinity column so formed used to isolate hybridoma immunoglobulin.

Materials and equipment

Anti-mouse immunoglobulin, goat or rabbit (Section 1.4.2)
Mouse immunoglobulin (Section 1.2.2)
Hybridoma derived antibody
Also as for Section 8.1.2

Method

1   Isolate the antibody (Section 8.1) or IgG (Section 7.3) fraction from the anti-mouse immunoglobulin serum.
2   Link anti-immunoglobulin to Sepharose (Section 8.1.1) and pack into a column.
3   Add 100 mg normal mouse immunoglobulin prepared by ammonium sulphate precipitation, (Section 1.2.2) and allow it to filter slowly through the column.
4   Elute with glycine-HCl buffer (Section 8.1.2) and re-equilibrate the column with PBS until the absorbancy of the effluent is less than 0·01 at 280 nm.

These columns are pre-cycled with normal mouse IgG and eluted with acid buffer to saturate the high affinity anti-immunoglobulin antibodies that would otherwise bind the expensive monoclonal antibody virtually irreversibly. In any case, these columns should always be pre-eluted with acid buffer and re-equilibrated before use to remove any loosely bound material.

5   Add solution containing hybridoma derived antibody, wash and elute as above.

To minimize denaturation elution should be accomplished with the most gentle conditions compatible with release of antibody (Section 8.1.5).

Mouse immunoglobulin may also be isolated by ion exchange chromatography (Section 7.3) or by affinity chromatography on staphylococcal protein A-Sepharose (subclasses IgG2a, IgG2b and IgG3—Section 8.5). (Rat immunoglobulin, with the exception of the minor subclass IgG2c, do not bind to protein A.)

11.9 PRACTICAL APPLICATIONS OF MONOCLONAL ANTIBODIES

The production, selection and maintenance of hybridoma clones synthesising antibody of a required specificity is so time consuming that before starting one must be convinced that hybridoma technology is the best way to achieve the desired result.

Under some circumstances, for example, for the production of antibodies for the class-specific precipitation of immunoglobulins, the restricted reactivity of monospecific antibody is a downright disadvantage. In general, these antibodies bind to only one determinant per molecule when used with nonpolymeric antigens, thus precluding the formation of a matrix for precipitation.

There are however, numerous examples where the availability of monoclonal antibody has greatly improved existing technology or has been fundamental for the generation of new techniques. This is to be expected when one considers their advantages compared with conventional antisera:

1 Because they are monospecific, hybridoma-derived antibodies can be used for the estimation of degree of structural homology between antigens. For example, with influenza virus, antibodies against chemically defined antigens have been used to investigate variant strains of virus for the presence of identical or closely related antigens.

2 In solid phase binding assays, these antibodies can be used at very low protein concentrations. This is of particular advantage because these assays are essentially affinity independent and can detect the very low affinity protein-protein interactions often found with conventional sera. Hence the degree of non-specific binding shown by an unrelated monoclonal antibody is much less than would be found with a normal control serum or unrelated antiserum;

3 The production of hybridoma-derived antibody is highly reproducible. If one prepares a hybrid cell using a non-synthesising plasmacytoma line, then the hybridoma line will produce only one type of antibody. Thus, whenever a new batch of antibody is produced

from the same cell line, it will have the same specificity. (Unless, of course, the cell line ceases to produce immunoglobulin or there is a mutation in the variable region immunoglobulin gene.)

Although in general the use of monospecific antibody is still at the research stage, several interesting developments have been reported. Of particular interest, is the use of monospecific antibodies for the definition of cell surface markers for the investigation of specialised or abnormal cell function. This should yield new information on the development and control of the immune system, and perhaps, also on the process of tumourogenesis.

Monospecific antibodies might have a therapeutic application in clinical medicine once a suitable human plasmacytoma parent line has been discovered. (This application was previously discounted because of the possible co-purification of viral oncogenes from hybridoma supernatants. However, an analogous situation now exists with the production of interferon from human cell lines. It is possible that the safeguards developed for the production and use of interferon might be applicable to hybridoma-derived antibodies).

Monospecific antibodies produced by mouse fusion hybrids have many immediate applications in the clinical laboratory as diagnostic or immunoassay reagents:

1   Tissue typing. Current typing techniques rely on antisera derived from multiparous women or from patients who have received multiple blood transfusions. They are of low titre and often contain several specificities. A programme has been established in the United States for the production of typing reagents using hybridoma techniques.

2   Immunoassay of hormones, etc. Fusions can be performed with cells from mice immunised with relatively unpure antigen. The need for antigen purification is circumvented by the selection of appropriate cell lines from cloned populations. This, and the mono-specificity of the antibody thus obtained, has greatly enhanced the range and sensitivity of potential immunoassay techniques. For example, an improved 'pregnancy test' has recently been developed using hybridoma-derived antibody for the radioimmunoassay of human chorionic gonadotrophin (HCG). It is claimed that this test can detect HCG in the urine of pregnant women within a few days of conception.

3   Immunodiagnosis of infectious disease. It is probable that radio-immunoassays using monoclonal antibodies will be sufficiently sensitive to allow the diagnosis of infectious disease by the detection (and perhaps quantitation) of microbial antigen rather than antibody. This is of much greater clinical value as it is a direct measure of the actual parasitaemic status of the patient. Antibody detection has the disadvantage that it is virtually impossible to distinguish between a past or present infection using a single blood sample. Again,

325

the monospecificity of the antibody used should avoid the imprecision of present immunodiagnostic techniques.

11.10   SUMMARY AND CONCLUSIONS

Although the production of antibody by hybridisation techniques is *very* time consuming, it is technically no more demanding than normal *in vitro* cell culture.

Unless the antigen of interest is valuable or in short supply, there is little to be gained by starting hybridization experiments with irrelevant antigens such as sheep erythrocytes or keyhole limpet haemocyanin. Almost invariably, the most difficult and rate limiting step in the isolation of antibody synthesising hybridoma lines is the need to screen large numbers of culture supernatants. For this reason, it is essential to establish and standardise the screening assay before attempting to produce hybrids.

On a practical level, the maintenance of hybridoma lines requires:

1   A well ordered technique to enable the operator to maintain several lines without cross-contamination, otherwise all lines will eventually be overtaken by the one with the fastest growth rate.

2   Facilities for the cryopreservation of cells. This is essential as a source of new cells, if cultures are lost by microbial contamination or overgrowth by non-secreting variations, and also to avoid having to maintain the many hundreds of hybridoma lines that are rapidly produced.

FURTHER READING

KNUTTON S. & PASTERNAK C.A. (1979) The mechanism of cell-cell fusion. *Trends in Biomed. Sci.* **41**, 220.
KÖHLER G. & MILSTEIN C. (1975) Derivation of specific antibody-producing tissue culture and tumour lines by cell fusion. *Eur. J. Immunol.* **61**, 511.
LITTLEFIELD J.W. (1964) Selection of hybrids from matings of fibroblasts *in vitro* and their presumed recombinants. *Science* **145**, 709.
MELCHERS F., POTTER M. & WARNER N.L. (1978) Lymphocyte hybridomas. In *Current Topics Microbiol. Immunol.* **81.** Springer-Verlag, Berlin.
NABHOLZ M.V., MIGGIANO W. & BODMER W. (1969) Genetic analysis with human-mouse somatic cell hybrids. *Nature* **223**, 358.
PARKS D.R., BRYAN V.M. OI V.T. & HERZENBERG L.A. (1979) Antigen specific identification and cloning of hybridomas with a fluorescence-activated cell sorter (FACS). *Proc. Nat. Acad. Sci.* **76**, 1962.
SHARON J., MORRISON S.J. & KABAT E.A. (1979) Detection of specific hybridoma clones by replica immunoadsorption of their secreted antibodies. *Proc. Nat. Acad. Sci.* **76**, 1420.

STÄHLI C., STAEHELIN T., MIGGIANO V., SCHMIDT J. & HARING P. (1980) High frequencies of antigen-specific hybridomas: Dependence on immunisation parameters and prediction by spleen cell analysis. *J. Imm. Methods* **32**(3), 297.

STOCKER J.W. & HEUSSER C.H. (1979) Methods for binding cells to plastic: application to a solid phase radioimmunoassay for cell surface antigens. *J. Imm. Methods* **26,** 87.

—— (1979) Hybrid myeloma monoclonal antibodies against MHC products. *Immunological Reviews* **49.** Munksgaard, Copenhagen.

Appendixes
I Buffers and media

All solutions must be made up in deionized, double- or triple-glass distilled water.

Acetate-acetic acid buffer, pH 4·0, ionic strength 0·1

Materials

Sodium acetate, 0·6 M (49·2 g l^{-1})
Acetic acid, 0·6 M (34·4 ml glacial acetic acid in 1 litre distilled water)

Method

Mix 435 ml 0·6 M acetic acid with 130 ml 0·6 M sodium acetate and adjust to 1 litre with distilled water.

Acetate-acetic buffer 0·001 M pH 4·4

Materials

Sodium acetate, CH_3COONa, 8·20 g l^{-1}
Acetic acid 6·0 g l^{-1}

Method

Mix $\frac{1}{3}$ sodium acetate solution with $\frac{2}{3}$ acetic acid solution.
Dilute 1 : 1000 to give 1 mM

Balanced salt solution (BSS)

Materials

Calcium chloride 0·14 g l^{-1}
Sodium chloride 8·00 g l^{-1}
Potassium chloride 0·40 g l^{-1}
Magnesium sulphate, $MgSO_4$ $7H_2O$ (0·8 mM) 0·20 g l^{-1}
Magnesium chloride, $MgCl_2$ $6H_2O$ (1·0 mM) 0·20 g l^{-1}
Potassium di-hydrogen phosphate (0·4 mM) 0·06 g l^{-1}
Di-sodium hydrogen phosphate, Na_2HPO_4 $2H_2O$ (1·4 mM) 0·24 g l^{-1}

Method

1   If required 1 g of glucose may be added l^{-1}.
2   Dissolve all components in 1000 ml.
3   Membrane filter, if required sterile.

Barbitone buffer, pH 8·2, ionic strength 0·08

Materials

Barbital sodium (5'5 Diethylbarbituric acid, Na salt)
Barbital (5'5 Diethylbarbituric acid)
Sodium hydroxide 5 M
Merthiolate

Method

1   Dissolve 12·00 g sodium barbital in 800 ml distilled water.
2   Dissolve 4·40 g barbital in 150 ml distilled water at 95°.

   Mix solutions 1 and 2 and adjust pH to 8·2 with concentrated sodium hydroxide. Add 0·15 g merthiolate (preservative) and adjust final volume to 1000 ml.

Note (cellulose acetate membranes)

For electrophoresis on cellulose acetate membranes we normally use barbitone buffer, pH 8·6, 0·05–0·07 M. The exact buffer composition and concentration can be adjusted according to requirements. At lower concentrations, the protein bands are wider and their mobility increased. A higher buffer concentration produces the reverse effect with crowding of the bands.
Diethylbarbituric acid 7·36 g.
Barbital sodium 41·2 g.
Distilled water to 4 litres.

Barbitone buffered saline, pH 7·6, 0·15 m, for complement fixation test

Materials

Sodium chloride
Barbital (5'5 Diethylbarbituric acid)
Barbital sodium (5'5 Diethylbarbituric acid, Na salt)
Magnesium chloride
Calcium chloride 1·0 M ($111·1 \text{ g } l^{-1}$)

Stock solutions

A   85·0 g sodium chloride + 2·75 g sodium diethylbarbiturate in 1400 ml of distilled water.

B   5·75 g diethylbarbituric acid in 500 ml hot distilled water.

C   20·3 g $MgCl_2$ $6H_2O$ (2·0 M) dissolved in 50 ml distilled water + 30 ml 1·0 M calcium chloride solution. Adjust to 100 ml with distilled water. (Final concentrations $MgCl_2$ 1·0 M, $CaCl_2$ 0·3 M.)

1   Mix solutions A and B, and cool to room temperature.

2   Add 5 ml of C.

3   Adjust final volume to 2 litres with distilled water and store at 4°.

This buffer is 5 × the concentration used in the text. Dilute just before use.

Borate buffer, pH 7·4, 0·1 M

Materials

Disodium tetraborate $N_2B_4O_7$ $10H_2O$ 9·54 g in 250 ml distilled water

Boric acid 24·73 g in 4 litres distilled water.

Method

Add approximately 115 ml borate solution to 4 litres boric acid solution until pH reaches 7·4.

Borate saline buffer, pH 8·3–8·5, ionic strength 0·1

Materials

Boric acid, 6·18 g l^{-1}
Sodium tetraborate (borax) 9·54 g l^{-1}
Sodium chloride 4·38 g l^{-1}
Make up to 1000 ml with distilled water

Borate-succinate buffer, pH 7·5, 0·15 M (*for tanning erythrocytes*)

Solution A—Sodium tetraborate $Na_2B_4O_7$: $1OHO_2O$, 0·05 M (19·0 g l^{-1})

Solution B—Succinic acid, 0·05 M (5·9 g l^{-1})

Sodium chloride
Horse serum (Appendix II)

Method

1   Take 1 litre of A and add B until pH 7·5.

2   Add sodium chloride to 0·14 M and 1% horse serum (final concentration) previously heat inactivated (56° for 45 min).

Cacodylate buffer, pH 6·9, 0·28 M

Materials

Sodium cacodylate
Hydrochloric acid 3 M

Method

1   Dissolve sodium cacodylate (60 g l^{-1}) in distilled water.
2   Titrate to pH 6·9 with 3 M HCl.
3   Adjust to 1 l with distilled water.

Carbonate buffer, pH 9·6, 0·05 M

Materials

Sodium carbonate Na_2CO_3 1·59 g
Sodium hydrogen carbonate $NaHCO_3$ 2·93 g

Method

Dissolve in 1 litre of distilled water

Carbonate buffer, pH 9·5, 0·2 M (*for peroxidase conjugation*)

Materials

Sodium carbonate Na_2CO_3 21·2 g l^{-1}
Sodium hydrogen carbonate $NaHCO_3$ 16·8 g l^{-1}

Method

Add sodium carbonate solution to sodium hydrogen carbonate solution to pH 9·5 (approx. 6·4 ml to 18·6 ml).

Carbonate-bicarbonate buffer, pH 9·0

Materials

Sodium carbonate, anhydrous
Sodium bicarbonate
Saline (0·14 M sodium chloride in water)

Method

1   Prepare stock solutions of 1 M carbonate and 1 M bicarbonate.
2   Mix carbonate and bicarbonate in the proportions 1 : 9 (v/v) and titrate pH to 9·0 with one of the stock solutions (carbonate raises pH, bicarbonate lowers pH).

3 Dilute buffer to the required molarity with saline.

Note: The bicarbonate solution will not keep.

Citrate buffer, pH 3·0–7·0, 0·1 M

Materials

Citric acid $(C_6H_8O_7 \cdot 1H_2O)$ 0·1 M $(21·01$ g l$^{-1})$
Di-sodium hydrogen phosphate $(Na_2HPO_4 \cdot 2H_2O)$ 0·1 M $(17·80$ g l$^{-1})$

Method

pH 5·0, is approximately a 50 : 50 mixture of citric to phosphate.
Below pH 5·0: titrate pH of citric acid with phosphate.
Above pH 5·0: titrate pH of phosphate with citric acid.

Citrate-phosphate buffer, pH 5·0, 0·15 M

Materials

Citric acid 21·0 g l^{-1}
Disodium hydrogen phosphate $Na_2HPO_4 \cdot 2H_2O$ 35·6 g l^{-1}

Method

Mix approximately 49 ml citric acid solution with 51 ml of phosphate solution until pH 5·0.

C1q buffers

Buffer 1

Ethyleneglycol-bis-(β-amino-ethyl ether) N, N^1 tetra acetic acid (EGTA) 19·76 g. Add 1500 ml distilled water. Slowly add strong NaOH (about 8 ml of 11 M NaOH) to both dissolve the EGTA and bring the pH to 7·5. Add distilled water to a total volume of 2 litres.

Buffer 2

Sodium acetate 0·02 M 1·64 g in 1 litre distilled water.
Acetic acid 0·02 M 1·14 ml glacial acetic acid in 1 litre distilled water.
Ethylene diamine tetra acetic acid (Na$_3$) EDTA 1·79 g.
Sodium chloride 21·91 g.
   Add the EDTA and sodium chloride to 300 ml of the acetic acid. When dissolved add further acetic acid and sodium acetate-solution until a pH of 5·0 and a volume of 500 ml is reached.

332

Buffer 3

EDTA (Na$_3$) 86 g
Hydrochloric acid
Dissolve the EDTA in 3·5 litres distilled water. Add concentrated HCl to pH 5·0 and then make up to a total volume of 4 litres with distilled water.

Buffer 4

Potassium dihydrogen phosphate 0·34 g in 500 ml distilled water
Disodium hydrogen phosphate 0·355 g in 500 ml distilled water
Sodium chloride 21·91 g
EDTA (Na$_3$) 1·79 g
Dissolve the sodium chloride and EDTA in about 200 ml of the disodium hydrogen phosphate solution. Add further disodium hydrogen phosphate and potassium dihydrogen phosphate solutions to a pH of 7·5 and volume of 500 ml.

Buffer 5

EDTA (Na$_3$) 50·15 g
Hydrochloric acid
Dissolve the EDTA in 3·51 litres distilled water. Add concentrated HCl to pH 7·5. Make up the volume to 4 litres with distilled water.

Buffer 6

Ingredients as for buffer 2
Dissolve EDTA and the sodium chloride in 300 ml sodium acetate solution. Adjust the pH to 7·5 and the volume to 500 ml with further sodium acetate and acetic acid solutions.

Cryopreservation of cells

Cells may be stored for an indefinite period in a frozen state under liquid nitrogen. Freeze viable, actively growing cells whenever possible.
Cryoprotective solution; by volume
Fetal bovine serum (FBS) 50%
Dimethyl sulphoxide (DMSO) 20%
Tissue culture medium 30%

Method

1   Harvest the cells by centrifugation (150 g for 10 min at 4°), count and adjust to 1×10^7 ml^{-1}.

2 Add cell suspension dropwise to an equal volume of cryoprotective solution.

3 Dispense convenient volumes into ampoules suitable for storage in liquid nitrogen.

4 Freeze slowly (at about 1° min^{-1}) down to at least $-20°$ and then immerse in liquid nitrogen. *DMSO (or alternatively, glycerol) allows water to go from a liquid to a solid state without the formation of ice crystals.*

Cells may be recovered from liquid nitrogen storage by thawing rapidly to 37° (in a water bath) and washing three times in tissue culture medium by centrifugation (150 *g* for 10 min at room temperature).

Diamino ethane–acetic acid buffer, pH 7·0, ionic strength 0·1

Materials

Diamino ethane
Acetic acid 1 M (57·3 ml glacial acetic acid in 1 litre distilled water)

Method

Mix 2·88 g diamino ethane with 73·0 ml 1 M acetic acid and make up to 1 litre with distilled water.

Giemsa buffer (*for May–Grünwald/Giemsa staining*)

Materials

Citric acid 0·1 M (21·01 g l^{-1})
Di-sodium hydrogen phosphate 0·2 M (Na_2HPO_4, 28·39 g l^{-1})

Method

Mix 85 ml 0·1 M citric acid with 115 ml 0·2 M di-sodium hydrogen phosphate and adjust pH to 5·75. Make up to 1000 ml.

Glycine–hydrochloric acid buffer, pH 2·5 or 2·8, 0·1 M (*for acid elution of antibodies from immunoadsorbents*)

Materials

Glycine 0·2 M (15·01 g l^{-1})
Hydrochloric acid 0·2 M

FOR 1000 ML BUFFER

Titrate pH of 500 ml of 0·2 M glycine to 2·5–2·8 as required, with 0·2 M hydrocyloric acid. Make up to 1 litre.

Glycine saline buffer, pH 8·6, 0·5 M (*for immunofluorescence mountant and latex agglutination*)

Materials

Glycine 14·00 g
Sodium hydroxide, solid 0·7 g
Sodium chloride 17 g
Sodium azide (preservative) 1 g

Method

Dissolve in 500 ml of distilled water and adjust pH to 8·6. Make up to 1000 ml.

Mounting medium made as follows: 30 ml above buffer plus 70 ml glycerol.

Hank's saline (*there are other formulations for this medium*)

Materials

Sodium chloride, 8·00 g l^{-1}
Calcium chloride, 0·20 g l^{-1}
Magnesium sulphate, 0·20 g l^{-1}
Potassium chloride, 0·40 h l^{-1}
Potassium di-hydrogen phosphate (KH_2PO_4), 0·10 g l^{-1}
Sodium bicarbonate, 1·27 g l^{-1}
Glucose, 2·00 g l^{-1}

Method

Dissolve in 1000 ml of distilled water. (Concentrated Hank's saline is sold commercially, but often has phenol red added as a pH indicator. This makes visualization of haemolytic plaques difficult.)

Phosphate buffer, pH 8·0, 0·5 M

Materials

Sodium di-hydrogen phosphate 1 hydrate (NaH_2PO_4 H_2O) 69·0 g l^{-1}
Di-sodium hydrogen phosphate, anhydrous (Na_2HPO_4) 71·0 g l^{-1}

Method

Prepare stock solutions of each salt in water and add one drop of chloroform as a preservative. Store at room temperature.

Mix the two solutions to obtain the required pH using a pH meter and then adjust to the desired molarity.

Take care not to add too much chloroform especially if the buffer is to be used with plastic chromatography columns.

Phosphate buffer pH 7·4, 0·08 M phosphate, containing 0·077 M or 1·1 M sodium chloride, pH 7·4 (*for IgM preparation*)

Materials

Potassium dihydrogen phosphate KH_2PO_4, 2·14 g
Disodium hydrogen phosphate Na_2HPO_4, $2H_2O$, 11·46 g
Sodium chloride, 4·50 g for 0·077 M and 64·28 g for 1·1 M
Sodium azide 0·2 g

Method

Dissolve in distilled water and make up to 1 litre with distilled water.

Phosphate buffered saline (PBS), pH 7·2, 0·15 M

Materials

Sodium chloride, 8·00 g l^{-1}
Potassium chloride 0·20 g l^{-1}
Di-sodium hydrogen phosphate (Na_2HPO_4) (0·008 M) 1·15 g l^{-1}
Potassium di-hydrogen phosphate, 0·20 g l^{-1}

Method

Dissolve in 1000 ml of distilled water.
   It is convenient to make up a × 10 solution for storage and dilute as required.

Phosphate saline buffer, pH 7·2, 0·20 M (*for tanning erythrocytes*)

Materials

Potassium di-hydrogen phosphate (KH_2PO_4) 0·02 M (12·2 g)
Di-sodium hydrogen phosphate (Na_2HPO_4) 0·06 M (40·4 g)
Sodium chloride 0·12 M (36·0 g)

Method

Dissolve in 5 litres of distilled water

Saline—physiological or 'normal' saline, 0·14 M

Sodium chloride 8·5 g l^{-1}
   Store at a × 10 concentration solution and dilute as required.

Scintillation fluid

2,5-Diphenyloxazole (PPO) 6 g
2,2'-p-Phenylene-bis (5-phenyloxazole) (POPOP) 0·05 g
Toluene 1 litre

Tissue-culture media

Many different culture media are available, each usually in an 'old' and 'new' or 'improved' formulation. For general use we suggest Eagle's Minimal Essential Medium (EMEM), or as Dulbecco's modification (DMEM).

Buffers for culture media

A good argument can be made for using sodium bicarbonate (2·2 g l^{-1}) buffered by CO_2 in air, as this is at least physiological under closed-culture conditions (5% CO_2 in air in a gassed incubator). Recently, double-buffering systems have been used to good effect, for example, RPMI containing bicarbonate and HEPES, 30 mM (N-2-hydroxyethylpiperazine N-2-ethanesulphonic acid). In this case, under low CO_2 tension, the pH is maintained by the interaction of the bicarbonate with the HEPES; and in culture, under high CO_2 tension, the bicarbonate also acts as a buffer, as described above.

To avoid the expense of large volumes of this relatively expensive medium, cells may be prepared from the animal in PBS and washed in medium before culture.

For *in vitro* handling of lymphocytes, not involving culture, we have used DMEM containing HEPES, 20 mM, adjusting the pH to 7·2 with 1 M sodium hydroxide.

Antibiotics for culture media

Again many workers have their own recipe; we suggest:
penicillin 200 units ml^{-1}.
streptomycin 100 $\mu g \, ml^{-1}$.

If there is persistent yeast contamination it is possible to add Fungizone (amphotericin B) at 10 $\mu g \, ml^{-1}$ (final concentration).

Serum supplements

For murine cells:

10% fetal bovine serum (FBS). It is necessary to select a 'good' batch of serum, i.e. giving acceptable cell survival, without a high background of incorporation of the DNA analogue due to mitogenic stimulation by the FBS.

The proportion of FBS required may be reduced by adding 2 mercaptoethanol. The medium listed below was developed for murine mixed lymphocyte cultures, but it may be used for the maintenance of mouse cell lines (including hybridoma lines).

Dulbecco's modification of EMEM containing:

arginine 200 mg l^{-1}
folic acid 12 mg l^{-1}
asparagine 36 mg l^{-1}
2 mercaptoethanol 5×10^{-5} mol l^{-1}
HEPES 1×10^{-2} mol l^{-1}
FBS 5% v/v

This section is by no means a guide to *in vitro* culture techniques. Many improvements have been made in the whole technology of cell culture, particularly with the advent of microculture plates (microtitre plates, Appendix II) and micro-microcultures using Terasaki plates. The basic systems we have described will work, but for research purposes it is necessary to consult the literature.

Tris-ammonium chloride (*for erythrocyte lysis*)

Materials

Tris(hydroxymethyl)aminomethane 0·17 M (20·60 g l^{-1})
Ammonium chloride 0·16 M (8·30 g l^{-1})

Method

Add 10 ml of 0·17 M tris to 90 ml of 0·16 M ammonium chloride and adjust to pH 7·2.

This buffer induces red-cell lysis without reducing lymphocyte viability, unlike 1·0% acetic acid which is also used to lyse erythrocytes during white-cell counts.

Tris-buffered saline pH 8·0 (*for IgM preparation*)

Materials

Tris (hydroxy methyl) aminoethane 12·1 g
Sodium chloride 29·22 g
Glycine 0·75 g
Sodium azide 0·2 g
Hydrochloric acid 1·0 M

Method

Dissolve ingredients in 800 ml distilled water and adjust pH to 8·0 with HCl. Make up volume to 1 litre with distilled water.

Tris-glycine buffer, pH 8·3, 0·25 M tris, 1·92 M glycine

Materials

Tris(hydroxymethyl)aminoethane 30·3 g
Glycine 134·6 g
Sodium dodecyl sulphate 10 g

Method

Dissolve materials in water and make up to 1000 ml.

Tris-hydrochloric acid buffer, pH 8·2, 0·15 M

Materials

Tris(hydroxymethyl)aminomethane 0·15 M (18·15 g l^{-1}).
Hydrochloric acid, 1 M

Method

1   Dissolve 18·15 g tris in 500 ml of water.
2   Titrate tris solution to pH 8·2 with 1 M HCl and adjust final volume to 1 litre.

Tris-hydrochloric acid buffer, pH 7·4, 0·1 M (*for protein iodination*)

Materials

Tris(hydroxymethyl)aminomethane 0·1 M (12·1 g l^{-1})
Hydrochloric acid, 1 M

Method

1   Dissolve 12·1 g tris in 500 ml water.
2   Titrate tris solution to pH 7·4 with 1 M HCl and adjust final volume to 1 litre.

Tris-hydrochloric acid buffer, pH 6·8, 0·5 M

Materials

Tris(hydroxymethyl)aminoethane 30·3 g
Hydrochloric acid 1 M

Method

1   Dissolve tris in 100 ml water.
2   Titrate tris solution to pH 6·8 with 1 M HCl and adjust volume to 500 ml.

Tris-hydrochloric acid buffer, pH 8·5, 9·0, 1·0 M

Materials

Tris(hydroxymethyl)aminomethane 1 M (121 g l^{-1})
Hydrochloric acid 1 M

Method

pH 8·5—Mix 25·0 ml 1 M tris with 7·2 ml 1 M HCl.
pH 9·0—Mix 25·0 ml 1 M tris with 2.5 ml 1 M HCl.

Tris-hydrochloric acid buffer, pH 8·8, 1·5 M

Materials

Tris(hydroxymethyl)aminoethane 45·51 g
Hydrochloric acid 1 M approx. 66 ml

Method

1 Dissolve Tris in 100 ml water.
2 Titrate this solution to pH 8·8 with 1 M HCl and adjust final volume to 250 ml.

Veronal buffered saline (*for PEG precipitation*)

Materials

Sodium chloride 85 g
Sodium barbitone 3·75 g
Barbitone 5·75 g

Method

Dissolve and make up to 2 litres with distilled water.
This buffer is 5 times the concentration used in the text, as it is more stable as a concentrated solution. Dilute just before use.

II Equipment and manufacturers' index

Terminal code number(s) indicates listing in address index.

MANUFACTURER'S ADDRESS INDEX

1 Aldrich Chemical Co, The Old Brickyard, New Road, Gillingham, Dorset, SP8 4JL.

2 Animals for Research, Directory of Sources, National Academy of Science, Washington, USA.

3 Arnold Horwell, 2 Grange Way, Kilburn High Road, London NW6 2BP. Clay Adams, Division of Becton, Dickinson and Company, Cockeysville, Maryland 21030, USA.

4 Autowrappers (Sales) Ltd, 23/25 Brunel Road, East Acton, London W3 7UR 3M Company, St. Paul, Minnesota, USA.

5 BDH Chemicals Ltd, Baird Road, Enfield, Middlesex EN1 1SH. E. Merck, Darmstadt, W. Germany.

6 Becton Dickinson (UK) Ltd, York House, Empire Way, Wembley, Middlesex; BBL, Box 243, Cockeysville, Maryland 21030, USA.

7 Biological Standards Division, National Institute for Medical Research, Mill Hill, London NW7.

8 Bionetics, Uniscience Ltd, Uniscience House, 8 Jesus Lane, Cambridge CB5 8BA.

9 Biorad Laboratories Ltd, Caxton Way, Holywell Industrial Estate, Watford, Herts WD1 8RP; Bio-rad Laboratories, 2200 Wright Avenue, Richmond, California 94804, USA.

10 British Food Manufacturing Industries Research Association, Randalls Road, Leatherhead, Surrey.

11 Central Veterinary Laboratories, Weybridge, Surrey.

12 Cheesebrough-Pond's or Johnson Ltd, London.

13 CP Laboratories Ltd, PO Box 22, Bishops Stortford, Herts; Calbiochem-Behring Corp, PO Box 12087, San Diego, California 92112, USA.

14 Degussa AG, Abt. Russ, 6 Frankfurt am Main 1, Postfach 3993, Germany.

15 Difco Laboratories Ltd, PO Box 14B, Central Avenue, East Molesey, Surrey; Difco Laboratories, Box 1058-A Detroit, Michigan 48232, USA.

16 Dynatech, Daux Road, Billingshurst, Sussex; Cooke Engineering Company, 900 Slater's Lane, Alexandria, Virginia 22314, USA.

17 Ethicon GmbH, Hamburg-Noderstedt, W. Germany.

18 Flow Laboratories Ltd, Victoria Park, Heatherhouse Road, Irvine, Ayrshire, Scotland; 7655, Old Springhouse Road, McLean, Va 22102, USA.

19 Fluorochem Ltd, Dinton Vale Trading Estate, Dinton Vale, Glossop, Derbyshire; Fluka AG, Buchs SG, Switzerland.

20 Gallenkamp, PO Box 290, Technico House, Christopher Street, London EC2.

21 Gelman Hawksley, 10 Harrowden Road, Brackmills, Northampton NN4 0EB.

22 Gibco Bio-cult Ltd, Washington Road, Sandyford Industrial Estate, Paisley PA3 4EP, Renfrewshire, Scotland; 3175, Staley Road, Grand Island, NY 14072.

23 Günther Wagner AG, Pelikan Werk, Adliswil, Zurich, Switzerland.

24 V. A. Howe & Co. Ltd, 88 Peterborough Road, London SW6. Heraeus Christ GmbH, D3360 Osterode an Harz, Postfach 1220, W. Germany.

25 Hopkins and Williams, Freshwater Road, Chadwell Heath, Essex.

26 Ilford Ltd, Plate Production Dept, Town Lane, Mobberly, Cheshire.

27 Jackson Laboratories, Bar Harbour, Maine 04609, USA.

28 Jencons Scientific Ltd, Mark Road, Hemel Hampstead, Herts HP2 7DE.

29 Koch-Light Laboratories Ltd, Colnbrook, Buckinghamshire.

30 Kodak Research Chemicals, Kirkby, Liverpool; Eastman Kodak Ltd, Rochester, NY 14650, USA.

31 E. Leitz (Instr) Ltd, 48 Park Street, Luton, Bedfordshire; Ernst Leitz, 6330 Wetzlar, W. Germany.

32 LH Engineering, Bells Hill, Stoke Poges, Buchinghamshire; Bioassay systems, 100 Inman Street, Cambridge, Mass 02139, USA.

33 LKB Instrument Ltd, 232 Addington Road, Selsdon, South Croydon, Surrey; LKB-Produkter AB, S161 25 Bromma 1, Sweden.

34 Luckham Ltd, Victoria Gardens, Burgess Hill, Sussex.

35 Measuring and Scientific Equipment Ltd, 33 Manor Royal, Crawley, Sussex.

36 Medical Research Council Laboratory Animals Centre, Carshalton, Surrey. International Index for Laboratory Animals.

37 Medicell, 239 Liverpool Road, London N1 1LX; Union Carbide Corporation, Foods Products Division, 6733 West 65 Street, Chicago, Illinois 60638, USA.

38 Mercia Brocades Ltd, Brocades House, Pyrford Road, West Byfleet, Weybridge, Surrey.

39 Miles Laboratories Ltd, Research Products Division, PO Box 37, Stoke Court, Stoke Poges, Slough SL2 4LV; Miles Laboratories Inc., Research Products Division, Box 2000, Elkhart, Indiana 46515, USA.

40 Millipore (UK) Ltd, Abbey Road, Park Royal, London NW10 7SP; Worthington Biochemical Corporation, Freehold, New Jersey 07728, USA.

41 Nordic Immunological Laboratories, 60 King Street, Maidenhead, Berks SL6 1EQ; Nordic Immunological Laboratories, Langestraat 57-61, Tilburg, Holland.

42 Olac (1976) Ltd, Shaw's Farm, Blackthorn, Bicester, Oxon OX6 0TP.

43 Organon Laboratories Ltd, Crown House, London Road, Morden, Surrey.

44 Ortho Pharmaceuticals, Saunderton, High Wycombe, Buckinghamshire.

45. Pierce & Wariner (UK) Ltd, 44 Upper Northgate Street, Chester, Cheshire CH1 4EF.

46 Pharmacia (GB) Ltd, Prince Regent Road, Hounslow, Middlesex TW3 1NE; Pharmacia Fine Chemicals AB, Uppsala, Sweden; 800 Centennial Avenue, Piscataway, NJ 08854, USA.

47 Porvair Ltd, Kings Lynn, Norfolk.

48 Radiochemicals Centre, Amersham, Buckinghamshire; Amersham Corporation, 2636 S, Clearbrook Drive, Arlington Heights, Illinois 60005, USA.

49 Raven Scientific Ltd, Sturmer End, Haverhill, Suffolk CB9 7UU.

50 Salisbury Laboratories Ltd, Salisbury, Wiltshire.

51 Scientific Supplies, Vine Hill, London EC1; Falcon Plastics, Division of Becton, Dickinson and Company, Oxnard, California 93030, USA.

52 Seward Laboratory, UAC House, Blackfriars Road, London SE1 9UG.

53 Shandon Southern Products Ltd, 93-96 Chadwick Road, Astmoor Industrial Estate, Runcorn, Cheshire.

54 Sigma London Chem. Co Ltd, Fancy Road, Poole, Dorset BH17 7NH; Sigma Chemical Co, Box 14508, St. Louis, Missouri 63178, USA.

55 Travenol Laboratories Ltd, Thetford, Norfolk; Hyland Therapeutics Div. Travenol Laboratories, 3300 Hyland Avenue, PO Box 2214, Costa Mesa. California 92626, USA.

56 Vestric Ltd, PO Box 21, Lockfield Avenue, Enfield, Middlesex; Nyegaard and Co AS, Oslo, Norway.

57 Wellcome Reagents Ltd, 303 Hither Green Lane, Hither Green, London SE13 6TL; Burroughs Wellcome Co, 3030 Cornwallis Road, Research Triangle Park, NC 27709, USA.

58 Whatman Biochemicals Ltd, Springfield Mill, Maidstone, Kent.

59 Wright Scientific Ltd, Upper Mill, Stonehouse, Glos. GL10 2BJ.

III Summary tables of useful immunochemical data

SERUM CONCENTRATIONS OF HUMAN IMMUNOGLOBULINS

Class	Concentration (mg ml^{-1})
IgG	8–16
IgA	1·4–4
IgM	0·5–2
IgD	0–0·4
IgE	17–450 ng ml^{-1}

DISTRIBUTION OF HUMAN IMMUNOGLOBULIN SUBCLASSES IN SERUM

Subclass	% of total in class
IgG 1	70
IgG 2	18
IgG 3	8
IgG 4	3
IgA 1	80
IgA 2	20

SERUM CONCENTRATIONS OF MOUSE (BALB/C) IMUNOGLOBULINS (15 WEEKS OLD)

Class	Concentration (μg ml^{-1})
IgG 1	6500
IgG 2a	4200
IgG 2b	1200
IgA	260
IgM	1000

Protein	Molecular Wt	$E_{1\,cm}^{1\%}$	Wavelength nm	Solvent
IgG	160 000	14·3	280	0·2 M NaCl pH 7·5
IgA	170 000	10·6	280	—
IgM	900 000	11·85	280	0·2 M NaCl pH 7·5
IgD	184 000			
IgE	188 000			
μ chain	73 814			
α chain	59 582	10·6	280	5 M guanidine HCl
γ chain	50 179	13·7	280	0·01 N HCl
light chain	25 170	11·8	280	0·01 N HCl
Fab$_\gamma$	50 000	15·3	278	PBS
F(ab$'_\gamma$)$_2$	104 000	14·8	280	PBS
Fc$_\gamma$	50 000	12·2	278	PBS
pFc$'_\gamma$	26 000	13·8	280	PBS
Ovalbumin	43 500	7·35	280	PBS
Human serum albumin	68 460	5·3	279	PBS
Bovine serum albumin	67 000	6·67	279	Water
Fowl gamma globulin		13·5	280	—
Keyhole limpet haemocyanin	3 000 000	(*Megathura crenulata*)		
Squid haemocyanin	611 800	(*Ommatostrephes sloani pacificus*)		
Murex haemocyanin		18·1	278	Water
Limulus haemocyanin		11·2	278	Water
2, 4 Dinitrophenol (DNP)	184	14 900 ($E_M^{1\,cm}$)	358	0·5 M phosphate pH 7·4
4, hydroxy, 3, nitro 5, iodo phenacetyl azide (NIP azide)	348	—	—	
Fluorescein	389	53 000 ($E_M^{1\,cm}$)	490	0·15 M NaCl, p·02 M K phosphate pH 7·4

Type	Fractionation range for globular proteins (molecular weight)
Sephadex	
G-10	−700
G-15	−1500
G-25	1000–5000
G-50	1500–30 000
G-75	3000–80 000
G-100	4000–150 000
G-150	500–300 000
G-200	5000–600 000
Sepharose	
2 B	$7 \times 10^4 - 40 \times 10^6$
4 B	$6 \times 10^4 - 20 \times 10^6$
6 B	$10^4 - 4 \times 10^6$
Sephacryl	
S 200	$5 \times 10^3 - 2 \cdot 5 \times 10^5$
S 300	$1 \times 10^4 - 1 \cdot 5 \times 10^6$

Dialysis

Visking tubing used for dialysis has a nominal exclusion value of 14,000 but this probably varies from batch to batch and for each size. The 8/32″ tubing holds approximately 1 ml per 3 cm. The 18/32″ tubing holds about 1 ml per cm.

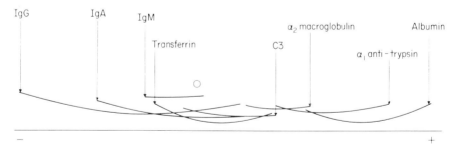

Fig. III.1. Immunoelectrophoresis of human serum in agar, sodium barbitone buffer pH 8·2
The main immunoglobulin classes are shown together with several other major proteins.

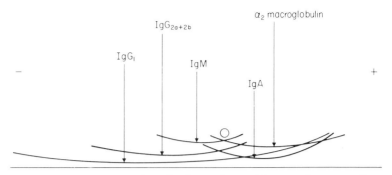

Fig. III.2. Immunoelectrophoresis of normal BALB/c serum in agar, sodium barbitone buffer pH 8·6
Proteins visualized with a rabbit antiserum to mouse immunoglobulin. Such antisera invariably contain antibodies to α-2 macroglobulin.

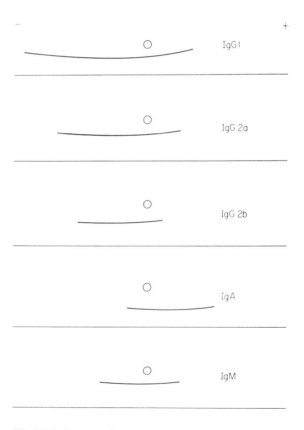

Fig. III.3. Immunoelectrophoresis of normal mouse serum (BALB/c) in agar, sodium barbitone buffer pH 8·2
Specific antisera to each class and subclass are placed in the antisera troughs.

349

Index

351

352

359